MW01205402

Springer Series on REHABILITATION

Editor: Thomas E. Backer, PhD
Human Interaction Research Institute, Los Angeles

Advisory Board: Carolyn L. Vash, PhD, Elizabeth L. Pan, PhD, Donald E. Galvin, PhD, Ray L. Jones, PhD, James F. Garrett, PhD, Patricia G. Forsythe, and Henry Viscardi, Jr.

Dennis R. Maki, PhD, CRC is a Professor, Division of Counselor Education, Graduate Programs in Rehabilitation, at The University of Iowa. Dr. Maki is a Past President of the American Rehabilitation Counseling Association and recipient of numerous awards including the National Council on Rehabilitation Education's Rehabilitation Educator of the Year. He has been a consistent contributor to the professional literature and with Dr. Riggar served as Co-Editor for Special Issues for the *Journal of Applied Rehabilitation Counseling* from 1983–1994. Drs. Riggar, Maki and Wolf co-edited a previous text in the Springer series, *Applied Rehabilitation Counseling*.

T. F. Riggar, EdD. is a Professor, Rehabilitation Institute, Southern Illinois University at Carbondale. Dr. Riggar, recipient of more than a dozen state, regional, and national awards, has published over 70 articles in professional rehabilitation journals. This is Dr. Riggar's thirteenth book.

Rehabilitation Counseling

Profession and Practice

Dennis R. Maki

T.F. Riggar

Editors

 SPRINGER PUBLISHING COMPANY

Springer Publishing Company, Inc.
536 Broadway
New York, NY 10012–3955

Cover design by Margaret Dunin
Production Editor: Kathleen Kelly

Second Printing
97 98 99 00 01 / 6 5 4 3 2

Library of Congress Cataloging-in-Publication Data

Rehabilitation counseling: profession and practice /
    Dennis R. Maki, T. F. Riggar, editors.
            p.   cm.—(Springer series on rehabilitation)
        Includes bibliographical references and index.
        ISBN 0-8261-9510-5
            1. Handicapped—Counseling of.   2. Handicapped—Rehabilitation.
    I.   Maki, Dennis R., 1938–   . II.   Riggar, T. F. III.   Series.
    HV1568.R435,   1996
    362.4' 0486—dc21   96-46426
                                                                   CIP

This work is dedicated to the American Rehabilitation Counseling Association whose mission is to enhance the lives of persons with disabilities and to advance the profession of rehabilitation counseling. The editors and authors would like to acknowledge the Presidents of the American Rehabilitation Counseling Association for their leadership and outstanding contributions to the profession over the years.

Salvatore DiMichael	1958–59	Frank Touchstone	1978–79
William Usdane	1959–60	Don Linkowski	1979–80
Abraham Jacobs	1960–61	Kenneth Reagles	1980–81
Lloyd Lofquist	1961–62	Dan McAlees	1981–82
C. H. Patterson	1962–63	Stanford Rubin	1982–83
William Gellman	1963–64	Ken Thomas	1983–84
Daniel Sinick	1964–65	Paul McCollum	1984–85
John McGowan	1965–66	Edna Szymanski	1985–86
John Muthard	1966–67	Randy Parker	1986–87
Marceline Jaques	1967–68	Brian McMahan	1987–88
Martin Acker	1968–69	John Thompson	1988–89
Leonard Miller	1969–70	Ross Lynch	1989–90
Gregory Miller	1970–71	Dennis R. Maki	1990–91
Richard Thoreson	1971–72	Martha Walker	1991–92
George Ayers	1972–73	Jeanne Patterson	1992–93
Lawrence Feinberg	1973–74	John Dolan	1993–94
George Wright	1974–75	Linda Shaw	1994–95
Tom Porter	1975–76	Michael Leahy	1995–96
Ray Ehrie	1976–77	Bill Richardson	1996–97
Bob Johnson	1977–78	Vilia Tarvydas	1997–98

Contents

Part 2. Practice

Foreword

Total rehabilitation as a human service philosophy is designed to attend to the physical, mental, emotional, spiritual, social, and vocational aspects of life. Its goal is to facilitate productivity and independent living as well as community integration of a wide variety and substantial population of persons who otherwise may be functionally and societally limited in fully realizing their potential.

The success of rehabilitation case work is remarkable considering the potential obstacles, such as the severity and range of client disablements, public prejudices, inadequate program funding and resources, including a shortage of well-trained professional personnel. Most noteworthy in today's helping services is the modern technology of rehabilitation as practiced by professionally qualified (master's-degree-prepared) rehabilitation counselors. These techniques for helping clients with disabilities have advanced with government-sponsored research and graduate training programs.

This book addresses modern technology and paradigms, as well as the information needed for contemporary professional rehabilitation practice. It focuses on the basic knowledge and skills essential for counseling and other professional services. In the last decade the rehabilitation disciplines witnessed great changes and substantial growth, which effected professional practice often altering its goals, clientele, and public endorsement of programs. This book provides comprehensive guidelines for rehabilitation professionals and students, including the basic information about the profession, persons with disabilities, professional practice, social values, and impact on recipients. It took many years for me to acquire the information that is contained in this volume. This knowledge was gained through personal experience as both a client and then a counselor in the state/federal vocational rehabilitation system, in addition to being a student, consultant, researcher, and professor of rehabilitation counseling. Given this experience I endorse this text as an excellent reference and resource for the practitioner, educator, and researcher.

As a text for preservice university courses, as well as continuing education and in-service training programs, this book provides a comprehensive reference of fundamental knowledge in the area of rehabilitation counseling. Both the editors, Professors Maki and Riggar, and the chapter authors are highly respected for their expertise in various aspects of the profession and practice of rehabilitation counseling.

Though no previous course work on this subject is a prerequisite for the reader of this text or the beginning student, this book provides concepts and principles that are essential for developing a comprehensive, in-depth understanding of the profession and practice of rehabilitation counseling. For allied professionals it contains useful knowledge on the basic principles of rehabilitation. A didactic editorial style provides clear, concise, and accurate information for students of rehabilitation counseling, as well as for those seeking the useful references it provides. For the practicing rehabilitation counselor, this text serves as a contemporary reference providing up-to-date discussions of current issues, research, and models of practice.

Rehabilitation Counseling: Profession and Practice is destined to be adopted by rehabilitation education programs everywhere, for its up-to-date, comprehensive coverage of rehabilitation practice. It was an honor to write a foreword for a book so well designed as to cover the modern processes and goals of rehabilitation. The editors and contributors are all highly respected professionals who deserve our utmost appreciation for shaping and articulating the many components of the modern rehabilitation process. The great value of this book will be in enabling future clients to attain a better life through well-informed professional rehabilitation practice.

On a personal note, I wish to congratulate the editors and chapter authors, all of whom I respect for this and their many other contributions to our literature and to the field of rehabilitation counseling. I would like to further acknowledge their generosity as all royalties generated by the sales of this text will be donated to the American Rehabilitation Counseling Association to further its mission.

GEORGE N. WRIGHT

Contributors

Norman L. Berven, PhD, is Professor in Rehabilitation Counseling/ Rehabilitation Psychology, Department of Rehabilitation Psychology and Special Education, University of Wisconsin—Madison.

Jack L. Cassell, PhD, is Associate Professor in the Rehabilitation, Deafness, and Human Services Unit, University of Tennessee—Knoxville.

Al Condeluci, PhD, is Executive Director of the UCP Center for Personal Development in Pittsburgh, PA. He is associated with the University of Pittsburgh and Community College of Allegheny County.

William Crimando, PhD, CRC, is Professor and Coordinator of Rehabilitation Administration and Services, Rehabilitation Institute, Southern Illinois University at Carbondale.

William G. Emener, PhD, CRC, is a Distinguished Research Professor in the Department of Rehabilitation Counseling, University of South Florida, Tampa.

Carrie Engen, RN, BSN, CCM, is the owner and Director of Case Management Operations for Advocare, Inc., in Naperville, IL. She is a past president of CMSA and past Chair of the Commission for Case Manager Certification.

Carl Flowers, RhD, is a Program Manager with the Region V Rehabilitation Continuing Education Program, Southern Illinois University at Carbondale.

Dennis D. Gilbride, PhD, is Associate Professor in Rehabilitation, Department of Special Education, Counseling, and Rehabilitation, Drake University.

Charlotte Griffin-Dixon, RhD, is Assistant Professor in the Department of Rehabilitation Counseling, University of South Florida, Tampa.

Rochelle Habeck, PhD, CRC, is a Professor in the Rehabilitation Counseling Program at Michigan State University.

James T. Herbert, PhD, CRC, is Associate Professor and Director of Rehabilitation Programs, Department of Counselor Education, Counseling Psychology, and Rehabilitation Services, The Pennsylvania State University.

Marvin D. Kuehn, EdD, is currently Professor and Director of Rehabilitation Programs in the Division of Counselor Education and Rehabilitation Programs, Emporia State University, Emporia.

Michael J. Leahy, PhD, CRC, is Associate Professor, Director of the Office of Rehabilitation and Disability Studies, and Coordinator of Doctoral Studies in Rehabilitation Counselor Education, Michigan State University.

Lisa Lopez Levers, PhD, CRC, LPCC, currently serves as Chair of the Counseling and Human Development Department at the Margaret Warner Graduate School of Education and Human Development, University of Rochester, Rochester, New York.

Ruth Torkelson Lynch, PhD, CRC, is an Associate Professor, Department of Rehabilitation Psychology and Special Education, University of Wisconsin—Madison.

Ralph E. Matkin, RhD, is Professor at California State University—Long Beach in the master of science in counseling degree program within the College of Education. Dr. Matkin is an NCC, CRC, CIRS, and Registered Professional Rehabilitation Counselor in California.

Michael J. Millington, PhD, is Assistant Professor in the Rehabilitation Counseling Program, Louisiana State University Medical Center, School of Allied Health, New Orleans, Louisiana.

S. Wayne Mulkey, PhD, CRC, is Associate Research Professor and Director of the Region IV Rehabilitation Continuing Education Program at the University of Tennessee—Knoxville.

Margaret Sebastian, MEd, is a doctoral student in the Rehabilitation Counselor Education Program at Michigan State University.

Robert Strensrud, EdD, is Associate Professor in Rehabilitation, Department of Special Education, Counseling, and Rehabilitation, Drake University.

Vilia M. Tarvydas, PhD, CRC, is Associate Professor and Coordinator of the Graduate Programs in Rehabilitation, University of Iowa.

Beatriz Treviño, PhD, is Assistant Professor, University of North Texas, Perton.

Martha Lentz Walker, EdD, CRC, is Emeritus Professor, Rehabilitation Counselor Education Program, Kent State University, Kent, OH.

Susan M. Wiegmann, PhD, CRC, is Assistant Professor, Rehabilitation Counselor Education Program, Kent State University, Kent, OH.

Janet M. Williams is President of communityworks, inc., Kansas City, Missouri. She is completing a Ph.D. in Family Studies and Disability, University of Kansas.

George N. Wright, PhD, CRC, is Professor Emeritus, Rehabilitation Counseling/Rehabilitation Psychology, Department of Rehabilitation Psychology and Special Education, University of Wisconsin—Madison.

PART 1

Profession

CHAPTER 1

Rehabilitation Counseling: Concepts and Paradigms

Dennis R. Maki and T. F. Riggar

R ehabilitation is a robust concept that is widely used in our society. It is used in diverse contexts with reference to the rehabilitation of persons, places, and even things. In each of these contexts, there is an implied connotation of restoration to a state of health or useful and constructive activity. As a concept, rehabilitation counseling is not as robust nor is it as generally understood. It is, however, used to refer to a profession, and a scope of practice within the health care and human service delivery systems. It is therefore critical to begin with definitions in order to provide a language through which the concepts and paradigms of rehabilitation and rehabilitation counseling may be presented. From this foundation, rehabilitation counseling may be articulated more clearly as both a profession and a practice.

The following definitions for these terms have been proposed. They provide an infrastructure for this and subsequent discussions. Therefore, it is important to first understand each definition independently and then to further consider each of these definitions in relation to the others. This will allow a better understanding of the direct, though complex relationship linking the terms and the importance of a shared language for the profession.

• Rehabilitation is defined as, "a holistic and integrated program of medical, physical, psychosocial, and vocational interventions that empower a person with disability to achieve a personally fulfilling, socially meaningful, and functionally effective interaction with the world" (Banja, 1990, p. 615).

• Rehabilitation within the context of the rehabilitation counseling process is "a comprehensive sequence of services, mutually planned by the consumer and rehabilitation counselor, to maximize employability, independence, integration, and participation of persons with disabilities in the work place and the community" (Jenkins, Patterson, & Szymanski, 1992, p. 2).

• Rehabilitation counseling is viewed "as a profession that assists persons with disabilities in adapting to the environment, assists environments in accommodating the needs of the individual and works toward full participation of persons with disabilities in all aspects of society, especially work" (Szymanski, 1985, p. 3).

• Rehabilitation counseling as a scope of practice is defined as " a systematic process which assists persons with physical, mental, developmental, cognitive, and emotional disabilities to achieve their personal, career, and independent living goals in the most integrated setting possible through the application of the counseling process. The counseling process involves communication, goal setting, and beneficial growth or change through self-advocacy, psychological, vocational, social, and behavioral interventions" [Commission on Rehabilitation Counselor Certification (CRCC,) 1994, p. 1].

The field of rehabilitation counseling is thus defined as a specialty within the rehabilitation professions with counseling at its core, and is differentiated from other related counseling fields. Therefore, rehabilitation counseling is a profession. It is also a practice that has evolved within the context of changing legislative mandates (Appendix A), societal perspectives, as well as technological and medical advances. Clearly defined terminology, as well as those concepts and paradigms that operationalize the terms are critical to an understanding of this profession and its practice. Therefore, definitions of terms are provided throughout the text, Appendix B provides a listing of acronyms commonly used in rehabilitation as a reference to expand a shared language. An underlying philosophy is embedded within each of the above definitions of fundamental terms. This philosophy is equally as important to understanding the profession as all the definitions themselves.

REHABILITATION PHILOSOPHY

The philosophy of rehabilitation is premised in a belief in the dignity and worth of all people. It values independence, integration, and the inclusion of people with and without disabilities in employment and in their communities. Rehabilitation represents the philosophy that whenever possible persons with a disability will be integrated into the least restrictive environments. Inherent in this philosophy is a commitment to equalize the opportunities to participate in all rights and privileges available to all people and to provide a sense of equal justice based on a model of accommodation. In addition, there is a commitment to supporting persons with disabilities in advocacy activities in order to enable them to achieve this status and thus further empower themselves.

Simultaneously, within this philosophy there is a commitment to models of service delivery that emphasize integrated, comprehensive services that are mutually planned by the consumer and the rehabilitation counselor. Throughout rehabilitation emphasis is given to choice and the holistic nature of people. This serves to define the philosophy of rehabilitation as one that is existential and systemic. Individuals are conceptualized as interacting within multiple contexts of life, especially those of their family and cultural systems. The philosophy is solution-focused and stresses the assets of the person and the resources of the environment. The focus is on adaptation and accommodation from an ecological perspective that is directed toward achieving a meaningful quality of life for the person with a disability.

Contemporary rehabilitation philosophy is reflected in several paradigm shifts. These shifts include a movement from an individual problem-solving approach to an ecological solution-focused approach, from institutionalization to community participation; from charity to civil rights; from segregated vocational training models to community-integrated or community-supported employment and independent living models, and from a medical model with an illness and pathology focus to a wellness model focusing on development and life stages. The philosophy of rehabilitation advocates for consumer choice and empowerment. Embedded within this philosophy is the principle of informed consent; full consideration must be given to the individual's right to fail as one potential outcome involved with choice, growth, and risk. The philosophy of rehabilitation embraces a person's right to choose his or her relationships and goals, both personal and vocational.

This philosophy of rehabilitation has been articulated clearly within the underlying values of the rehabilitation counseling Scope of Practice (Appendix C). Maki and Murray (1995) provide a more complete discussion of the philosophy of rehabilitation. This reference and its source documents provide an excellent resource for further exploration of this topic as well as the discussion found herein.

PERSONS WITH DISABILITIES

Operationalizing the philosophy of rehabilitation begins with a belief in the dignity and worth of all people. The terms and language used in practice must reflect and reinforce this belief as well. Persons with disabilities are the recipients of rehabilitation services. Contemporary rehabilitation practice uses differing terms when making reference to these individuals. The medical model refers to the patient, whereas legal and mental health professionals refer to their clients. Traditionally, the term *client* has predominated in the rehabilitation counseling profession and its practice. The terms *consumer* or *customer* have been advocated as the preference among some persons within the disability communities. These terms are seen to reflect their empowered status and to reflect their position relative to the service delivery system and those who deliver services more adequately. All these terms will be used respectfully, yet interchangeably, throughout this text in reference to persons who seek or receive rehabilitation services.

In addition to the terms used in reference to persons with disability, it is important to be aware of and comply with basic principles of non-handicapping language. *The Publication Manual of the American Psychological Association [American Psychological Association (APA), 1994]* provides the standard reference style guidelines for the field. The following discussion related to "nonhandicapping" language is derived from this reference (APA, 1994). The guiding principle always is to use language that maintains the integrity and dignity of people as human beings. To this end, it is important to avoid language that (a) equates persons with their condition (e.g., the disabled or epileptics); (b) that has negative or superfluous overtones (e.g., AIDS victim); or (c) is regarded as a slur (e.g., cripple). Consistent with the conceptual framework of practice, use of the term *disability* should occur only to describe an attribute of a person, and *handicap* to describe the source of limitations, such as the attitudinal, legal, and architectural barriers. It is important to note that disability and handicap are not synoymous. In fact, the next section provides a detailed description of terms associated with these concepts. The terms "challenged" and "special" are often considered euphemistic and should be used only when the people you serve prefer them.

When communicating orally or in writing the American Psychological Association (1994, pp. 59–60) guidelines suggest the following rules with regard to reference to disabilities:

- Put people first, not their disability. Preferred expressions avoid the implication that the person as a whole is disabled.
- Do not label people by their disability or overextend its severity. Because the person is not the disability, the two concepts should be separate.
- Use emotionally neutral expressions. Terms such as victim, afflicted, suffering and confined are examples of problematic expressions which have excessive, negative overtones and suggest continued helplessness.

It is important to reiterate that the term of professional reference, be it client or consumer, as well as the language used to describe a person involved in our service is a critical consideration. The language chosen communicates a philosophical and attitudinal orientation at both a personal and professional level. Remember, it is preferable to put the person before the disability. Avoid using adjectives as nouns. Person-first language is the generally accepted rule. Therefore, "person with_____," "person living with_____," and "person who has_____" are neutral and preferred language. Referring to a client as retarded is inappropriate in contemporary rehabilitation practice. Therefore, reference would be made to a person with mental retardation. Persons with disability is to be used rather than disabled persons.

There are some persons with disabilities who may elect other language conventions. For example, there are members of the deaf community who prefer to be referred to collectively as the deaf or individually as a deaf person. This language preference is also found among some members within the blind community. Avoid use of the term "normal" in any regard. As professionals working with persons with and without disabilities, it is essential to communicate clearly and respectfully. An open discussion with the person with whom you are working usually provides a forum for selecting subsequent language to be used with each individual.

THE CONCEPT OF DISABILITY

Persons with disabilities may choose to present themselves for rehabilitation services. In the previous section, the importance of language respecting the dignity of persons with disabilities as people first was stressed. The next concept critical to this discussion of rehabilitation is to clarify what is meant by the term disability. Nagler and Wilson (1995) note that disability may be congenital, developmental, or acquired as well as defined from a medical, rehabilitation, legal, or social perspective. It is critial to understand these differences and to communicate accurately when making reference to disability and the associated concepts that serve to operationalize the medical and legal translation of a condition to society.

The following definitions and discussion are based on a conceptual model of the rehabilitation process presented by the National Center for Medical Rehabilitation Research (NCMRR, 1993). They are presented here as an attempt to promote a uniformity of language and conceptual framework to enhance communication and understanding among diverse professionals as well as those other persons with and without disabilities involved in rehabilitation.

• *Pathophysiology* An interruption or interference of normal physiological and developmental processes or structures. It is the diagnosed pathology, typically referred to as a medical condition (e.g., multiple sclerosis, neurological deficit).

• *Impairment* A loss and/or abnormality of cognitive, emotional, physiological, or anatomical structure or function; including secondary losses or pain, not just those attributable to the initial pathophysiology (e.g., perception, memory, processing)

• *Functional Limitation* A restriction or lack of ability to perform an action in the manner or within the range considered normal and consistent with the purpose of an organ or organ system that results from impairment (e.g., organize, climb, read, adapt).

• *Disability* An inability or limitation in performing socially defined tasks, activities, and roles to levels expected within physical and social environments as a result of internal or external factors and their interplay (e.g., self-care, leisure activities, education).

• *Societal Limitations* Restrictions attributable to social policy or barriers (structural or attitudinal), that limit fulfillment of roles or deny access to services and/or opportunities that are associated with full participation in society. These have historically been referred to as handicapping conditions (e.g., parent role, worker role, quality of life) (p. 33).

In everyday usage by laypersons, words and phrases such as pathophysiology, impairment, functional limitation, disability, and handicap or the more descriptive societal limitations are often used interchangeably. However, these terms are used with specific meanings and precise reference by different rehabilitation agencies and allied professions. The rehabilitation counselor must be sensitive to the existence of these different perspectives and terms, their varied usages, and the relationships among them. For example, from a legal perspective the Americans with Disabilities Act (ADA, 1990) specifically defines an individual with a disability as a person who: (1) has a physical or mental impairment that substantially limits one or more of the major life activities of that person, (2) has a record of such an impairment, or (3) is regarded as having such an impairment. Major life activities include caring for oneself, performing manual tasks, walking, seeing, hearing, breathing, learning, and working. This legal definition reflects a perspective that is congruent with that of the medical and rehabilitation conceptualization of disability proposed. It is also consistent with the ecological conceptualization of adaptation and accommodation philosophically proposed to systemically describe a social perspective embracing the culture and structure of societal institutions.

FUNCTIONAL LIMITATIONS AND THE REHABILITATION COUNSELOR

The definitions proposed in the previous section provide rehabilitation counselors with a language and conceptual reference regarding the medical aspects of disability as they translate to their functional impact within the environmental contexts wherein they assume meaning. Walker (1995) asserts, "The skills of rehabilitation counselors in returning persons with disabilities to communities to live, work, recreate, learn, and function actively as citizens, rather than as patients or inmates, are transferrable to all human service systems" (p. 620). Rehabilitation counselors work within diverse institutional and community-based settings, including public and private medical, educational, mental health, correctional, corporate, human resource, and social service programs and agencies. The professional role of the rehabilitation counselor remains constant over the various settings of practice although the specific functions performed may vary.

Maki, McCracken, Pape, and Scofield (1978) defined the effective role of the rehabilitation counselor as that of problem solver. The main characteristics of this role are the ability to perceive the problems of each client as they relate to his or her rehabilitation, and to help plan appropriate intervention strategies. The Scope of Practice Statement (Appendix C) operationalizes this role and articulates the functions and responsibilities of the rehabilitation counselor. It identifies the knowledge and skills required for the provision of effective rehabilitation counseling services to persons with physical, mental, developmental, cognitive, and emotional disabilities as embodied in the standards of the profession's credentialing organizations. The Code of Ethics (Appendix D) dictate that individual practitioners develop and maintain the necessary knowledge and skills to effectively function within their role and individual scope of practice.

As previously mentioned, the philosophy of rehabilitation has shifted to a solution-focused orientation based on client assets and preferences. The role of the rehabilitation counselor involves the translation of the impact of the medical condition through an analysis of the functional limitations, disability, and ultimately the societal limitations subsequently imposed. This provides the rehabilitation counselor with an effective and efficient case-work format. It is important to stress that although the identification of functional limitations is a necessary first step, it is the simultaneous identification of residual capacities, transferable skills, as well as the person's interests and preferences, that forms the basis of rehabilitation planning and placement activities in functional terms.

Nagler and Wilson (1995) stated that rehabilitation "focuses on functional limitations resulting from physical (e.g., mobility), sensory (e.g., vision, auditory), organic (e.g., diabetes, epilepsy, cerebral palsy), intellectual (e.g., learning), or psychiatric (e.g., schizophrenia, types of depression) impairment" (p. 257). A clearly specified limitation of function can help the counselor understand the actual and contextual limitations of the client. The work of the counselor is facilitated through a clear understanding of medical conditions stated in functional terms to describe the disability. Thus, functional limitations operationally define the disability and represent the intervening physical and/or behavioral variables considered in describing the nature and extent of the societal limitation or handicap. The following functional limitations are based on the work of G. N. Wright (1980) and were presented by Maki (1986). They can be used to assist in conceptualizing and planning interventions with persons who are seeking rehabilitation services. The rehabilitation counselor may consider whether any of the following limitations are involved.

- Sensory impairment refers to reduction in or incapacity to receive environmental stimuli in the visual, auditory, olfactory, tactile, or taste domains.
- Communication difficulty refers to reduced capacity or incapacity to receive, process, and/or transmit messages, either verbally or non-verbally, to or from other persons in the environment.
- Atypical appearance refers to physical or behavioral cues emitted by an individual that may be interpreted as significantly different from environmental normative standards to attract the attention of other persons in the environment.
- Emotional/behavioral considerations refer to those interpersonal, intrapersonal, or physical manifestations of affective and/or cognitive processes that interfere with an individual's ability to effectively function within his/her environment.
- Unapparent or invisible limitation refers to those situations in which, although disability is present, no cues are overtly transmitted to others in the environment. Thus, the disability is invisible and the person is considered to be without a disability by the general public.
- Cognitive/learning difficulty refers to an impaired ability to obtain, process, or retain information that has a potential impact on the individual's ability to attend, conceptualize, abstract, judge, problem solve, or gain from interaction with the environment.
- Substance dependency refers to the physical or psychological need for and the use/misuse of chemical agents over a period of time either on a prescribed or self-regulated basis.
- Pain sensitivity/intolerance refers to those situations in which the physical or psychological sensation of pain exceeds the individual's threshold of tolerance affecting his or her life-style and ability to concentrate, learn, effectively interact, or physically maneuver within the environment.
- Alteration of consciousness refers to an inability to maintain a condition of mental awareness of the environment at any given point in time.
- Debilitation refers to a progressive, though usually gradual deterioration of physical, emotional, or intellectual capacities.

- Motion deficit refers to partial or total restrictions in movement or coordination in the limbs or trunk of the body affecting the individual's ability to maneuver within and to manipulate his/her environment.
- Mobility refers to an impaired ability or the inability of an individual to independently move between points in his/her environment as a result of physical, psychological, sensory, or environmental factors.
- Restricted environment refers to a situation in which an individual is unable to interact within the total context of the environment as a result of physical barriers, when factors may be present that cause or exacerbate the disabling condition, when the individual would be a threat to self or others if permitted to interact, or if a controlled environment is required in the treatment of the disabling condition.
- Uncertain prognosis refers to the inability to predict with any degree of certainty the duration, severity, and/or probable final status of a disease or mental disorder.
- Special considerations refers to those unique implications of a situation which, if unattended to would result in less than optimal rehabilitation outcomes for any given individual (Maki, 1986, pp. 9–10).

The terms *pathophysiology* and *impairment* are direct references to medical aspects of disability. In considering the effects of the medical condition on the functioning of the individual, as well as the environmental variables operative in the situation, it is possible to assess the degree and types of limitations impinging on the individual. Rehabilitation counselors need expertise and access to consultation in the area of medical aspects of disabling conditions to work effectively with persons who have disabilities. It is the function of the rehabilitation counselor to apply this expertise when developing rehabilitation goals reflecting the functional limitations, residual capacities, transferable skills, as well as the interests, needs, and temperaments defining the rehabilitation potential of persons with disabilities. Realistic objectives for an individualized rehabilitation plan are ones that are within the client's physical, intellectual, and emotional capacities and reflect his or her interests, preferences, and temperaments.

Finally, in considering the establishment of realistic objectives, the NCMRR (1993) stated that there are three categories of personal background factors that influence an individual's response to a given situation. When considering the impact of pathology and impairment, the rehabilitation counselor should consider each of the following as they assess rehabilitation potential and those limitations surrounding disability:

1. Organic factors are those characteristics of the body and constitution that influence the reaction to disability onset and daily function, such as endurance, strength, general health status, genetic and family predisposition to certain disorders, and others aspects of physical function.
2. Psychosocial factors that may influence outcome include style of coping with stress, will to live, self-reliance, motivation, problem solving, judgment, locus of control, cultural and ethnic group, gender, social skills, belief system, and others.
3. The environment in which a person grew up and in which he or she lives also influences daily function and response to disability. These factors include, but are not limited to, income, family and interpersonal support, access to and payment for proper health care, availability of transportation and proper rehabilitation, availability of physical and behavioral assistance (if needed), and access to appropriate educational, recreational, and vocational resources.

All of these personal factors combine to make an individual's response to the condition or impairment unique. They are only one element affecting the ultimate functional level reached during a lifetime with disability, however. Any of these personal background factors may help or hinder the person's ability to adapt and live in the community at a satisfactory level of function.

Brodwin and Brodwin (1993) described the usefulness of Bandura's work on self-efficacy to the field of rehabilitation. They suggest that this growing body of research related to individual response tendencies supports the hypothesis that self-efficacy beliefs are cognitive mediators of assured, purposeful, and persistent behavior. These are behaviors that need to be developed and increased in persons with disabilities if they are to receive maximum benefit from the various rehabilitation systems. Self-efficacy theory is concerned with the personal self-judgments that influence the environments that people choose, the activities in which they engage, and the effort and persistence they demonstrate at a task in the face of obstacles. The theory provides an overall framework to explain why some clients are successful in rehabilitation efforts and others are not. It also addresses how counselors can most effectively help clients maximize rehabilitation potential.

Rehabilitation potential as defined by these same authors consists of three characteristics: (1) attaining increased functioning in the direction of maximizing physical and emotional growth, (2) having a sense of well-being, and (3) facilitating development of a personally satisfying level of independence. These authors note that different rehabilitation systems (e.g., worker's compensation, long-term disability, social security, state vocational rehabilitation, independent living) define a client's rehabilitation potential within the context of their specific organization's parameters. Crimando and Riggar (1991) stress that the counselors need to be aware of the differing requirements of each rehabilitation system(s) providing services.

PARADIGMS OF REHABILITATION PRACTICE

The individual is considered to be the primary focus of the medical model of the rehabilitation process. Each individual has a unique personality and life before disability, this has a significant impact on the process of rehabilitation. In addition, the human service and health care environments, as well as society as a whole effect the person and the rehabilitation process. A conceptual model proposed by Hershenson (1990), provides a rationale for distinguishing rehabilitation counseling from such other helping disciplines as medicine or psychotherapy. This system of categories involves primary, secondary, and tertiary prevention:

- Primary prevention is characterized by activities directed toward preventing the onset of disease or disability. This has been traditionally the mission of such fields as public health and occupational health and safety.
- Secondary prevention is characterized by activities directed toward preventing or, when that is not possible, limiting the effects of the disease or disability in cases in which primary prevention has failed. This has traditionally been the mission of medicine, psychotherapy, and similar curative fields.
- Tertiary prevention is characterized by activities directed toward preventing long-term residual conditions from having any greater disabling effects than necessary, once the secondary prevention fields have done all they can do to cure or limit the disease/disabling

process. This has traditionally been the mission of rehabilitation counseling and allied rehabilitation fields.

Hershenson (1990) described how the relative attention given to the individual and to the environment differs at each level. Primary prevention, for example, is heavily weighted toward the environment (e.g., drinking-water supply, worksite safety, automobile seat belts) and considers individuals only insofar as they are affected by that environment. Secondary prevention is heavily weighted toward the individual (e.g., curing or limiting the pathology that exists within the individual) and examines the environment only insofar as it facilitates or impedes the curative process within the individual. Tertiary prevention differs from both of the other categories of prevention in that it requires an equally balanced focus on both the environment and the individual. This dual focus is necessary because disability may stem as much from environmental barriers as from internal limitations. Thus, at each level the disciplines of public health, medicine, and rehabilitation counseling differ from each other in their basic science, focus, strategy for intervention, and goals.

PARADIGMS FOR REHABILITATION COUNSELING

For intentional, systematic practice to occur, it is critical that rehabilitation counselors have a conceptual model or paradigm to guide their work. It has been argued that rehabilitation counselors have at least three such orientations to conceptualize their teaching, research, and practice. These paradigms include the psychomedical model, the systems model, and the ecological model (Cottone & Emener, 1990). Each of these orientations have merit and distinguish themselves by the relative emphasis they place on the person, the environment, and the relationship between them. After a brief discussion of the psychomedical and systems model, a more detailed description of the ecological model will be presented.

The Psychomedical Model

The psychomedical model looks within the individual for a diagnosis of the problem, placing the patient in a "one-down position" relative to the expert, typically a medical doctor or psychiatrist. From this perspective the person with a disability is examined and treated relative to the extent and prognosis of his or her pathophysiology, impairment, and potentially his or her functional limitations. The psychomedical model represents a biomedical orientation toward the scientific representation of the person's condition and uses diagnostic categories to administratively classify and subsequently treat the underlying cause of a person's disability. This approach is valuable to understanding the medical and allied health professionals' contributions to the rehabilitation team. It underlies the restorative services offered in rehabilitation and is related to the secondary prevention model referred to above.

The Systems Model

Cottone and Cottone (1986) provide yet another perspective to conceptualizing rehabilitation counseling practice, that is, the systems approach. This perspective suggests that it is neither the person nor the environment that is the unit of analysis but the relationship between the two, specifically defined within interpersonal interaction style. This perspective suggests that to focus on either the individual (psychomedical) or the individual–environment transaction (ecological) is incomplete as the inherent nature of persons is systemic and the impact of disability affects all persons with relationship to the person and in the varied environments involved. This perspective argues for the inclusion of family counseling in the curriculum and competency of the rehabilitation counselor.

The Ecological Model

An ecological model reflects the tertiary prevention model and has been proposed by Cottone and Emener (1990) as an alternative to the psychomedical and systems perspectives. Historically, this perspective of rehabilitation has emerged from a trait-factor tradition, which measures traits within the individual and parallel factors within environmental contexts and further seeks to describe the extent of congruence between them. The Minnesota Theory of Work Adjustment (Lofquist & Dawis, 1969) has provided an empirically valid version of the trait-factor model for vocational rehabilitation practice, specifically with persons with disabilities. This model gives equal consideration to the person and the environment.

The tradition of the personnel management model in business and industry is reflected in this approach as it seeks selectively to match a person to a job for which he or she is qualified and would find satisfaction.

The personnel model in general does not adopt a developmental perspective; the latter perspective seeks to match persons to jobs with consideration of changing either the traits of the individual with or without a disability or accommodations within the essential functions of the job task or environmental reinforcers under consideration. Maki, McCracken, Pape, and Scofield (1979) suggested that an ecological perspective with a developmental orientation transformed a trait factor approach into a viable theoretical framework for vocational rehabilitation. Kosciulek (1993) supported the continuing validity of this approach to contemporary practice. It is assumed that the conceptual discussion that follows would apply to all people, as well as tasks or environments other than vocational, such as independent living and recreational pursuits.

Basically, this ecological model of individual differences provides a conceptual infrastructure for the profession of rehabilitation counseling and its model of practice. To better understand this paradigm the approach is briefly described. Traits refer to the underlying characteristics that exist in people. They account for the observed behavioral consistencies within people and for the stable and enduring differences among people in response to similar stimuli. All people are assumed to possess the same traits, but in differing amounts. In the process of measuring and evaluating the trait configurations of an individual, one must infer their presence from samples of behavior, as traits cannot be measured directly or in their pure form. The particular traits the rehabilitation counselor decides to evaluate depend on the purpose of the assessment. The professional must identify those traits most relevant to the client's objectives. The assessment techniques that have been demonstrated to provide the most valid and reliable evaluation of the individual's physical as well as cognitive capacities in terms of his or her aptitudes and achievements are then selected for use.

These individual traits are paralleled by factors describing the essential and marginal functions of an environmental context. In this way a vocational factor or job requirement, such as the ability to lift 50 pounds or read at the 6th-grade level, would need to be measured to see if these traits existed to the same extent within the trait structure of the person. If the traits of the individual correspond to the factor demands of the job, it is hypothesized that the person would be successfully placed in that job. Both traits and factors can be measured or assigned numbers to indicate the extent to which each is present in the individual and in the environment.

Job analysis is a process that is often used to define the functions of a job and the tasks that comprise it. The matching or congruence between the worker's performance and the job or task has been described as the level of satisfactoriness the worker is perceived to have as evaluated by the employer. The rehabilitation counselor may refer the person to a psychologist for psychometric or psychological measurement of aptitudes and achievement or have the physical capacities of a person evaluated by allied health professionals, such as a physical therapist. Both of these referrals represent a request for information based on a psychomedical paradigm of describing capacities within the individual. This information may be used within the ecological model, however.

The Minnesota Theory of Work Adjustment (Lofquist & Dawis, 1969) also emphasizes the importance of the individual's satisfaction with the work. The rehabilitation counselor may predict with enhanced accuracy the person's likelihood to remain on a particular job by evaluating this satisfaction. The behavioral consistency principle is applied with the assumption being made that past performance is the best indicator of future behavior. Therefore, the person's needs, interests, and personality must be identified as well as the reinforcers that are available to meet these needs in a given environment. In a parallel way, the individual's needs and the extent to which factors that meet these needs are present in the environment must be considered. It is therefore critical to consider both the person's interests and his or her ability to meet these needs, as well as his or her ability to do the job in order to enhance the person's tenure in a given job. Although in some instances referral to psychologists and other mental health professionals may be involved in this rehabilitation assessment gathering process, it is possible that rehabilitation counselors themselves would secure this information through interview, observation, and the occasional use of inventories. The question of who secures what information is a matter of the scope of practice of the individual professional and the available resources that define the functions performed by the staff in a particular human service or rehabilitation system.

The ecological perspective builds on this trait factor approach, however, it embraces more of a social learning orientation respectful of the reciprocal nature of both persons and environments. Scofield, Pape, McCracken, and Maki (1980) described an Ecological Adaptation Model, which conceptualizes this reciprocal relationship in describing: (1) the nature of the individual with a disability as he or she interacts and to various degrees adapts to various environments and (2) the simultaneous ability of environments to accommodate persons with a disability. This model highlights the importance of not only assessing traits and factors, but the transactions that dynamically describe the interactive nature of person(s) and environment(s). It is suggested that adaptation as a dynamic concept describing the extent to which a person accepts disability as one of his or her many characteristics is a preferred concept to adjustment, which infers a more enduring, static and categoric description when referring to a persons acceptance of their disability.

This model provides a basis for assessing the normative standards, frames of reference, and response tendencies of environments and persons at various levels of intimacy to the person with a disability. The model suggests that attitudes, defined as learned predispositions to respond in an evaluative manner, are especially critical to assess considering their potential impact. The model also assesses the individual's completeness and accuracy of reception of information (both overt and covert), his or her frame of reference (including self-concept and self-efficacy), and his or her response tendencies, or typical interaction style, with reference to particular persons and environments. This conceptualization acknowledges that only behaviors that are actually exhibited are public and observable. Nonetheless the model provides the ability to consider the individual's adaptation to disability and to conceptualize societal limitations. The Ecological Adaptation Model perspective also provides the rehabilitation counselor with a systematic framework to organize and conceptualize the complexities of his or her work with individuals with disabilities in relation to the significant persons and environments in which they live, work, and recreate.

THE REHABILITATION CONCEPT

Once the rehabilitation counselor has a clear respect for and understanding of the philosophy of rehabilitation, the concept of disability, his or her own role and scope of practice, as well as a systematic paradigm to guide that practice, it is possible to revisit the rehabilitation concept. Maki (1986) operationalized the rehabilitation philosophy defining the rehabilitation concept in terms of a comprehensive, individualized process, prescriptive in nature, and directed toward the development or restoration of functional independence and a quality of life. Vocational rehabilitation traditionally defines functional independence in terms of economic self-sufficiency, whereas independent living rehabilitation defines this in terms of community integration and autonomous living. Both vocational and independent living rehabilitation programs increasingly include quality of life indices in their definitions of successful outcome.

The following represent the key elements in understanding the concept of rehabilitation:

- *It is comprehensive in scope and holistic in nature.* The rehabilitation process is an orderly sequence of activities related to the total needs of the individual. Though comprehensive services will differ from client to client, there are certain basic dimensions relevant to understanding the total person. The most significant dimensions include the medical, psychological, personal–social, cultural, educational, vocational, as well as spiritual considerations. To understand the client or provide services relating to only one aspect of the person's life functioning, without considering the other aspects and their interdependency, would be ineffective and may result in the ultimate failure of the rehabilitation effort. Effective rehabilitation thus usually demands the coordinated efforts of a multidisciplinary or interdisciplinary team. The rehabilitation counselor is an integral member of this team.

- *It is an individualized process.* Each person is unique in terms of skills, residual capacities, functional limitations, resources, and personality. The manifestations of disability present themselves differently to each individual, with varying meanings and implications depending on the environmental context. Rehabilitation is thus a process based on the needs and assets of a particular client. Rehabilitation counselors must continually be aware of the pitfalls of labeling and stereotyping. Various authors (Feist-Price, 1995; Nathanson, 1979) have noted that counseling professionals are not immune to bias or prejudice regarding disability and must be aware of their own attitudes and expectations. Successful rehabilitation is based on individualized written rehabilitation plans (IWRP) developed with clients based on valid and meaningful data.

- *It is prescriptive in nature.* That is to say, a prescriptive course of action is developed with each individual. The type and amount of services provided are based on the needs and characteristics of the individual. Services are selected that will remove, reduce, or compensate for the functional and societal limitations of the individual in achieving the goals established in the individualized plan. Environmental accommodations and modifications must be considered, as well as client development and change through restoration or education programs.

• *It functions to develop or restore.* Habilitation is the term that denotes the development or acquisition of skills and functions previously not attained. This term is used commonly in reference to serving persons with developmental disabilities who, due to lack of training or experience, are initially developing their functional independence. Habilitation refers to an initial learning of skills and roles that allows an individual to function in society. Rehabilitation refers to the restoration or reacquisition of skills and functions lost through injury, disease, or trauma. The term rehabilitation is used here as well as throughout the text to generically describe either process resulting in functional independence.

• *Its goal is functional independence and a quality of life.* Functional independence is the capacity to take care of one's own affairs to the extent that one is capable. This is a broad goal; subsumed under the goal are economic self-sufficiency as well as personal, social, and community living skills (Morris, 1973). It also reflects the individualized orientation in defining success and functioning. Functional independence considers the total individual in his or her environments.

A quality of life (QOL) perspective on rehabilitation counseling integrates competing program goals such as client independence or employment into a higher-order, multidimensional rehabilitation outcome. Counselors committed to a QOL orientation work from a wellness and holistic position that addresses both the development of the individual and the environment in which the person lives. QOL is directly applicable to the long-standing criterion problem in rehabilitation. Rehabilitation professionals continue to disagree as to whether the primary goal of rehabilitation is promoting client independence or vocational placement. QOL offers a higher-order goal that subsumes both independence and employment as legitimate outcomes (Roessler,1990).

THE REHABILITATION PROCESS

Historically persons with disabilities have received services through a delivery system that contains the following ordered components: Intake, Assessment, Services, and Outcomes. This is a generic model that accommodates the interdisciplinary nature of rehabilitation. The model presented by Maki, et al. (1979) provides a framework for describing this rehabilitation process. It is important to note that this sequence does not represent supported employment and disability management services.

The client's entry into the service delivery system begins with intake procedures. Here administrative decisions are made regarding the client's eligibility for services based on predetermined criteria. Once eligibility is determined, the client proceeds to the assessment component. As clients' concerns become more complex and the range of services broadens, the need for comprehensive assessment becomes increasingly important. Without accurate and effective assessment there can be, at best, only marginal adaptation. From this base, the client and rehabilitation counselor work together in plan development using the skills of problem solving and resource analysis. Prescribed in the plan are those services necessary to assist the client in attaining the specified outcomes.

Services are selected that will allow the client to acquire skills and behaviors appropriate for the designed outcomes. Services are generally either in the area of education, restoration, or counseling. Education is usually prescribed for clients who lack the skills or knowledge necessary to reach their long- or short-term goal(s) and the objectives outlined in their individualized rehabilitation plan. Education may be formal or informal and generally lies outside the scope of practice of the rehabilitation counselor. Restoration services are usually prescribed when there is a need for enhancing the physical functioning of an individual; prothestics, work hardening, or speech therapy are examples of these services. As with education, these services are often coordinated or managed by the rehabilitation counselor as they generally lie outside this individual's scope of practice. Counseling as a therapeutic or psychoeducational service is often provided by the rehabilitation counselor within the relationship and parameters of the agency, organization, or facility in which a particular counselor functions. It is in the performance of this function that the rehabilitation counselor selects an individual, group, or family counseling theory to guide this aspect of their practice. A final service that the rehabilitation counselor provides is consultation and advocacy to those persons and environments relevant to the client's plan.

The final component of the service delivery system presented herein is outcome. During this stage placement and follow-up occur. These activities may be performed by the rehabilitation counselor or they may be referred to a professional who specializes in these functions. Even though the traditional outcome of vocational rehabilitation success is reflected in a case-closed Status 26, other outcomes related to independent living and quality of life are valued in contemporary rehabilitation practice. Table 1.1 provides Client Status Codes for the State–Federal Vocational Rehabilitation Process that demonstrate a typical case-flow process and expands

TABLE 1.1. Client Status Codes: The Vocational Rehabilitation Process

Referral processing status
00	Referral
02	Applicant
06	Extended evaluation

Preservice status
10I	IWRP development
12I	IWRP completed

In-service status
14	Counseling and guidance only
16	Physical and mental restoration
18	Training
20	Ready for employment
22	In employment
24	Service interrupted
32	Postemployment services

Closure status
08	Closed from referral (00), applicant (02), or extended evaluation (06)
26	Closed rehabilitated
28	Closed for other reasons after the IWRP was initiated (not rehabilitated)
30	Closed for other reasons before the IWRP was initiated (not rehabilitated from Status 10 or 12)
34	Closed from postemployment services

on the generic human services model presented in this section.

Throughout the rehabilitation process the rehabilitation counselor performs differing functions depending on the needs of the client and the resources available within the service delivery system and the community. Hershenson (1990) proposed the "C–C–C" Model of Rehabilitation Counseling, which prescribes the following functions:

- Coordinating is a function through which the counselor coordinates the "restoration or replacement of assets and skills . . . for example, coordinating the programs that provide needed physical, social, and vocational rehabilitation services."

- Counseling is a function through which the counselor uses "the processes of reintegrating the self-image and of reformulating goals."
- Consultation is a function through which the counselor engages in "the process of environmental restructuring and requires consultation with the client's family, employer, and community" (p. 275).

Counselors are direct-service providers, and the manner in which they manage their time and activities contributes significantly to the efficiency and effectiveness of the rehabilitation process. Therefore, the counselor needs to develop caseload management practices that result in effective allocation of time and services. The case management model of rehabilitation counseling presented by Greenwood (1992), requires the counselor to emphasize five functions: (1) intake interviewing; (2) counseling and rehabilitation planning; (3) arranging, coordinating, and/or purchasing rehabilitation services; (4) placement and follow-up; and (5) monitoring and problem solving. The counselor and client must mutually establish the goals to be accomplished within the parameters of the practice setting, which may occur in a public agency, a nonprofit program, or a private for-profit organization. The practice setting will affect the range of functions and tasks that are to be performed.

No matter what other functions and responsibilities are engaged in by the rehabilitation counselor, counseling is the central function that is provided continuously throughout the rehabilitation process. It should be repeated that counseling is inherent in rehabilitation. G. N. Wright (1980) stated that, "this is a nontransferable obligation of the rehabilitation counselor. Consultant and rehabilitation services of other kinds may or should be purchased, but the ultimate professional responsibility for the function of counseling cannot be delegated. Professional counseling is indispensable to the proper selection, provision, and utilization of the other rehabilitation services" (p. 55).

Goodwin (1992) has noted that the reality of present-day rehabilitation counseling practice is that the vast majority of rehabilitation counselors do specialize. He noted that they may specialize by employment settings, such as the state–federal rehabilitation agency, private-for-profit rehabilitation sector, mental hospitals, rehabilitation facilities, halfway houses, correctional programs, schools, and independent living centers. They may also specialize in working with people with particular types of disabilities, such as substance abuse, mental retardation, hearing impairment, visual impairment, head injury, and mental illness. Some rehabilitation counselors specialize in one aspect of the rehabilitation process or job function, such as job placement and development, vocational evaluation, and work adjustment, clinical mental health counseling, and administration. Other rehabilitation counselors specialize in rehabilitation counselor education including preservice, inservice, and continuing education. Rehabilitation counselor specialization is likely to continue and will probably increase in the future. Rehabilitation counselors will continue to become supervisors, administrators, researchers, and educators.

REHABILITATION OUTCOME

NCMRR (1993) defines successful outcomes of the process of rehabilitation in terms of restoring the individual to maximal functioning and provides the foundation for a fulfilling, productive life following rehabilitation. The areas that are considered include survival and productivity, as well as social and work relationships Survival issues include maintenance of health, prevention of unnecessary medical complications, capacity for mobility, and control of the activities of daily living (ADL).

The outcomes of the rehabilitation process are strategies, products, and treatments that enhance the probability that people with disabilities will participate more fully in society. Activities that enhance productivity and give a sense of purpose and enjoyment to life must be possible; these may include employment, education, recreation, family, and community involvement. This participation should provide meaning and dignity to life so that persons with disabilities have a reason to live, not merely to exist.

The focus of the rehabilitation counseling effort is the improvement of function of people with disabilities so that they can live satisfactory lives in their community. Function within this context encompasses not only physical performance, but emotional, and cognitive functioning as well. The ability to develop and maintain social relationships with family, friends, and coworkers is a fundamental skill. The ability to manage finances, personal and work life, and supervise personal-care attendants is critical to successful community life.

Concern for the developmental cycle of an individual with disability is an essential feature of rehabilitation counseling as intervention strategies, life activities, and quality of life outcomes will vary according to age. Rehabilitation counseling should incorporate knowledge of the person's developmental life stage when assessing interventions or outcomes in persons with disabilities. The model provides for the growing awareness that the initial impairment may be complicated by subsequent impairments across the life span. Problems unique to growing up and aging with disabilities are seen as relevant to the rehabilitation process. The resulting variations in, or losses of function across time are important considerations in building a conceptual model of rehabilitation.

PROFESSIONAL DEVELOPMENT

Any discussion of the development of professional competence begins with consideration of the individuals who have self-selected themselves for a career in rehabilitation counseling and have been selected by the faculty of an education program or the administration of a service program to be permitted to study or provide service to persons whose rehabilitation would be the focus of such a professional. Competence is the sum total of knowledge, skills, and attitudes considered necessary by the profession's standards and community sanctions, values, and expectations within the context of its social, political, and cultural mores.

Individuals who apply for, or choose to engage in the rehabilitation counselor role must be vigilant in their commitment to self-awareness and reflect on their beliefs, motives, needs, and competencies themselves as a person first. It requires an honest and on-going process of self-assessment and self-understanding of how they are alike and different in relation to other persons. This is a key first step in the adoption or induction into any role as either the provider or recipient. The following dimensions of self-assessment/definition are representative of those critical aspects of the self that need articulation: age, gender, learning style, socioeconomic status, sexual orientation, life-style, developmental life stage/tasks, disability status, ethnic/cultural identity, occupation, and values, beliefs, and attitudes toward the role being considered. By definition, this introspection is self-focused and phenomenological. From this awareness perspective, consideration of others as individuals and the roles they may be engaged in, such as supervisor or client, is a prerequisite to ethical practice. This stance is also a prerequisite for the person to adopt and practice the various roles he or she is called on to play, such as parent, child, student, professional or client, or some combination thereof.

In consideration of the role of an individual as a professional rehabilitation counselor, it is therefore important to understand and to first be aware of his or her own personhood. Given this, it is then possible to select and systematically practice as a professional through an adopted theory of practice that is compatible with a personal belief system and that the individual integrates into his or her role as counselor. That is to say that a professional counselor engages in an ethical and defined relationship based on the articulated philosophy and theory, which guides the content and process of his or her work.

Specifically, the role and responsibilities of the counselor and the reciprocal role and responsibilities of the person seeking his or her services (client, patient, consumer) are, by design, established through the adoption of a theory or paradigm of practice appropriate to the profession and reflected in the mission and staffing patterns of their agency. From this perspective, the person-to-person relationship that may reflect a social interaction is differentiated from the professional theoretically role-defined relationship between a counselor and a client. This ethical and theoretical dimension defining the role parameters and principles of practice differentiates professional relationships from those defined as friendship or social as well as peer-counseling relationships. These latter relationships occur on a person-to-person level without the theoretical or ethical constructions invoked in a professional relationship between two individuals engaged in intentional role-defined interactions.

Graduate education in rehabilitation counseling imparts the knowledge of ethics and theory through didactic coursework, whereas qualified clinical supervision is critical to role induction and skill development. Research has shown that clinical supervision is critical to the development and maintenance of clinical competence. The translation of the natural helping skills that may have drawn an individual to seek a career as a professional counselor needs to be developed and a combination of didactic and experiential/clinical aspects further define the professional preparation standards of the rehabilitation counseling profession [Council on Rehabilitation Education (CORE),1991].

It is necessary to have a conceptual framework for understanding the developmental process involved in becoming and maintaining competence and integrity as a professional rehabilitation counselor. Prior to presenting such a model, however, a definition of clinical supervision is required. The following definition has been suggested as functional and appropriate for our profession and this discussion. Clinical supervision is defined as:

> An intervention that is provided by a senior member of a profession to
> a junior member(s) of that same profession. This relationship is evalua-
> tive, extends over time, and has the simultaneous purposes of enhancing
> the professional functioning of the junior member(s) monitoring the
> quality of professional services offered to the clients, she, he, or they
> see(s), and serving as a gatekeeper for those who are to enter the par-
> ticular profession. (Bernard & Goodyear, 1992, p. 4)

Clinical supervision as defined is therefore a distinct intervention that
requires a trained supervisor. Specialized education in the area of clinical
supervision is thus essential. Such supervision is critical at the preservice
level. It is equally as necessary at the continuing education and professional practice levels, however. To not engage in appropriate clinical
supervision does a disservice to the counselor and potentially places the
client at risk.

Maki and Delworth (1995) have proposed the Structured Developmental Model (SDM) as a robust and relevant paradigm to understand
counselor development. The SDM refines the Integrated Developmental
Model (IDM) proposed by Stoltenberg and Delworth (1987), through an
organization of the eight domains that reflect counseling practice.
Stoltenberg and Delworth assumed that progression from Level-1 counselor to Level-3 Integrated proceeds in a relatively systematic manner
through eight domains or areas of professional competence. The SDM
categorizes these domains into two main categories: (1) three primary
domains and (2) five process domains. The primary domains, essential
for every counselor, are sensitivity to individual differences, theoretical
orientation, and professional ethics. These first three domains serve as
metadomains and will continue to be addressed as counselors work
through the levels as well as through each of the remaining five process
domains. The preceeding discussion was based on these metadomains.

The five process domains parallel the functions of the rehabilitation
counselor and are presented in the traditional sequence of case service
delivery as follows: (1) interpersonal assessment, which uses the counseling relationship to evaluate the social skills, personality characteristics,
and interaction style of the client; (2) individual client assessment in his
or her environment, which focuses on the person and the functional
impact of disability and incorporates psychometric procedures and medical consultation; (3) case conceptualization, which requires the integration of interpersonal assessment and individual client-assessment data to

generate a working image of the client as a whole person; (4) treatment goals and plans; and (5) intervention strategies. Each of these process domains contains specific knowledge and skills that are interrelated and become integrated as the counselor reaches the fourth and final level proposed by this model, Level-3 Integrated. The model presented herein provides the supervisor with a format to achieve the dual goals of clinical supervision: enhancing the therapeutic competence of the counselor while simultaneously monitoring the client's welfare.

The following is a brief description outlining a modal developmental sequence defining the levels referred to previously. It is believed that a shared understanding of these levels and the developmental process involved will be of benefit to both the supervisior and counselor-in-training or in-practice who may be in the role of supervisee. This conceptual framework may serve to normalize and make more efficient this complex and often difficult process.

The developmental model assumes that counselors-in-training progress through four levels while learning to function clinically. According to Stoltenberg and Delworth's (1987) Integrated Developmental Model, as individuals progress across these levels, change occurs in a continuous manner with regard to the following: self and other awareness, motivation, and autonomy. As the individual moves through the levels, increased competence in each of the process domains can be observed.

At Level One counselors are both highly dependent on their supervisor and highly motivated to learn. They are concerned with their counseling performance to such an extent that they seem largely self-focused on their own behavior instead of their clients. Counselors at this level are also influenced by their supervisor's method or technique and will most likely function from an imitative or recipe-oriented approach to counseling.

At Level Two the counselor is less method bound, more client focused, and concerned with investing his or her own personality style into the counseling work. Counselors begin to experience in greater depth the emotional and cognitive states of the client. Developing insight and differentiating personal reactions from client realities are recurring struggles during this level. This dynamic may result in the counselor's vacillating motivational level. Because of the increase in skill base, Level-Two counselors also seem to vacillate between the need for supervision and the need for autonomy.

Level-Three counselors are more likely to assume a collegial relationship with their supervisor and other professionals. At this level, the counselor is able to ask for what he or she needs without feeling inadequate or that his or her competency will be called into question through such requests. Supervision becomes consultative in nature and counselor initiated. The Level-Three counselor also tends to have developed the ability to be empathetic with clients and to have a simultaneous sense of self-awareness, which allows for clear, professional boundaries. Having developed a balanced sense of personal and professional identity usually reflects itself in a fairly stable level of motivation.

The goal of a CORE-accredited rehabilitation counselor education programs is to provide the preservice foundation for the counselor to become a Level-Three Integrated professional who is able to function independently. It is believed that this level can occur with supervised experience and continuing education after graduation.

SUMMARY

In a manner consistent with the holistic nature of rehabilitation counseling, this chapter addressed the philosophy of rehabilitation and its attendant components, the concept of disability, various paradigms of both rehabilitation practice and rehabilitation counseling, the sequential process involved, and the centrality of the person with a disability throughout the rehabilitation-counseling intervention. Issues related to appropriate and respectful language and terminology were emphasized, along with a discussion of the importance of rehabilitation outcomes, including quality of life.

Professional preparation of rehabilitation counselors is also included in order to address the critical importance of adequate and ethical rehabilitation counselor supervision that ultimately serves to guide professional practice. As mentioned above and throughout this chapter, it is important to recognize not only the centrality of the person with a disability throughout this rehabilitation process, but also the integrative and reciprocal nature inherent in this process. The rehabilitation counselor becomes a key component in the enrivonment of the person with a disability once services commence, and the domains discussed in the Structured Developmental Model (Maki & Delworth, 1995), serve to enhance both the development of the rehabilitation counselor as a professional and the quality of services provided to those who seek rehabilitation services from qualified professionals. Both in terms of practice and professional development, it is important to remember, "without theory to direct tasks and duties rehabilitation counseling becomes more a technical occupation than a profession" (Emener & Cottone, 1989, p. 577).

CHAPTER 2

Paradigms of Practice: Theory and Philosophies

William G. Emener

"W hy?" *Why questions* are the most difficult kinds of questions people are ever asked by themselves or others. Consider, for example, the following three bogus, yet typical case illustrations.

Linda, a rehabilitation client, who, at the age of 23, a college senior, engaged, and a member of her college's diving team, slipped on the 3-meter board and hit her head. She woke up in the hospital and was informed that she had T-3 quadriplegia. Two months later she says: "I know what happened, I watched the videotape. I know *when* and *where* it happened, I read the newspaper story. I know *how* it happened, the orthopedic surgeon explained it to me. But, *why*? I never did anything to deserve this. *Why* me? That's the question I am struggling with!

John, Linda's rehabilitation counselor, a 31-year-old university graduate, says to his supervisor: "I know *what* to do to help Linda, I had good orientation training. I know *when* and *where* I need to do things, I've been with the agency for 3 years. I know *how* to be a rehabilitation counselor. But *why* will I be doing what I plan to be doing in order to help Linda? *Why* will it be helpful to her?

Terry, John's agency director, a 53-year-old administrator with 25 years of experience in the field, says to his colleagues: "I know that we have to prioritize our funds from the state. Money is very tight right now. And I have reviewed the data you provided for me. Do I increase the funding of our mental-retardation program? I care about those kids. Do I increase the funding of our spinal-cord-injury program?—I feel for the Linda's of the world. *Why* should we decide what we have to decide? *Why* will we do what we will do?

When people are faced with difficult *why questions* such as these, even in the presence or absence of relevant data, two things usually occur: (1) they find answers to their why questions; and (2) they wittingly or unwittingly rely on theoretical and philosophical bases for their answers. And when we find a commonality, linkage, or pattern to our theoretical and philosophical tenants, the overall consideration is called a paradigm. Thus, it indeed would appear imperative for rehabilitation professionals to remain aware of and sensitive to the theoretical and philosophical tenants, as well as the overall paradigm, underlying their thoughts, feelings, actions, and decisions with and on behalf of individuals with disabilities.

Three terms critical to these above considerations were defined rather well by Webster (1983): *theory*—"an idea or mental plan of the way to do something . . . a formulation of apparent relationships or underlying principles of certain observed phenomena which has been verified to some degree" (p. 1983); *philosophy*—"the general principles or laws of a field of knowledge, activity, etc; as the *philosophy* of economics" (p. 1347); and *paradigm*—"a pattern, example or model" (p. 1298). And from a historical perspective, society has witnessed identifiable shifts in rehabilitation's theoretical, philosophical, and paradigmic cannons and social Zeitgeists as shown in the following example:

> For example, the Greek philosophy of the unity of body and soul circa 300 b.c. to 1000 a.d. (Dickinson, 1961; Garrett, 1969; Nichtern, 1974), the demonology of the Middle Ages (Obermann, 1965), the Humanistic, Empiricist, and Secularist movements of the Renaissance and Reformation (Rubin, & Roessler, 1978), America's Social Darwinism and the Social Gospel Movements (Obermann, 1965), the theory of Eugenics (Kanner, 1964), the Charity Organization Movement (Lubove, 1965), and the current era [the 1980s] of Rights and Entitlement. (Emener & Ferrandino, 1983, p. 62)

The 1990s, it would appear, has been influenced primarily by what might be considered the Era of Empowerment (Banja, 1990; Beck, 1994; Emener, 1991; Olney & Salomone, 1992). For a professional rehabilitation counselor to be an integral part of his or her profession, to efficiently and effectively serve individuals with disabilities, and to be a direct and/or indirect force in shaping rehabilitation's future, an in-depth understanding and appreciation for the theoretical, philosophical, and paradigmic cannons and tenants of rehabilitation and rehabilitation counseling is minimally necessary.

PHILOSOPHICAL QUESTIONS

One of the first and early uses of philosophical questioning was vested in the query: "What is reality?" Indeed, there have been many "answers" to this question, "ranging from the view that what we experience every day, because of its transience, is an imitation of a greater Reality in the form of Ideas (a type of Idealism), to the view that what we experience every day is all there is (a type of Materialism)" (Emener & Ferrandino, 1983, p. 63). This philosophical question unquestionably interfaces with disability and rehabilitation. For example, DeLoach and Greer (1981) discussed adjustment to disability (which they called "stigma incorporation," p. 221) as involving a two-phase process. The first phase occurs when the individual with the disability employs his or her psychological defense mechanisms (e.g., denial, rationalization, projection), followed by the second phase (which they called "utilizing task oriented mechanisms," p. 25) in which the individual employs a problem-solving approach in order to ameliorate some of his or her difficulties and get on with his or her life. Phase one, in effect, suggests that the individual is a pawn of the universe, akin to "I am a victim and have no control over what has and is happening." In phase two, however, the individual begins to see himself or herself as a "creator of reality" and therefore he or she can be more proactive (and less reactive) concerning his or her life's experiences.

When I discuss this foregoing, philosophical, "reality" concept in my graduate classes, I affectionately tell my "Three Umpires Story."

At a national baseball umpires convention, there were three umpires on a panel discussing the calling of balls and strikes. The first umpire, a recent graduate of umpiring school, said: "I call 'em what they are. If it's a ball, I call it a ball. If it's a strike, I call it a strike." The second umpire, who had upwards of 15 years experience in the major leagues, said: "I call 'em what I think they are. If I think it's a ball, I call it a ball. If I think it's a strike, I call it a strike." The third umpire, whose leather-like skin and almost permanent squinting eyes revealed many many years of experience behind home plate, said: "They ain't nothin' till I call 'em. If I say it's a ball, it's a ball. If I say it's a strike, it's a strike."

In this example, the first umpire is saying, in effect, "reality exists in the world, it's my job *to recognize* it and say what it is." The second umpire is suggesting that "reality exists in the world, it is my job *to try to recognize* it and say what it is." And the third umpire is suggesting a dramatically different philosophical tenant from the first two, "I create the reality of the world merely by what I say it is."

In the field of rehabilitation, it is not uncommon to meet a person with T-3 quadriplegia who says, "I am here in this hospital and my life now is doomed. I am unable to do anything. I just have to live with it and bear it." On the other hand, it also is not uncommon to meet a person with T-3 quadriplegia who says, "I know that there are many things that I no longer can do, but I can't wait to get out of this hospital so I can get on with my life." Clearly, the philosophical considerations of "reality," "freedom," "choice," "commitment," and "responsibility," to name a few, are intricately interwoven in every person's life—those who have a disability and those who do not have a disability. (Yet again, philosophically speaking, "What is disability?") Existential philosophers address these issues and collectively suggest that "there is no given meaning or abstract meaning, people make meaning in the world through the vehicles of responsibility, choice, and commitment" (Emener & Ferrandino, 1983, p. 64). Although Kierkegaard stated, "The most tremendous thing which has been granted to man is: the choice, freedom" (Kierkegaard, in Winn, 1960, p. 15), Sartre said: "If existence really precedes essence, man is responsible for what he is. Thus existentialism's first move is to make every man aware of what he is and to make the full responsibility of his existence rest on him" (Sartre, in Spanos, 1966, p. 279).

Other philosophical questions critically germane to rehabilitation and rehabilitation counseling (in addition to "What is Reality?"), include "What is Truth?," "What is Meaning?," "What is Responsibility?," "What is Choice?" and "What is Freedom?"

APPLIED PHILOSOPHICAL CONCEPTS

The direct and indirect application of philosophical considerations to rehabilitation and rehabilitation counseling can be illustratively delineated by Existential considerations regarding "What is Reality?" Kierkegaard's statement that "man is responsible for what he is" implies that the person (i.e., the client with T-3 quadriplegia) is himself or herself the individual responsible for defining who he or she is, for maximizing his or her potential as a person. Commensurately, Sartre's statement "to make every man aware that he is to make the full responsibility of his existence rest upon him" implies that the rehabilitation counselor working with the client with T-3 quadriplegia is responsible for helping the client to realize his or her responsibility (i.e., to be responsible for him or herself) and to facilitate the client's acceptance of, and ultimately acting on, his or her self-responsibility. In the main, a rehabilitation counselor's philosophical beliefs regarding "the basic nature of man" provide the a priori assumptions on which can rest his or her theory of counseling.

PHILOSOPHY AND THEORY OF COUNSELING

If a rehabilitation counselor's believes, philosophically, that the human being is born basically ''good'' and "strives toward being good," then he or she may be in a position to subscribe to a Rogerian or client-centered theory of counseling. [For example, "People know what is best for themselves and will ultimately do what is good and in their best interest."] On the other hand, if a rehabilitation counselor's a priori belief is that the human being is born basically "bad" and must learn to be "good," he or she may prefer considering a Freudian or NeoFreudian theory of counseling. [For example, "People are born with one main purpose—to satisfy the id, and they eventually must develop a superego and ego structure in order to be uncontrollably less self-serving and less self-centered."] If a rehabilitation counselor subscribes to John Locke's Tabula Rasa theory (i.e., people are neither born good nor bad but "with a clean slate—people learn to be good or bad"), then he or she may be more inclined to subscribe to a learning theory model of counseling. The most important concept for rehabilitation counselors to remember is that whatever their theoretical orientation to their work as counselors or therapists may be, their theoretical orientation ultimately rests on their a priori, philosophical assumptions and beliefs regarding life, the human being, and the nature of human existence.

FUTURISTIC CONSIDERATIONS

Our modern medical and technological revolutions currently are approaching their zeniths. More and more people are avoiding and/or surviving heretofore life-ending diseases and traumas. Just around the corner, however, American society will be boldly confronted with Dowd and Emener's (1978) prediction that "on a global scale, large numbers of people may be able to survive. Humanity would probably survive, but the decision may be: who would be able to survive and under what conditions?" (p. 35). From a macro perspective, to whom we will be providing our preciously available rehabilitation services as our technological capabilities increasingly exceed our diminishing resources (aka, "I feel for the Linda's of the world")? Indeed, our society's social philosophies shall be stretched and tested with social-euthanasian questions such as these. From a micro perspective, how will health care professionals respond when a person, such as an acquired immune deficiency syndrone (AIDS) patient or an individual with T-3 quadriplegia in severe physical and/or psychological pain, says, "I do not want to live this way any longer. I do not want to live any longer. Will you help me do what I want to do?" Professional rehabilitation counselors, if not already, will be confronted with decisions such as these (Emener, 1986). And as Dowd and Emener (1978) suggested over a decade and a half ago, "These decisions are already upon us. If we do not involve ourselves in these decisions, others will make them for us. These others may not be nearly as enlightened as we" (p.36).

A number of years ago in a graduate seminar, one of my doctoral students suggested that modern technological advances will make our jobs and pertinent decisions easier. With a wry smile, one of the other students said, "Or make them harder." As an aspiring rehabilitation professional, it is imperative for you to be a lifetime student of philosophical and theoretical aspects of rehabilitation. In many ways, the future is now and we have only scratched the surface of these aforementioned questions, issues, and questions. And as Emener and Ferrandino (1983) fittingly offered,

"Although philosophy per se will not solve rehabilitation's problems, philosophically enlightened individuals might better pave the way toward enlightened solutions" (p. 67).

CHAPTER 3

History and Systems: Mostly Mavericks

Martha L. Walker and Susan M. Wiegmann

PLAYWRIGHTS' NOTES

The history of rehabilitation counseling was shaped by social, political, and economic changes of the twentieth century. Rehabilitation counselors were called "mostly mavericks" by Mary Switzer, the architect of rehabilitation in this country. Most of these heroes and heroines are unknown, and we have combined their stories into a handful of characters. We hope this history will be read aloud, with today's students taking on these collective voices from the past. The story is also about our society and how our view of disability has changed over the last century. It begins with public rehabilitation, referred to as "VR" in the play. Join us in the retelling, then sample the references for more understanding.

CAST IN ORDER OF APPEARANCE

Martha and Susan, rehabilitation counselor educators
Rita, rehabilitation counseling student
Mary Switzer, federal administrator of rehabilitation in the United States
Tracy Copp, one of five original U.S. rehabilitation "agents"
Bell Greve, originator of rehabilitation center concept

Don Dabelstein, rehabilitation counselor/philosopher
Jim Garrett, administrator of research and training programs
Cecile Hillyer, developer of training programs
Simon Olshansky, workshop director
Clayton Morgan, rehabilitation counselor educator
Ed Roberts, independent-living leader
Herbert Rusalem, rehabilitation researcher and educator

*   *   *

(The stage is divided into two levels of action, an elevated level at the rear of the stage where simple office furniture is in evidence, and a large room where the principal action occurs. As the curtain rises, Martha and Susan are putting on their coats inside the office. Rita knocks. With coat in hand, Susan opens the office door.)

*   *   *

Rita: I see you are on your way out. I just needed to talk to someone. Maybe it will wait . . . when will you be back?

(Susan and Martha look at each other.)

Susan: We hadn't planned to be back today, but come in—we're not in that much of a rush.

Martha: What's up? (Susan and Martha sit down, Rita moves into the room and sits, shaking her head.)

Rita: I've just been in class, and I'm totally confused. We heard a consumer say you can't be a rehab counselor if you don't have a disability. I chose this field because I wanted to help, and now it seems my help isn't wanted.

Susan: Do you have any idea what was behind that statement?

Rita: Not really, but it was pretty clear that she was angry at the rehab counselors she had known!

Susan: There's a history to her view . . .

Rita: But, I've also heard that the state VR program may no longer exist. It just seems like everything is changing. Will there be a job for me when I finish this program?

Martha: We can't guarantee that. But, this country has come a long way in its commitment to people with disabilities.

Susan: You know, we were just leaving for an important gathering. Sort of a once-in-a-lifetime event. If you'd like to come, you might learn how we got to this point. The guests' careers spanned the development of a federal rehabilitation program, the growth of modern medicine, and the emergence of many rehabilitation professionals.

Martha: Many of them shaped the role and function of rehabilitation counselors. They can tell you what they thought was important at turning points in our history.

Rita: But today has been such a downer. I wouldn't want to rain on their parade.

Susan: I'd count on them to be pretty hardy—and glad to meet someone who's asking good questions.

Martha: What do you say? Shall we go?

Rita: At this point, I've got nothing to lose . . .

* * *

(The three move out of the office. The spotlight shifts to the front of the stage. The buzz of multiple conversations fill the large room. Small groups of guests are standing around the edge of the room. A tall, smiling woman approaches as Rita, Susan, and Martha enter the room.)

* * *

Martha: This is Mary Switzer who was the head of the federal rehabilitation program from 1950 until 1970. She created the research and training components of the rehabilitation program in 1954. Mary, this is Rita, a first-year student in rehabilitation counseling.

Mary: Welcome. We're glad you're here to help us celebrate. As I look around the room, we could be celebrating the emergence of rehabilitation counseling. *(She turns to face Rita.)* Are you just starting your journey?

Rita: Yes, I'm in my first semester of study. *(She glances at Martha and Susan.)* My professors invited me to come along. I've got lots of questions. How did you become interested in rehabilitation counseling?

Mary: When I came to Washington in 1920 one of the first people I met was a rehabilitation counselor, Tracy Copp. I stayed as a permanent guest at a woman's club on H Street, and just happened to meet Tracy, who also lived there. Over many a breakfast, she talked with me about her work trying to interest states in beginning a rehabilitation program. They called her a rehabilitation agent, and she was one of five people in the federal office. The program was tiny then, but love of the program was contagious. *(She turns and scans the room.)* I see her over here. Let me introduce you to her. *(Mary moves toward a very erect, slim woman nearby, swooping up Rita, Martha, and Susan.)*

Mary: Tracy, I'd like you to meet someone who is studying to be a rehabilitation counselor. I was trying to tell her what was going on in 1920. It must be hard for someone new to rehabilitation counseling to imagine that this country had just decided that disability was its responsibility, not just the individual or the family whose child had a disability. What did those first rehabilitation counselors do?

Tracy: You must remember that the federal office of vocational rehabilitation was placed within vocational education then, and rehabilitation was virtually seen as reeducation. The first rehabilitation counselors had little experience with persons with physical disabilities, and their efforts in the first 3 years were experimental. The work was tested by concrete casework. It was apparent to all of us that rehabilitation of people with disabilities was a highly complex, personalized service. *(She speaks more rapidly, a little angrily.)* It wasn't long before a basic incompatibility between what was needed and what vocational education could provide developed. Vocational education was based on a classroom approach to training, while rehabilitation was a highly personalized service. *(She slows, and looks for a moment at Mary.)* And, also, many of the first rehabilitation counselors had been school principals. Counselors usually had 2 to 3 days getting familiar with state and federal laws, 2 weeks of traveling with the senior supervisor, and then were assigned a territory to travel in a Model-T Ford. They were expected to cover the state, and to be in each of the counties at least once a month. *(She gestures broadly.)* When the counselor arrived at the meeting place there would be a room filled with clients and their friends and families. The would-be clients had varied needs, but they had one thing in common. They wanted to work and to be independent. At that time, the counselor couldn't pay for medical treatment of any kind. If the client needed to go away for vocational training, the counselor couldn't pay for room or board. There were few organized charities in these communities for the counselor to use as resources. The counselor spent a great deal of time begging individuals and clubs to help the clients. *(She looks directly at Rita.)* You see, originally, the rehabilitation process was developed for adult males with physical disabilities. Rehabilitation called for the "highest types of workers". Many thought it was important to recruit mature people with industrial experience. Rehabilitation was seen as remaking a person. Although this was seen as a complex process, there was no specialized training required during the first 10 years of the vocational rehabilitation program.

Rita: Were there no qualifications for the job?

Tracy: It depended on the state, even as it does today, but by and large, rehabilitation counselors were male and were political appointees who had worked in the school system.

Mary: You see, Rita, by the time most states were offering rehabilitation programs, we were in the midst of a terrible depression. Jobs were very scarce. In the early 30s Franklin Roosevelt was elected on the basis of the "New Deal"—that government should act as the guarantor of the common good within the existing economic system—and that system wasn't working for so many Americans. I can remember traveling with Eleanor Roosevelt to visit the Arthurdale Mining Resettlement in West Virginia. This was just one national project to put people back to work. I think of Eleanor Roosevelt as a rehabilitationist, because of her basic belief: that we care enough to come, to remember what we see, and to keep our promises. She became a beacon of hope to many impoverished families. A nation's expectations of government were changing.

Tracy: *(Tracy nods at Mary)* Yes, it was remarkable that rehabilitation programs survived the Depression, and that rehabilitation counselors with little training themselves were able to find work for citizens with disabilities. Perhaps it was the message of hope and the enlarged role of government in people's lives that kept it alive. When World War II began in 1940, the vocational rehabilitation program was well-rounded, and the war emergency brought public attention to the fact that people with physical impairments can make in the production work of the nation. The country needed workers on the homefront, as all its "able-bodied men" went to war. The nation learned how profligate it had been in the waste of human resources. Both women and people with disabilities became a valuable part of the workforce almost overnight.

Mary: *(Mary turns, extending her hand to Bell.)* Tracy, before you go on, here's Bell Greve, whom you introduced me to many years ago. While the nation was struggling with the Depression and the war, Bell was in Cleveland showing that difficult problems of people with chronic conditions were best approached through comprehensive medical, social, psychological, and vocational programs. Bell, Tracy has been telling Rita, who has just started her study of rehabilitation counseling, about the developing role of the rehabilitation counselor. At the local level, what were you trying to accomplish?

Bell: (Bell smiles at Rita.) I was convinced that public and private agencies could deliver community services to people with disabilities. Dr. George Deaver, of the Institute for the Crippled and Disabled in New York, had begun a program of physical restoration to reinforce the social and vocational elements of the Institute's program. He didn't have to rely on the willingness of city hospitals and clinics for services to people with disabilities. I wanted Cleveland citizens to have that same opportunity at the Cleveland Rehabilitation Center.

Mary: You were a pathfinder for the workshops and facilities that grew rapidly over the next 20 years. It was the combined forces of the unmet needs of people with disabilities as well as their potential as untapped manpower that led to change in the legislation in 1943. Twenty years had passed before vocational rehabilitation was "liberated" from the Department of Vocational Education. There were only 300 rehabilitation counselors in the country at that time, and just less than 20,000 citizens were being rehabilitated each year. The stage was set to enact legislation that provided the possibility of physical restoration. Rehabilitation counselors no longer had to train around a disability, they could provide medical services to remove or minimize the impairment.

Rita: Do you mean that before 1943, rehabilitation counselors only had training or retraining to offer? That physical restoration wasn't authorized?

Mary: Yes, and what was very obvious to us at this time was that rehabilitation counseling was a vertical segment of many fields. Rehabilitation as a multidisciplinary program needed to be able to move across professional and administrative boundaries. *(Mary beckons to two men who are talking nearby, who walk toward Rita, Mary, Bell, Martha, and Tracy.)* Now here's Don Dabelstein and Jim Garrett who were working as rehabilitation counselors after World War II. Jim, Dabs— how do you explain the change in the work of rehabilitation counselors that resulted from administrative relocations and legislation that provided for a comprehensive rehabilitation program? *(Mary motions to Rita.)* We're trying to fill Rita in on how rehabilitation counseling developed. She's just begun her study.

Dabs: (Dabs smiles at Rita.) I'm glad to meet you, Rita. You see, we really needed trained personnel in federal–state vocational rehabilitation programs. The 1943 legislation gave us authority to provide medical services—the first time in our history that the public paid for medical services for individuals. Even after the 1943 legislation, training for professional rehabilitation counselors was limited to 6 weeks, and most of the personnel had been recruited from vocational education. Rehabilitation counselors had neither an understanding of physical restoration nor of psychological services. A great deal of research was now available from the Veterans Administration work with readjustment of veterans to civilian life, and vocational counseling, assessment, and guidance were now valued approaches. We were struggling with how to train rehabilitation counselors.

Tracy: I remember that period, Dabs. Counselors needed to interpret reports of medical personnel so they could integrate physical restoration services with vocational adjustment. They had to make use of psychological tests without being a psychologist or psychiatrist. Add to that the knowledge of regulations and risk of injury and other services, and you have quite an educational challenge.

Jim: (Interrupts.) It was more than an educational challenge! Rehabilitation was booming in the private sector and the need for trained personnel was *critical.* I was working with the Institute for the Crippled and Disabled in New York, and joined Howard Rusk in 1948 at his Institute for Physical and Rehabilitation Medicine. At the Institute, we combined psychological and social service components that worked. It seemed to us that the federal–state program was not helping anyone by the end of the 40s. In fact, we went for over a year without a single referral from the New York Department of Vocational Rehabilitation. We were getting plenty of referrals from the United Mine Workers—they saw that our comprehensive treatment worked. Severely injured miners were being rehabilitated.

Mary: (Nods to Jim.) Howard Rusk made sure that did not go unnoticed. I think the unwillingness of the federal–state program to work with clients with severe disabilities, using rehabilitation medicine approaches accounted largely for my being asked to become the Director of the

Office of Vocational Rehabilitation in 1950. When I recruited you, Jim, in 1951, 85% of persons who were considered rehabilitation counselors did not come from psychology or social-work backgrounds, but from classroom teaching. Your job was to organize a research and training effort at the federal level. *(Turns to a woman nearby.)* Here's Cecile Hillyer. *(Cecile joins the group.)* Cecile was in charge of the training after the 1954 legislation that established research and training as part of the Rehabilitation Act. What was training like after 1954, Cecile?

Cecile: I was brought in with the responsibility to enlarge the supply of trained personnel. In 1955, 35% of VR training grants were to the field of rehabilitation counseling. The other VR training programs included rehabilitation medicine, nursing, occupational and physical therapy, speech and hearing, visually and orally handicapped, and rehabilitation-facilities direction. Still, a major policy was channeling funds to meet the needs of state vocational rehabilitation agencies for qualified personnel. *(She looks at Jim.)* Jim, you and I differed about the disciplinary basis for the program, probably because you were a clinical psychologist and I was a social worker. So we decided to let each of the universities determine where the rehabilitation counseling courses would be offered, believing that the job contains elements of social work, psychology, and vocational guidance. In fact, one of our criteria for awarding rehabilitation counseling grants was evidence of interdisciplinary planning in the curriculum. You remember, Jim and Dabs, that we convened a workshop in Charlottesville, Virginia in 1955 and produced a document that shaped the curriculum of all rehabilitation counseling training programs.

Mary: And I got news of some of the controversy! Meetings of educators and administrators didn't always go well. But, Cecile, you encouraged joint committees between educators and state agency personnel to align university curriculum.

Jim: Before we had any programs, basic principles had been established that became the core of the programs. The concept of eligibility and feasibility of casework, process, and standards, along with counseling and guidance were the backbone of rehabilitation practice. The individually written rehabilitation program came from those basic principles, with a person-to-person working relationship between the counselor and the person with a disability.

Dabs: Those basics allowed rehabilitation counselors to serve newly targeted populations. We were just learning about working with people with developmental and psychiatric disabilities. We were growing so fast with an organic Act that provided services, research, training, expansion, innovation, and facility support.

Mary: (Interrupts.) I remember once trying to sell you on improving mental health for the deaf. You listened patiently and then said, "Carry on your justification speech if you must, but you really don't have to sell human need to me. I have met it in so many forms. I know what it is. Just explain to me the form it takes in deafness." I'll never forget that. It was an explosion of opportunity for rehabilitation in those days, and we were busy beyond belief.

Rita: Excuse me, but I'm just beginning to realize how fast things were happening then. The authority to provide physical restoration services created an acute training need. And added to that was the new appreciation of psychological aspects of disability, and the importance of research with new populations. But no one insisted that having a disability was a prerequisite to being a rehabilitation counselor?

Bell: No, Rita. This was a period of growth for many professions, and persons with disabilities were still viewed as entities to be changed. Expertise seemed to be the answer, and capacity building meant improving treatment and clinical skills.

Jim: (Interrupts.) But something was emerging during this period of growth. Because the 1954 Amendments allowed expansion of facilities in local communities, facilities led the way, not only in dealing with people with severe disabilities, but in reinforcing a team approach. Counselors who worked for state agencies were more familiar with individualizing services, but rehabilitation counselors in facilities worked on and through teams. I don't know where we would be without facilities, places that could do things for clients that needed to be done. The rehabilitation facility was a place where people could see what was going on in rehabilitation in the 1960s.

Dabs: You're right, Jim. Rehabilitation counselors who were working in rehabilitation facilities and psychiatric hospitals were on teams, developing relationships with employers in the hiring of persons with disabilities. It was a visible team, extending beyond the facility to include the community.

Rita: Were these facilities workshops? I thought workshops segregated people.

Mary: (Motions to a nearby person) There's Simon Olshansky. Now he can tell you about workshops. He directed many workshops during this time of facility expansion. Simon, this is Rita, and she has asked about workshops and effects on clients.

Simon: (Nods and speaks directly to Rita.) I can tell you that they've taken a bum rap! Was there any historical context given to what you read about them?

Rita: Only that they became dead ends for clients.

Simon: (Sharply.) But that ignores the original idea behind workshops, which was to provide a positive environment for a client's experiences as a worker. Those experiences were to emphasize competence and a sense of worth. Some clients who entered workshops had very severe disabilities—those who might not develop the speed or stamina to enter regular employment, and some who preferred sheltered employment. Theories of work adjustment and work evaluation were developed within facilities with the goal of encouraging easy exit to regular employment, while continuing to provide sheltered employment for those who might not improve much or stay improved for long.

Mary: We needed a place to show that clients, who earlier were thought incapable of working, could make it. Facilities were the place where extended evaluation happened, and this opened the door for our serving persons with very severe disabilities.

Cecile: It also prompted the creation of new training programs in vocational evaluation and adjustment training, and facility administration.

Jim: In the 1960s, we were ready with facility programs including skill training, work habit development, psychological testing, and job placement to help wage a war on poverty. Congress passed the Public Welfare Amendments, which included an attempt to inject a work orientation into the welfare program. Unemployment, decay in cities, and economic upheavals led to a sense of uneasiness in our country, and rehabilitation was seen as the preferred treatment for persons with socially disadvantaged backgrounds. Legislators reasoned that if rehabilitation had worked so well with persons who had physical or mental disabilities, it could be extended to serve public assistance recipients, public offenders, substance abusers, and others who were "job handicapped."

Mary: (Interrupts.) It was an outreach opportunity to multiply the effectiveness of the rehabilitation program over the past 15 or 20 years. For a brief time, Vocational Rehabilitation was called "the Marine Corps" of the Department of Health, Education, and Welfare. *(A tall, thin man steps into the group.)* It seemed to me that I had witnessed the change in public attitudes from compassion without action, to willingness to act for economic reasons, followed by a willingness to act for social reasons. I'm sorry, but Tracy, Bell, and I must leave now. It's been so good to meet you, Rita. As you can see, we've had many different personalities involved in rehabilitation over the years. Now, Clayton Morgan *(Mary gestures toward the man who just joined the group)* is just the man to tell you what happened next—he knows rehabilitation counseling and its history! Best wishes for your career, Rita. You are the future of rehabilitation. *(Nods to all the group and walks toward the door with Bell and Tracy.)*

Clayton: Thanks, Mary. That's a tall order. We really believed in the Great Society. President Kennedy's family had stimulated renewed efforts in rehabilitating people with developmental disabilities, and we were proving that anyone could work—with training and support. Meanwhile, the welfare program was in a mess. There were great expectations of the federal–state rehabilitation program to rehabilitate an unemployed group whose problems did not yield to standard procedures of education, training, and hiring. We soon learned that traditional counseling approaches were ineffective with clients from disadvantaged backgrounds, who had minimal education and underdeveloped self-concepts. These clients needed help coping with everyday problems of living while planning a future. They needed concrete services. In 1968, the Rehabilitation Act Amendments expanded eligibility to include disadvantaged persons, and individuals with a history of addiction became possible candidates for services. This tested the basic philosophy of the vocational rehabilitation process, a process that takes time. Addicts in treatment were in a hurry. Counselors working in this area were in a hurry. Public attitudes weren't as positive toward drug abusers or prison inmates as they were toward citizens with physical disabilities. Just to give you an idea of the job we faced, in 1967, nearly 50% of the entire population of several large state prisons were persons with mental retardation.

Cecile: We tried to help with training programs for counselors to learn new skills for new populations. Some saw the commitment to the vocational rehabilitation of drug abusers as a revitalization of vocational rehabilitation as a profession. Others thought the seeds of ruin had been sown when eligibility was expanded to persons with nonphysical disabilities.

Clayton: Rehabilitation counselors were coming of age as a profession then, also. Some rehabilitation counselors were feeling uncertain about their knowledge base being unique. The graduate field of rehabilitation counseling training had rapidly increased from graduating 12 counselors in 1954 to 1,000 in 1971. Students saw their role as lacking autonomy and as including "dirty work"; uncertain that rehabilitation counseling was a profession. Researchers and educators produced over 1,000 documents related to the roles and functions of rehabilitation counselors in the 60s. The specialized knowledge base of rehabilitation counseling was distilled through studies on competencies and skills, and accreditation and certification efforts were organized. Rehabilitation counselors were part of two national organizations. Outcome studies confirmed that clients were more satisfied with counselors who had graduate training in rehabilitation counseling. Just as rehabilitation counseling was meeting the criteria of a profession, we entered the crises of the 70s.

Jim: (Speaks loudly.) Rehabilitation suffered a setback when the Department of Health, Education, and Welfare was reorganized and rehabilitation techniques were brought to bear on disadvantaged populations. Something got lost along the way. The gospel of cost effectiveness swept away the Great Society. We retreated from the humanitarian frontier and took refuge in a scientific and technologic age.

Simon: (Speaks even more loudly.) And look how quickly we abandoned the rehabilitation facility as a primary community resource. When deinstitutionalization became the watchword, it was carried to the extreme. Anytime more than 10 persons with disabilities were gathered together, we were accused of creating restrictive environments. "Facilities" became a dirty word. People were returned to places where there was no community.

Clayton: I'd agree that with every advance, there was a loss. And it's a history of polarization. I agree that VR turned in on itself and developed ornate procedural rules, checks, and audits. After 1970 it moved away from the nation's agenda of solving the problem of poverty to the safety of clinical preoccupation, elaborate case planning, and monitoring. Front-line counselors were sapped of their vitality. *(Looks over Rita's shoulder.)* I see Ed Roberts over there. Let's see if we can get him to pick up the story in about 1972. *(Clayton moves toward a man seated in a wheelchair and using a ventilator.)* Ed, I'd like you to meet Rita, a student who has some very good questions.

Ed: Hi, Rita. I'll bet the 70's seem like ancient history to you.

Rita: But interesting history. Especially when I try to understand what my role as a rehabilitation counselor might be today. What happened in the 70s? Others see that period as a real turning point.

Ed: Well, I was at Berkeley in 1972 where we had a very active center for independent living. We weren't the first, because 10 years earlier the University of Illinois had an expanded program of independent living for persons with severe physical impairments. What "severely disabled persons" had going for us was the push for mainstreaming children and adults with developmental disabilities. Actually, the rehabilitation establishment was worried because the failed "War on Poverty" was about to drag rehabilitation down. So, the 1973 legislation shifted the emphasis to providing rehabilitation services to individuals with severe disabilities, despite two vetoes by President Nixon.

Rita: What happened to persons without severe disabilities?

Clayton: Often they were not served by the public rehabilitation program. Rehabilitation began to splinter at this point. Federally supported training programs emphasized architectural and transportation barriers, advanced technologies and assistive devices, and populations requiring intensive and more costly services. Meanwhile, rehabilitation programs for older adults and for persons with narcotic addictions, alcoholism, psychiatric disabilities, developmental disabilities, and work-related injuries were established independent of public rehabilitation structures. Rehabilitation counselors whose primary interests were with those disabilities groups felt marginalized, neither belonging to rehabilitation counseling nor to their specialized areas.

Cecile: (Tosses her head.) A very small group of people developed rehabilitation from a small and relatively unimportant part of the welfare–health structure of our country, and others wanted those programs.

Dabs: (Looks at Cecile.) Mary said that the greatest tragedy that could happen to rehabilitation would be to train people who became profession-centered or agency-centered, or centered anywhere except on the people they were supposed to be serving.

Jim: (Speaks to Cecile and Dabs.) I have to meet my car pool. But what you can't lose sight of is the leadership of the federal government in saying what a qualified professional should know. If we hadn't done that, rehabilitation counselors would still be state political appointees.

Cecile: Dabs and I wanted to talk with you about something, Jim. We'll walk over with you. *(Jim, Dabs, and Cecile say goodbye to all, shake hands and leave together.)*

Simon: I'd best shove off as well. *(Speaks to Rita.)* Just keep asking questions—keep us all on target, because each of us tells this history from our own point of view.

Ed: (Looks at Rita and Clayton.) Let's go back to the "dismemberment of the rehabilitation establishment." What I think was really happening is that a traditional program, which depended on professional expertise to reach well-defined medical and vocational goals was facing a new reality—consumer choice. The 1973 legislation required client participation through an individually written rehabilitation plan.

Clayton: The irony is that many state-federal agencies did not hire graduates of rehabilitation counseling programs, so they had few "professionals" to establish relationships based on mutual respect, a principle of counseling. In fact, existing staff and administrators sometimes viewed graduates as overtrained in psychological theory and undertrained in practical aspects of the job. The definition of a qualified rehabilitation professional didn't even appear in the Rehabilitation Act until 1984.

Ed: There was a price to be paid for that delay. By 1991, consumers reshaped the Rehabilitation Act to rest upon consumer control.

Rita: How does the Americans with Disabilities Act figure into this?

Ed: It made the clear point that asking the client to make all of the adjustments was unjust—society had some changes to make also. That meant counselors had to know about environmental barriers.

Clayton: The sharpened focus of the public rehabilitation program had other consequences. I see one of the prophets of the effects of the Rehabilitation Act of 1973, Herbert Rusalem. Herb, how about joining us for a minute? *(A man joins the group.)* I think you know Ed Roberts, and this is Rita, a student in rehabilitation counseling. I remember your saying that all rehabilitation professionals should be more aggressive in seeing that the rehabilitation movement served all persons with disabilities with understanding and dignity.

Herbert: (Lowers his head.) I was distressed in the late 1970s with play-it-safe bureaucrats who pulled back from the expansion of the program to disadvantaged clients. And I was also aware of occasional counselor callousness and stereotyping, such as limiting rehabilitation goals to early employment rather than career development. In 1991, when consumers insisted on careers versus entry-level jobs, this seemed a just inheritance. It was also no surprise to me when applicable rehabilitation services became available through private for-profit agencies.

Rita: I don't understand.

Herbert: (Faces Rita directly, speaks slowly.) With the mandate of public agencies to give priority to clients with severe disabilities, individuals with work-related injuries were not being served adequately through the state–federal system. When they were determined eligible for services, the agency process was often time-consuming, which was costly for employers. So employers' insurance companies began to hire rehabilitation counselors to provide vocational rehabilitation services. By the mid-1970s there were approximately 10,000 rehabilitation counselors working in the private sector.

Ed: You know what's interesting? Although public and private rehabilitation went separate ways after 1973, the passage of the Americans with Disabilities Act in 1990 resulted in reuniting the sectors, at least in functions. Now, whether a rehabilitation counselor works in a private or a public sector, the focus is on eliminating discriminatory practices in any aspect of an employment relationship.

Clayton: (Speaks thoughtfully.) Yes, and there's also a heritage from the public program's emphasis on finding ways to include persons with severe disabilities in community life and employment. Assistive technology and supported employment are being used in both public and private rehabilitation services.

Herbert: But look at the down side of those decisions of the 70s! The cost of serving clients with severe disabilities has resulted in people who are "only" economically disadvantaged being discarded. We know that vocational rehabilitation pays off, and especially for those who are culturally and economically disadvantaged. But after 1970 our research, training, and service efforts were focused on those who met an arbitrary definition of severe disability. We have subsidized employment for those who may always require the most expensive and extensive services to maintain employment. How can that decision be justified in view of today's societal problems?

Rita: (Speaks quietly.) The questions I started out asking seem much simpler than the ones I have now. . . . It seems that the same questions keep coming up: Whose problem is disability? What is a disability? What are we willing to pay for? What is required of a professional rehabilitation counselor? *(Looks at Martha and Susan.)* Maybe what you wanted me to see was that if I am going to have a job as a rehabilitation counselor, I'll always be asking these questions from chapter 3.

Clayton: (Turns to face Rita.) But there are some answers—answers crafted by mavericks who had a vision and stayed with it. John Lewis, a Georgia rehabilitation counselor who is blind, wrote his answer in 1970 for all of us. *(Clayton hands Rita a letter, which she opens and reads it aloud.)*

"I believe people can withstand any amount of physical and material poverty, but none of us can long endure the ravages of a benevolent paternalism which refuses to accept us as productive and responsible members of the human family. Rehabilitation is the voice of America to all people across the land. 'Never mind your loss; use what you have and it will multiply a hundredfold and more.' I've often said that what we achieve in rehabilitation is secondary to what we attempt to achieve. If we fail, we can try again, but if we never try, we become a bankrupt people and though our pockets may jingle, we bake a bitter bread."

*   *   *

(The lights dim, as all stand perfectly still.)

CHAPTER 4

Parameters of Practice:
Policy and Law

Marvin D. Kuehn

T he priorities and mandates of federal disability legislation and the implementation policies that have been established have resulted in an implicit yet significant impact on the professional practice of rehabilitation counseling. This practice has also been influenced by numerous issues of professionalism, rehabilitation agency priorities, and federal program initiatives.

Numerous articles discussing the role and functions (practice) of rehabilitation counselors in various work settings verify the diversity and uniqueness of rehabilitation counseling practice (Emener, Patrick, & Hollingsworth, 1984; Kuehn, 1991; Leahy, Szymanski, & Linkowski, 1993; Rubin & Roessler, 1995; Thomas, 1991a; Thomas & Parker, 1984; G. N. Wright, 1980). These articles frequently identify new skill and knowledge competencies or expanding responsibilities for counselors and generally reflect the functions that counselors perform and the employment settings in which they work. This chapter, however, will focus on the general factors that influence rehabilitation counseling practice that are related to agency priorities and policies, professionalization issues, and mandated legislation versus roles and functions per se.

Evaluating rehabilitation counseling practice and the parameters that have influenced service goals is difficult because of the inability of professionals, and persons with disabilities themselves, to agree on a set of operational concepts for defining the scope of professional practice and rehabilitation counseling programs. It is important to understand how changing priorities and political issues have determined the various parameters that impact the scope of rehabilitation services, employment settings, populations to be served, advocacy efforts, and intervention strategies to be utilized. Further, influences on professional practice must be examined from the perspective of the events and decisions that have occurred over time, for example, a series of transitional factors involving change, rather than discrete priorities or laws that suggest simple directions and parameters for rehabilitation counseling practice.

Earlier chapters reviewed the history and philosophies that have formed the foundation of the profession of rehabilitation counseling; however, some important historical influences and service delivery priorities need to be revisited briefly in order to understand the issues and limitations that policies and laws have created for service provision. Evidence of these influences on rehabilitation counseling practice can be seen most clearly in the differing interpretations of the term "disability," the types and purposes of different government agencies and programs, and the emphases identified in federal legislation (Noble, 1985; Weaver, 1994; G. N. Wright, 1980). These three factors have all had an indirect and implied impact on rehabilitation counseling practice in spite of the fact the broad scope and intent of vocational rehabilitation services have been clearly articulated.

IMPLICATIONS OF DISABILITY DEFINITIONS

A substantial roadblock to more effective rehabilitation counseling practice lies in the fact that "disability" has different meanings depending on the eligibility requirements or purposes of programs that are dealing with this factor. This definition problem continues to influence professional practice and delays the articulation of a strong, rational, national disability policy.

Policy definitions of disability, even though general and unique to individual programs, are also very important because they often have the impact of law. Legal and governmental definitions tend to be formal and specific, depending on legislative, regulatory, or judicial interpretation. These expanded or restricted definitions add to the complexity of the issues in service delivery. The definition of disability may be based on only one perspective, and can create frustration and misunderstanding as agencies attempt to determine whether a person or a population is disabled (Kuehn, Crystal, & Ursprung, 1988). To qualify for payments such as Workers' Compensation, Disability Insurance, and Supplemental Security Income, an individual's disabling condition must meet certain medical, psychological, or vocational criteria. Laws are made by elected officials who are influenced by lobbyists and the changing public mood; judges who respond to evidence presented by health and social experts, advocates, and the personal condition of the individual may not interpret these laws in accord with the intent of lawmakers (Hahn, 1985; Scotch, 1984).

Individuals entering the rehabilitation field to become service providers must learn the differences and implications of the definition of disability used in their respective work settings. In the worker's compensation program and in the courts, disability means the damages that one person collects from another as a result of an insult or injury. In the Social Security Disability Insurance (SSDI) program, disability refers to a condition that links ill health and unemployment. In addition, policy analysts have spent a great deal of time puzzling over the distinctions among such terms as "functional limitations," "impairment," "disability," and "handicap." Despite the scholarly efforts to explain the relationships among the terms, different programs use the terms inconsistently or, in some cases, interchangeably (Berkowitz, 1987; National Council on the Handicapped, 1986). This definition or interpretation issue dictates the focus and breadth of rehabilitation counseling practice.

PARAMETERS INFLUENCING REHABILITATION SERVICES

Many disability programs reflect overlapping priorities and service delivery initiatives that have, at times, caused duplication of services and uncertainty in purpose and administrative vision and confusion in decision making. Ultimately, the lack of a consistent disability policy has led to unneeded competition, conflict, a splintering of professional preparation disciplines, program administration inconsistency, and vagueness regarding professional role identity. Some programs rely on the court system and the private sector to award benefits to persons with disabilities, whereas others operate through the tax system and the public sector to provide needed services. Some programs compensate people who have severe physical limitations; others attempt to minimize disability through training and other rehabilitation services (Berkowitz, 1987; Kuehn, 1991; Meili, 1993).

In establishing priorities for rehabilitation services, both state and federal politicians and other decision makers consider a multitude of relevant factors. They examine the available and projected resources, ascertain the needs and aspirations of their constituents, identify other targeted populations, and establish funding levels to accomplish desired outcomes. In addition, several other environmental-, assessment-, and service-delivery-trend influences determine the type and quality of rehabilitation services provided.

Changes in the nature and availability of jobs have and will continue to accompany economic changes in society and influence rehabilitation counseling services and disability policy. Jobs in the service sector will tend to be highly technological, labor intensive, interpersonally interactive, and increasingly complex. It is projected that many jobs will be greatly dependent on communication skills, they will be information based, and will require new expertise related to technology and computer applications (Roessler & Schriner, 1991; Roth, 1985).

The use of psychological testing as a tool in vocational placement along with other vocational-assessment techniques has shaped a distinctive approach toward rehabilitation counseling services. In workers' compensation, emphasis has been placed on the use of legal criteria and physical-functioning tests to determine the degree of a person's disability. In contrast, in public vocational rehabilitation programs, functional-assessment techniques and psychological tests have been used to determine a person's potential for successful employment.

The availability of sophisticated emergency medical and trauma services, advances in neonatal care, and improvements in medical therapeutics and diagnostics are also having substantial impact on the alternative and intervention services available and the quality of disability services provided and needed (Pope & Tarlov, 1991; Zola, 1989). These services are frequently involve expensive technology, for example, incorporating ventilators for breathing, electric wheelchairs for mobility, and computer systems for communication and life-skills management.

Acquired immuno deficiency syndrome (AIDS) is emerging as a disabling condition for which individuals are accorded rights under the Rehabilitation Act of 1973. Counselors are challenged to provide an array of services to meet the multifaceted needs of this consumer population.

Cohen (1990) has suggested that counselors will face unique and substantial ethical and policy dilemmas about confidentiality and disclosure. Some rehabilitation agencies may be confronted with increased costs for long-term medical benefits with the growing incidence of AIDS.

The importance of transition-to-work programs has become a major issue that, because of the size of the population to be served, could have significant policy implications related to resource allocation and case-service (time) obligations of counselors. Transition programs are a variant of supported employment, which relies heavily on the strategies of job coaching, industrial enclaves, and mobile work crews. Successful implementation of transition programs requires multidisciplinary cooperation of schools, rehabilitation counselors, employers, parent groups, and consumers. Rehabilitation counselors and educators may need to develop new intervention strategies and to relinquish previously held notions about professional roles in order to provide optimal services (Benshoff, 1990).

Supported work initiatives have also increased the scope of rehabilitation services available, and the continued growth of these programs may have major monetary implications for service delivery. Supported employment programs are characterized by intensive skill training and ongoing support services delivered at the employment site after initial job placement. These functions have significantly expanded the roles of the counselor in ways many professionals believe are not desirable (Thomas, 1991a). These factors may have only an indirect influence on the day-to-day responsibilities of counselors, but they have a significant impact on the priority and funding available for rehabilitation counseling services that are provided to consumers.

Legislation that has funded the application of new technologies, especially ergonomics, has great potential to prevent or reduce job-related injuries. Many agency policies have encouraged or mandated the use of computer technology; however, some studies have found an escalation of visual, neuromuscular, and headache difficulties resulting from prolonged use of keyboards and video display terminals (Kiernan, Sanchez, & Schalock, 1989; Whitehead, 1989). This suggests that curricula modifications related to assistive and computer technology may be needed in academic programs in rehabilitation counseling.

The development of both medical-model and vocational-model approaches in private-sector rehabilitation has pointed out two different philosophical orientations that have created planning and outcome inconsistencies for rehabilitation counselors. The medical model centers on the provision of medical case management, generally provided by a rehabilitation nurse. This model suggests that intensive, efficient medical service will result in a more timely return to work. The vocational model, more closely akin to traditional rehabilitation endeavors, stresses the importance of vocational rehabilitation services offered by a rehabilitation counselor as a complement to medical and other services. This model assumes that the rehabilitation process will be more closely synchronized to the needs of the employer and individual with a disability, resulting in greater mutual satisfaction (Benshoff, 1990).

Perhaps one of the most significant issues that affects disability policy and professional practice is litigation. Issues of economic feasibility, use of technology, and discrimination have received new attention since passage of the Americans with Disabilities Act (ADA). Because aspects of the process can be time-consuming, litigation frequently delays rehabilitation services (Holmes, Hull, & Karst, 1989). Because of inconsistency and fragmentation of disability policy, the trend toward more litigation is often not adequately addressed in academic training programs, nor is it recognized as a problem by many program administrators and Congressmen.

PROFESSIONALISM AND POLICY EVOLUTION

Professionalization in public vocational rehabilitation and in the delivery of services has become a vital component in agency growth and program evaluation and success. The emergence of the rehabilitation counseling profession, unlike some of the other established human-service professions, has been tied to federal legislative mandates, and its development has been closely related to the expansion of the state–federal system of vocational rehabilitation (Jenkins, Patterson, & Szymanski, 1992; Thomas, 1991a). Like other factors, concerns about professional services and quality were apparent quite early in the developmental years of public vocational rehabilitation (Berkowitz, 1987; Boschen, 1989; Roessler & Schriner, 1991). Even as state vocational-rehabilitation-program administrators struggled with changing federal initiatives every few years, they strove to adopt an ethical and professional approach to the rehabilitation process. As the profession of rehabilitation counseling has grown and evolved, the importance of expanded and relevant counselor competencies and services to be provided specific groups of clients/ consumers has strengthened the need for a focused disability policy in America.

Passage of vocational rehabilitation legislation in 1954 was a major event that fostered professional counseling services in the public rehabilitation delivery system. That year, the federal government, through the Rehabilitation Services Administration (RSA), authorized grants to public and nonprofit agencies and organizations, including institutions of higher education, to establish master's- and doctoral-level rehabilitation counseling programs. The purpose was to improve the quality of professional practice which would result in employment of persons with disabilities (Kuehn, et al., 1988). This legislation also initiated new types of federal grants to subsidize rehabilitation research and to enable counselors to attend new professional development and education programs at public expense. The impact on professional practice was profound. In essence, rehabilitation counseling was elevated to a profession that had been defined, created, and paid for by the federal government. A significant consequence of the 1954 law has been that the profession grew and expanded due to the efforts of professional organizations that helped develop academic preparation standards for counselors. The result of the emerging status and importance of professional practice is that the professional rehabilitation counselor is now required, in most states, to have a relevant master's degree.

Cost–benefit analysis (i.e., accommodation to the politics of disability), the creation of a self-sustaining professional culture, and the ability to purchase or deny services from other agencies have also helped to define the scope of practice for the professional vocational rehabilitation counselor. Each of these factors reinforces the natural appeal of the public vocational rehabilitation program as a source of hope rather than a cause of consumer dependency. However, the result of the interplay of these factors has, in effect, created agency policy that evolved out of self-interest rather than from a well-thought-out, rational plan (Berkowitz, 1987). In the early 1970s, the vocational rehabilitation program, like many social welfare programs, reached a time of transition; this transition period is noteworthy because it fostered negative attitudes about funding rehabilitation programs and the value of counseling services. Failure of the economy to grow as rapidly as it had before limited the number of new jobs available and put pressure on the federal budget. The increasing participation of women and members of the baby-boom generation in the labor force exacerbated the problem. Protected entitlement programs such as social security laid claim to diminishing federal funds. Vocational rehabilitation, not an open-ended entitlement in the federal or state budgets, was far more vulnerable to financial constraints than were the other disability programs, such as workers' compensation and disability insurance (Berkowitz, 1987). These issues clearly resulted in low morale and pessimistic attitudes of service providers.

Another trend that emerged in the 1970s involved the manner in which rehabilitation counselors selected their caseloads. Typically, counselors favored consumers with mild impairments in contrast to consumers with more severe disabilities (Berkowitz, 1987). In 1973 Congress produced a new vocational rehabilitation bill that signaled a major change in who should be served in the public program. Emphasis was to be placed on the vocational rehabilitation of the severely disabled rather than on those individuals who could readily be placed in employment. In addition, attention was given to serving individuals with mental retardation and those with other developmental disabilities, as well as persons with severe neurotic and psychotic conditions. The focus on the severely disabled was an attempt to eliminate "creaming" (i.e., the practice of serving only those individuals from the applicant pool most likely to be employed) and to shift the focus to more difficult cases.

The 1973 Rehabilitation Act also mandated the use of an individualized written rehabilitation plan (IWRP) signed by the counselor and the consumer; this new policy became a very significant requirement that influenced the planning process and collaborative involvement between consumers and counselors. Congress also initiated client-assistance projects that established ombudsmen in the rehabilitation agencies to protect the rights of the consumer. Furthermore, these programs were required to be independent of the vocational rehabilitation program itself. In this manner, some client-assistance programs (CAP) became a source of legal advice that a disgruntled consumer could use to pursue a grievance through the courts (Whitehead, 1989). Legislated priority on employment and consumer involvement in rehabilitation plan development in the past few years has helped to define more clearly the scope and mission of the practice of rehabilitation counseling (Rubin & Roessler, 1995). Overall, the 1973 law facilitated a new relationship between the individual with a disability and the vocational rehabilitation counselor.

The implications for professional practice became obvious. Contrary to the intent of the 1973 law, some program administrators became concerned primarily with the number of people successfully served, and individuals with severe limitations noticed their frequent exclusion from the vocational rehabilitation program (Coudroglou & Poole, 1984). Consumers argued that they were being "screened out" and denied services; agencies, on the other hand, called this practice "screening out the undermotivated." Individuals also objected to the way in which counselors consigned them to low-paying or low-status jobs (Percy, 1989; Schriner, 1990).

Declining numbers of successful rehabilitations (i.e., individuals who obtain employment) create new challenges for counselors and make inherent conflicts more visible and more difficult to resolve. At times program goals have seemed to be incongruent and often incompatible with the needs of individuals with severe disabilities or those interested in independent living issues. This situation creates pressures on counselors as "quantity," in contrast to needed services, seems to be the goal driving many programs (Schriner, 1990).

The development of the rehabilitation counseling profession was also stimulated by the growing variety of work settings available and expanding specialized functions rehabilitation counselors were expected to perform. The varied roles include case manager, coordinator of services, job developer, consultant/advocate, placement specialist, client-assessment specialist, therapeutic counselor/facilitator, and vocational evaluator. With complex, wide-ranging responsibilities, rehabilitation counselors were also given a great deal of power and control over the options available to consumers, the goals of programs, and the services that may be provided.

The influence of certification and accreditation procedures has generally facilitated clarification of professional identity issues for counseling practice (Szymanski, Linkowski, Leahy, Diamond, & Thoreson, 1993). However, Thomas (1991b) suggests that in establishing professional standards for practice and directions for the future, the roles and influence of practitioners, educators, policymakers, and professional organizations have often been controversial and created conflict. The ultimate issue appears to relate to curriculum control. The fear that special-interest groups or new federal priorities will mandate standards that could dictate a change in the roles and functions of counselors has been viewed as the key concern.

Finally, professional practice will always need to respond to the unique work settings and the multifaceted needs of consumers. Therefore, to promote a concise, simplistic description of disability policy and the future of rehabilitation counseling is probably not desirable or realistic. Vigilance and periodic reassessment of federal legislative intent must be practiced, however, to maintain the philosophical assumptions that form the framework of rehabilitation counseling practice.

DELIVERY SYSTEM OBJECTIVES

Albrecht (1976) suggested that publicly articulated goals of rehabilitation have largely reflected the values of American society. A major goal of vocational rehabilitation agencies is to get individuals with disabilities working on a paying job. It is noted, however, that the utilitarian side of rehabilitation services receives more attention because most industries are in business to make money, and government is accountable to Congress and the voting public.

Beyond the philosophical assumptions of rehabilitation counseling are additional objectives. Employment is primary, but assisting the individual in improving one's self-image and promoting the importance of respect for and dignity of each person are also of value in our society. In the United States, these goals have been approached through a variety of disability policies and programs, many of which have been oriented around the medical-care system. Unfortunately, the services and behaviors of some well-meaning professionals are motivated primarily by money. The attainment of appropriate rehabilitation goals and the pursuit of vocational and psychological adjustment by consumers are frequently influenced by the economic benefits that accrue to service providers.

As new disability policies are proposed that affect professional practice, their importance and impact must be weighed against the goals that agencies promote. Practice issues must be examined in light of the need for early intervention programs in the schools that might assist special educators, high-school counselors, and vocational educators (Boschen, 1989). The use of computer technology and its advantages and disadvantages must be rationally evaluated. Finally, the impact of policy decisions on special populations must be continually reviewed (Bowe, 1993; Emener, et al., 1984; Haber, 1985).

The use of cost–benefit analysis and cost effectiveness evaluations have become widely accepted tools in assessing the goals and values of disability policies and rehabilitation counseling services. Because of the concern about costs and outcomes, rehabilitation efforts must be quantified to validate the use of these assessment tools. A positive, justifiable "numbers game" plays a most important role in making policy and program decisions. The bottom line usually equates to the number of persons served, evaluated, and placed in employment; these criteria greatly influence policies in the rehabilitation delivery system and the day-to-day practice of a counselor.

Currently, public vocational rehabilitation programs attempt to restore the productivity of persons with disabilities by job placement and job training, this costs the federal government a little over $1 billion a year (Berkowitz, 1992). It is by far the least expensive of the major disability programs, whereas SSDI has emerged as the nation's most expensive (Bowe, 1993; Kiernan et al., 1989).

There is little evidence at the present time, other than discussions about national health care, that major disability policy reforms are forthcoming. Both state and federal government continue to authorize and fund programs with overlapping objectives and services without regard to program ramifications and to the discrepant system that is being created (Kuehn, 1991).

LEGISLATIVE AND POLITICAL INFLUENCES

The formulation and implementation of national policies and the passage of federal and state laws regulating disability programs and needed services are not major public issues when there is satisfaction with the economy. Declining job opportunities, increasing taxes, and the perceived inequitable allocation of resources are the bases of societal change, however (Hahn, 1985). When limited financial resources are not sufficient to meet increasing demands, it is imperative to establish policies that are justifiable and critical for addressing discrimination and service-delivery issues.

Broadly conceived, disability policy is comprised of three general components that affect professional practice in rehabilitation counseling: (1) civil rights laws and regulations; (2) income and in-kind assistance programs (e.g., medical); and (3) skill-enhancement programs, such as education and vocational rehabilitation (Berkowitz, 1987; Scotch & Berkowitz, 1990). Unfortunately, these components are not synchronous and often do not reflect current professional beliefs about the role of people with disabilities as productive citizens who desire respect and dignity.

A significant policy influence, with political overtones, on rehabilitation counseling practice and services is the debilitating effect of new governmental initiatives for special-interest groups. Ever-changing federal training priorities and guidelines calling for new program "emphases" are often vivid examples of politically motivated priorities. The challenge for academic training programs has been to respond to these changes in a timely manner and to understand the rationale for the changes in priorities. Sometimes the responses to these emphases, which are often reflected in grant applications, illustrate a typical "political" reaction to changing federal priorities, that is, write what is needed to get funded.

Another critical factor relates to the lack of adequate national recognition of the profession of rehabilitation counseling. This illustrates why disability programs have never attracted a political following and partially explains why it has been difficult to establish a comprehensive, national disability policy. The contrast with programs such as aid for the elderly is a striking example of this phenomenon. Highly visible congressional committees monitor public policy toward the elderly, but few congressional committees air the grievances and publicize the problems of individuals with severe disabilities (Berkowitz, 1987; DeJong & Batavia, 1990). Until the passage of the ADA in 1990, few leaders of the disability community had risen to national prominence, nor had people with disabilities received the sustained attention from media as had other special groups.

An illustration of how policies (priorities and services) are influenced by politics (power) can be seen in some disability programs, such as public vocational rehabilitation, which formulated policies and procedures for reasons that often had little to do with the people and agencies served (Berkowitz, 1985). People with disabilities have, therefore, tried to gain control over disability policy, to take power away from professional administrators, and to assume both of these themselves. This effort led to the creation of independent living centers, which are largely run by persons with disabilities, rather than by professional administrators and able-bodied, direct-service providers.

There have been several recent laws and policies enacted that have emphasized or suggested new priorities for professional practice. Kuehn, et al. (1988) suggest that in the 1970s, when agencies began to serve the consumer who was severely physically disabled, state rehabilitation agency caseload size began declining due to the complexity of services and the length of time often necessary to meet consumer needs. In addition to the various antidiscrimination laws passed in the 1980s, federal legislation was passed that increased the value and viability of vocational rehabilitation programs (i.e., client-assistance services). The rehabilitation legislation of 1986 fostered the establishment of rehabilitation engineering services that could expand options for individuals as well as encourage the development of collaborative programs leading to supported employment services. Consumer involvement was given new attention in the 1992 Amendments with the emphasis on "choice" and increased control in development of rehabilitation goals, the provision for annual review of IWRPs, handling of applications and eligibility determination, expeditious provision of expanded transition services, personal-assistance services, expanded supported-employment services, and expansion of services through renewed commitments to interagency cooperation (Rubin & Roessler, 1995). All of these new initiatives have forced counselors and agencies to reevaluate priorities and related day-to-day responsibilities.

The passage of the ADA, which reflects a new thrust in American disability policy, emphasizes discrimination issues. The ADA offers an opportunity for both the administration and the Congress to act positively in the face of the changing needs and aspirations of an increasingly politicized disabled population and to do so at a relatively low cost to the federal government. The political unwillingness to make fundamental changes in our disability-assistance programs made the passage of the ADA all the more urgent. Even if the legal requirements of ADA and efforts to eliminate discrimination are enforced vigorously, the law cannot adequately substitute for other policy changes that need to be made (DeJong & Batavia, 1990). Important policy issues that predate the passage of ADA still remain unresolved.

The confusing state of disability policy in this country can be attributed in part to the fact that many of the nation's disability programs were conceived in earlier periods when the social preconception and policy presumption inferred that disabilities necessarily precluded employability and participation in the social life of the community. Social policies were usually developed in relation to perceived problems; policies were generally not formulated and implemented until a problem became salient (Haveman, Halberstadt, & Burkhauser, 1984). The confusion has had some positive benefits in that it has served as the focus for articulating efforts directed to the justification and value of vocational rehabilitation services.

Even though discrimination and policy issues persist, the philosophy and changing attitudes regarding the purpose of vocational rehabilitation have had a positive influence on the professional rehabilitation counselor as well as a positive political impact on federal policymakers.

FUTURE OF REHABILITATION COUNSELING PRACTICE

To identify a clear picture for professional practice in the 1990s is difficult at best. No one person has all the necessary expertise to comprehend the diverse legal, economic, and social phenomena encompassed by disability policy and legislation. Few people understand all the parameters, and most do not have sufficient background to view the entire rehabilitation system from a holistic perspective. Legislators, for example, operate by means of subcommittees that are heavily dependent on experts, special-interest groups, and others who have learned the specialized language of policy discourse. Rarely does the level of analysis rise above individual programs to include the larger picture. The focus often becomes "justification of program," rather than "development of rational disability policy" (Schriner, 1990).

There are strong economic reasons to suspect that a disability and rehabilitation delivery system composed of professionally trained personnel will not go out of existence. Although disability costs may be becoming a national problem and social policies for rehabilitation are being developed and tested, at the same time, there are social and political reasons to suggest that disability services will not be eradicated; many businesses and industries ultimately depend on the misfortunes of individuals to justify or guarantee their existence. Disability-benefit programs sometimes provide a stable source of income to consumers that often surpasses the amount one could have earned through employment, creating discouragement for individuals to seek work. Professionally trained counselors are therefore needed to minimize the disincentives that are created.

One possible focus for professional practice is to encourage employers to accept the obligation to prevent disability by instituting disability-management principles in the workplace. The importance of prompt employer intervention after an accident or illness must be emphasized. The slower and less coordinated the intervention, the more likely an employee will progress from temporary illness to long-term or chronic disability (Habeck, Williams, Dugan, & Ewing, 1989).

Another way to improve the practice of rehabilitation counseling and to make it more responsive to consumer needs might be to introduce innovative approaches to the delivery of rehabilitation services involving more competition in the marketplace. This could provide the consumer with more options on the types, level, and location of service that one is receiving. Federal government funding of innovative delivery approaches has received considerable support in the 1990s. An open market for rehabilitation counseling services could force both the consumer and the providers of services to dramatically reassess the priorities, needs, and services in the rehabilitation process. This approach could also allow the consumer to be maximally independent in the decision-making process from the beginning. The implications of successful alternative services could have major ramifications for state and federal policies in regard to the use of monies allocated for implementation of programs specified in federal laws.

DeJong and Batavia (1990) suggested that to facilitate changes in disability policy and to support the improvement of professional practice, several additional alternatives should be considered:

- Provide greater economic incentives and financial deductions for persons with disabilities to obtain employment. Modify tax policy to offer greater deductibility of, or tax credits for, disability-related expenses.
- Eliminate any assumption in policy decisions that a person is, or is not, totally disabled. Disability may be a nonstatic condition.
- Alter the assumption that a disability necessarily reduces the capability to work. Rely less on medical eligibility criteria and give more consideration to individual functional capacity and to environmental accommodations that a person with a disability may require.
- Create incentives to work and separate employment status from program eligibility status. Assistive devices and health care benefits should be available regardless of employment status.

These ideas are not particularly radical or new. They reflect traditional American values that emphasize individual initiative, self-determination, private responsibility, and community support (Berkowitz, 1987; DeJong & Batavia, 1990). All persons who can contribute productively to our society must be encouraged to do so. The scope of professional practice can easily embrace these values, and practitioners can focus rehabilitation efforts on the dignity, independence, and employment of consumers.

The perception of the importance and value of rehabilitation counseling in America seems to be at a turning point. With recent concerns regarding the federal budget deficit concerns, the social policy agenda has basically been placed on hold. Finally, in the midst of economic recession, the threat of unemployment, and an exorbitant cost of living, there has been a strong public outcry for fiscal conservatism and a political backlash against programs making demands on the public purse. Individuals with disabilities who might benefit from rehabilitation counseling services are not exempt from the outcry and backlash. Because priority changes in the funding of programs often involve unanticipated consequences, the administration and Congress have been unwilling to risk changes that will require additional funds in the short run even though such changes would be likely to stimulate greater economic productivity in the long run (Thomas & Parker, 1984). Prospects for expanding disability programs have also been made worse by a slow-growth economy, the nation's unwillingness to accept new taxes, the financial fiasco of the savings-and-loan industry, and the continued rapid growth in health care costs (DeJong & Batavia, 1990).

SUMMARY

The factors that have influenced the practice of rehabilitation counseling have become the parameters that in some ways are controlling the development and viability of the profession. The impact of factors such as public policy, legislation, and a national health care program has been significant; all have contributed to the goal of reintegrating persons with disabilities into mainstream society. However, only vocational rehabilitation programs have employability as their stated aim.

Although the rehabilitation counseling profession places great value on the dignity of the individual, it recognizes the importance of the Protestant work ethic, the value of individual independence, and individual satisfaction that can occur when a person obtains employment. In some cases, however, these values come into conflict because of changes in or indecision about process or delivery issues, eligibility, and outcome policies.

In the 1990s it is virtually impossible for any one person to be current on all of the disability-service programs that exist, let alone the ways in which they interact. Disability policy and new legislation should form a coherent rationale for rehabilitation counseling practice. It may be difficult to agree on a common definition of disability and therefore to create a disability policy that bridges the uniqueness of individual programs. Because these programs have been frequently conceived and administered in isolation from one another, they have perpetuated a service structure that has been described as stagnant and resistant to change. Rehabilitation counseling programs could be stimulated and made more effective if the collection of insulated service programs were replaced by a cohesive disability policy that reflects the aspirations and values that people with disabilities have for themselves (Schriner, 1990).

It is clear that the parameters that could influence the professional practice of rehabilitation counseling in the 1990s are thought provoking, comprehensive, and possibly overwhelming. Awareness of the possibilities, challenges, and opportunities presented by these various alternatives will we hope be addressed by the profession (Kuehn, 1991). The strength of professional practice is a commitment to the inherent value, dignity, and uniqueness of each individual with a disability.

Integrated disability policy and well-conceived legislation, in concert with the development of comprehensive disability and health care systems, will foster a positive, optimistic future desired by all individuals experiencing disability. The ultimate result will be more responsive rehabilitation counseling services that reflect innovative, creative professional practices that are consistent with federal disability law and policies.

CHAPTER 5

Standards of Practice: Ethical and Legal

Vilia M. Tarvydas

Increased quality of life for clients with disabilities depends on professional rehabilitation counselors heeding the caution embodied in the words of the historical figure, Samuel Johnson: "Integrity without knowledge is weak and useless; Knowledge without integrity is dangerous and dreadful." The development of a strong professional identity rests on clear professional standards of practice. Rehabilitation counseling's unique legislative genesis as a profession over 80 years ago constitutes a covenant with both the society and its citizens with disabilities to exercise knowledge with integrity. The sociopolitical history of rehabilitation and research findings in the rehabilitation literature have demonstrated that the rehabilitation counselor's clients often must deal with social, political, and legal oppression. Therefore, they particularly need solution-focused, respectful, nonexploitative, empowering, and ethical relationships with their counselors.

Unrecognized ethical issues occur on a daily basis in rehabilitation and often have a powerful effect on counselors and clients alike. Witness three situations that would not be unusual and might occur anywhere. In these situations the rehabilitation counselors engage in unethical practice and their clients are placed in difficult, or even harmful, circumstances:

• *Scenario A.* Mary A. subtly pressures her clients with developmental disabilities to have reproductive sterilizations as a "condition" of placing them in a supervised apartment living program.

• *Scenario B.* Greg T.'s supervisor tells him to go back into old case records and write progress notes and initial assessment reports on several clients with whom he had not worked until last week. The supervisor states that these case files must be updated for the accreditation survey next month and these clients' old counselor left her job with agency and moved out of state. Greg is uncomfortable, but did this update. He thinks he knows the clients well enough, and he would like to make a good impression on his new supervisor.

• *Scenario C.* Sonja B. decides that she will not report Bob A., her partner in a private practice, for overbilling insurance companies for client services and intentionally misinterpreting test data to accommodate the referring account representative. She tried to persuade him to cease these practices, but he pointed out how much business it is bringing the firm, and that the workers' compensation market is becoming so highly competitive that their small firm would not be able to compete without this "edge." Bob notes that even the highly respected rehabilitation counselor who trained them at a larger firm has had to resort to such practices. Sonja dislikes these practices, but is secretly glad that Bob is willing to "shoulder the load" for their firm in this manner, thus freeing her to conduct her own portion of the practice in the manner she prefers.

Clearly, persons with disabilities require the services of professionals who are grounded firmly in the awareness of their value-laden mission and who are willing and able to assist persons with disabilities through appropriate knowledge and competencies (Gatens-Robinson & Rubin, 1995). The unusually strong tradition of explicit philosophical foundations is critical to the profession of rehabilitation counseling, and has led to an early recognition of the value based nature of rehabilitation counseling (B. A. Wright, 1986). This treasured legacy provides a strong basis for understanding the ethical principles at the heart of the ethical decision-making skills needed within the practice of rehabilitation counseling.

COMPONENTS OF PROFESSIONAL STANDARDS

The practice of rehabilitation counseling is both an art and a science, requiring the practitioner to make both value-laden and rational decisions. Rather than being incompatible stances, both facts and values must be considered in juxtaposition to engage in rational decisions (Gatens-Robinson & Rubin, 1995). Within ethical deliberation, the practitioner blends such elements as personal moral sensitivities and philosophies of practice with clinical behavioral objectivity and the quest for efficient care of clients.

The nature and complexity of standards of practice for all of the professions have changed and grown over the last several decades. The phrase *professional standards* no longer simply means specifically the ethical standards of the profession. This term is a general term meaning professional criteria indicating acceptable professional performance (Powell & Wekell, 1996). There are three types of standards relevant to describing professional practice: (1) the *internal standards* of the profession; (2) *clinical standards* for the individual practitioners within a profession; and (3) *external, regulatory standards*. Taken together these professional standards increase the status of the profession, and its ability for self-governance; they also enhance the external representation and accountability for the profession's competence with the clients, the general public, employers, external regulators, and payers (Rinas & Clyne-Jackson, 1988). These types of standards, their major characteristics, and principal components are depicted in Figure 5.1 below.

Internal Standards

First, the internal standards of the profession form the underpinnings of the appropriate role and functions of the profession. Internal standards are characterized by being focused on advancing the professionalism of the group in question, having the intent of setting a profession-wide standard of practice, and assisting individual practitioners through defining their professional identity and obligations. Prominent examples are the profession's code of ethics and any guidelines for specialty practice relevant to the discipline.

Clinical Standards

The next type of standards are the clinical standards for professional practitioners. These standards are close in locus to the internal standards described in that both are directly relevant to services delivered to the individual client or patient. Additional characteristics include focusing on a single disciplinary or multidisciplinary standard of clinical care, these

FIGURE 5.1 The Structure of Professional Standards for Rehabilitation Counseling

Purpose: To enhance
- Ethical Responsibility to the Client, the Profession, and Society
  - Self Advocacy for the Profession

Internal Standards of the Profession	Clinical Standards for the Professional Practitioner	External Regulatory Standards
Characteristics	**Characteristics**	**Characteristics**
• Professional Focused	• Clinically Focused	• Regulatory or Institutionally Focused
• Profession-wide Standard	• Disciplinary or Multidisciplinary Standards Used	• Concerns Legal or Risk Management Perspective
• Individual Professional's Identity & Obligation	• May be Setting or Client Specific	• Concerns Funding or Institutional Fiduciary Perspective
Related Components	• Evaluates Competency of Individual Professional(s)' Performance	**Related Components**
• Codes of Ethics	• Measuring Outcomes	• Judicial
aspirational (principles) mandatory (standards)	**Related Components**	*community standards of professional group*
• Guidelines for Specialty Practice	• Peer Review	*legally adopted codes of ethics*
	• Peer Review Standards Organization	• Institutional
	• Clinical Care Pathways	*Quality Assurance Review (QA)*
	• Clinical Best Practices Stanards	*Utilization Review (UR)*

ethical standards may be specific to a particular setting or client population, they evaluate the competency of individual professionals based on the specific care rendered, and have a client or patient-care outcome measurement focus. Peer-review processes and standards as well as clinical care pathways are examples of this type of standard.

External Regulatory Bodies

The last component of the professional standards trio involves the standards of external regulatory bodies of diverse sorts. They are focused on regulatory or institutional-level concerns. They usually involve legal or risk-management questions; and deal with funding or institutional fiduciary perspectives. There is a judicial type of component in which legal or quasi-legal processes are at play, such as community standards of a professional group being used in a malpractice suit, or a code of ethics adopted by a licensure board to discipline licensees. It is important to note that general social values underlie both the law and the values of the profession, making them generally compatible. The society would not long tolerate a profession that routinely operates in a manner significantly at variance with its core value structure. Corey, Corey, and Callanan (1993) note that law and ethics are similar in that they both constitute guidelines for practice and in some sense are regulatory in nature. However, law can be seen as representing the minimum standards that society will tolerate, and ethics involves the ideal standards set by the profession itself. The law also informs the counselor of what is likely to happen if the professional is caught performing a prohibited act. The other component of external regulatory standards involves institutional standards used to judge the effectiveness and efficiency of an entire institutional unit, as is typically done in quality assurance or utilization review.

This chapter is concerned with the *ethical standards of rehabilitation counseling,* but it is important to note the synergistic relationship among the three types of professional standards described earlier. *Ethics* are the moral principles that are adopted by a group to provide rules for right conduct (Corey, et al., 1993). The *code of ethics* for a professional organization is a specific document formally adopted by the organization that is an attempt to capture the profession's current consensus regarding what types of professional conduct are appropriate or inappropriate; they are normative statements rather than absolute dictates of situational guidance, however.

ETHICS GOVERNANCE

Effective processes used to govern ethics practice are necessary to give meaning to professional standards of practice and to enhance the societal stature of the profession. These governance processes guide the profession's practitioners through education and socialization into the professional role, and subsequently discipline them if they do not practice within the proscribed standards established. Ethical components of the standards of practice can be thought of as being either *mandatory or aspirational* in the level of direction they provide the practitioner (Corey, et al., 1993). The most basic level of ethical functioning is guided by *mandatory* ethics. At this level, the individuals focus on compliance with the law and the dictates of the professional codes of ethics that apply to their practice. They are concerned with remaining safe from legal action and professional censure. The more ethically sophisticated level is the *aspirational* level. At this level individuals additionally reflect on the effects of the situation on the welfare of their clients, and the effects of their actions on the profession as a whole.

These same concepts of mandatory and aspirational ethics can be applied to the overall structure of governance for a profession's ethical standards of practice as a whole. It is important to note that codes of ethics are binding only on persons who hold that particular credential [e.g., certification through the Commission on Rehabilitation Counselor Certification (CRCC)], or have membership in that organization [e.g., member of the American Counseling Association (ACA)]. Those professionals so governed must take ethical guidance and sanctions may be applied based on the specific ethical codes and disciplinary process of the specific professional entity. The disciplinary process of CRCC is an example of such a process applicable to rehabilitation counseling practice (see Appendix D). If a credential holder or member of a particular professional entity violates its code of ethics, the entity has the responsibility to provide a disciplinary procedure to enforce its standards. After due process, the entity applies an appropriate sanction to the violator. In the case of a professional organization the ultimate sanction would typically be removal from membership, with possible referral of the findings to other professional or legal jurisdictions. For a credentialing entity such as CRCC or a counselor licensure board, the violator could face the more serious option of certificate or license revocation, thus possibly removing an individual's ability to practice. Less serious levels of sanction, such as reprimand or probation, are also available and utilized. Often these statuses are coupled with significant educational or rehabilitative conditions, such as taking an ethics course, treating of an addiction, or supervised practice, so as to assist practitioners in regaining appropriate ethical standards of practice while at the same time protecting their clients. The assessment of the level of seriousness of the ethical violation will affect the actual choice of sanction once the individual is adjudicated as being in violation of the code of ethics. Factors often considered include intentionality, degree of risk or actual harm to the client, motivation or ability of violator to change, and recidivism of the violator (Keith-Spiegel & Koocher, 1985).

Responsible practitioners supplement this elementary mandatory level of practitioner ethics with advanced knowledge of the clinical wisdom and scholarly literature on the best practices in ethics. In addition they will gain guidance from other codes of ethics and specialty guidelines for ethical practice which present relevant guidance to them. These sources should be sought to supplement the required mandatory ethical standards with the more aspirational principles and ethical concepts to which the more sophisticated practitioner should aspire. In fact, for certain situations the course of action suggested by the aspirational ethics perspective may contradict that required by the dictates of mandatory ethics. Such a situation leaves the practitioner in the stressful position of needing to responsibly reconcile the two directions.

The contemporary structure of ethics governance for rehabilitation counselors is presented in Figure 5.2. This representation depicts types of professional organizational entities in rehabilitation counseling organized hierarchically in the shape of a pyramid. The levels of ethical functioning are represented by the vertical line to the side of the pyramid, depicting the entities as existing roughly on a continuum from a primarily aspirational to a primarily mandatory level of function.

Educational Institutions

Colleges and universities are *educational institutions* that provide professional education and research services, doing so under the review and credentialing bodies such as the Commission on Rehabilitation Education (CORE) or the Commission on the Accreditation of Counseling and Related Educational Programs (CACREP). As such they are entities that have the broadest function to provide aspirational education and guidance in ethics, and represent the foundation of the structure of ethics governance. Additionally, they build the theoretical and research base for understanding ethical issues, decision-making processes, and ethics educational methods. These aspects of the aspirational knowledge base are needed to support ethical development of the profession. Colleges and universities also ensure that proper preservice education and professional socialization occurs to inculcate future practitioners and educators with a proper ethics base from which to conduct their future practice of rehabilitation counseling. Importantly, this obligation includes active role-modeling and

FIGURE 5.2 Model of Ethics Governance for Rehabilitation Counselors

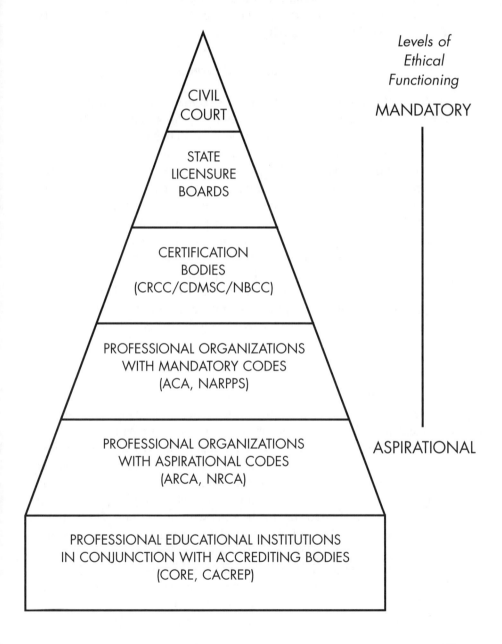

Levels of
Ethical
Functioning

MANDATORY

ASPIRATIONAL

CIVIL
COURT

STATE
LICENSURE
BOARDS

CERTIFICATION
BODIES
(CRCC/CDMSC/NBCC)

PROFESSIONAL ORGANIZATIONS
WITH MANDATORY CODES
(ACA, NARPPS)

PROFESSIONAL ORGANIZATIONS
WITH ASPIRATIONAL CODES
(ARCA, NRCA)

PROFESSIONAL EDUCATIONAL INSTITUTIONS
IN CONJUNCTION WITH ACCREDITING BODIES
(CORE, CACREP)

support of ethical analysis and behavior in teaching, supervision, and actual clinical practice. Lastly, educational institutions serve as a resource to other professional organizations and regulatory bodies to provide teaching, research, and service supporting aspirational and mandatory ethical practice in the community.

Codes of Professional Organizations

At the next level sit the *professional organizations with aspirational codes* of ethics that have no internal mandatory enforcement mechanisms. In rehabilitation counseling, the American Rehabilitation Counseling Association (ARCA) and the National Rehabilitation Counseling Association (NRCA) occupy this position. For such organizations the primary task is to encourage aspirational ethical levels of function in their members. Mandatory enforcement tasks are not undertaken by such professional organizations due to factors such as lack of appropriate consumer access and protection in the disciplinary process; appropriate remedies for serious infractions; and the substantial financial, staff, and professional resources necessary for responsible enforcement. In some cases the mandatory enforcement function of the organization is referred to a parent organization (e.g., to ACA in the case of ARCA), or the complainant is referred to another appropriate jurisdiction to initiate a disciplinary process.

Nonetheless, professional organizations with aspirational codes perform several significant functions within the ethics governance structure. They may provide supplemental, complementary codes of ethics for their members that extend and explicate other more general codes of ethics. Such a document provides guidelines for ethical practice for particular special issues frequently encountered or of particular concern to these professionals. For rehabilitation counselors examples of such issues might be: assessment of persons with functional limitations due to disability, interdisciplinary team practice relationship issues, managed care practice, and the responsibility of advocacy for persons with disabilities. This supplementary code may take the form of specialty guidelines for practices that address specialty setting or population-specific issues. One example of this type of guideline is the *Standards for Psychologists and Social Workers in SCI Rehabilitation* formulated by the American Association of Spinal Cord Injury Psychologists and Social Workers.

The *Code of Ethics for Rehabilitation Counselors* is a unified code of ethical standards for this entire profession (Tarvydas & Pape, 1988) (see Appendix D to review this code); and it has been endorsed by ARCA, NRCA, and the CRCC. Interestingly and uniquely, it functions both as a specialty aspirational code for NRCA and ARCA members, and as a mandatory code of ethics for any rehabilitation counselor who is certified by the CRCC. This unified code has 10 Canons, which are "general standards of an aspirational and inspirational nature reflecting the fundamental spirit of caring and respect which professionals share. They are maxims which service as models of exemplary professional conduct" (CRCC, Preamble, p. 2). The canons address general moral and legal standards, the counselor–client relationship, client advocacy, professional relationships, public statements/fees, confidentiality, assessment, research activities, competence, and use of the CRC credential. To supplement the canons for clarification and enforcement, the Code contains rules that are "more exacting standards that provide guidance in specific circumstances" (CRCC, Preamble, p. 2).

In addition to maintaining supplementary, specialty ethical standards for practice, professional organizations with aspirational ethical levels of function collect information regarding ethical trends and needs for revision of either the specialty or generalist ethics codes. Their leadership also should participate in the code revision and writing processes for both types of codes. These organizations should identify and supply qualified professionals to serve on the various mandatory enforcement bodies. They provide educational programs to further knowledge and the quality of ethical practice, performing significant educational and socialization functions. A new and innovative role, yet one that is potentially most meaningful, is the provision of mechanisms and expertise to offer remediation or rehabilitation programs for impaired professionals who have been found in violation (or are at risk of violation) of ethical standards.

Mandatory Codes

At the third level of ethical governance are professional organizations that maintain and enforce a *mandatory code* of ethics, such as ACA and the National Association of Rehabilitation Professionals in the Private Sector (NARPPS). These organizations provide an entry-level mandatory code of ethics and enforcement process for their members, and in the case of ACA, the enforcement for referred complaints of its specialty memberships. This level of organization consults with certification and licensing bodies and the specialty professional organizations to ensure active participation of all parties in the ethics-enforcement process and attempts to incorporate specialty viewpoints into a compatible and continually revised master code of ethics. They provide referral for complaints against accused parties to other jurisdictions when appropriate. They may provide important educational programs to increase practitioner expertise in ethical practice.

Professional Regulatory Bodies

At the next two levels of ethics governance are *professional regulatory bodies* that either certify or license professionals and constitute the preeminent enforcers of *the mandatory code*. National certification bodies, such as CRCC and the National Board for Counselor Certification (NBCC), as well as the state counselor licensure boards operate at this level. They perform a pivotal role in the promulgation and enforcement of ethical standards. However, they draw their specific codes of ethical standards from the professional organizations in that they do not constitute the profession, but rather regulate it based on the profession's own internal standards. They may provide information and consultation to the professional organizations in revising and maintaining the current codes of ethics. Beyond the ethical regulatory function, the regulatory bodies encourage ethical proficiency of their licensees and certificants through requiring preservice education and continuing education in the area of ethics.

As a practical matter, the states that license professional counselors usually adopt the ACA code of ethics, as does NBCC, and a rehabilitation counselor licensed in a state that has adopted the ACA code would be governed by that code. Additionally, CRCC (as described above) has endorsed the NRCA/ARCA/CRCC unified code. Therefore, the rehabilitation counselor licensed in the case above would also be governed by the unified code if she or he is a CRC. Fortunately, most of the core concepts and provisions of these codes are highly compatible because both are based on broader ethical traditions within the mental health professions. Generally, the rehabilitation counseling code provides more specific comment in some areas or consideration of specialty issues not considered in the ACA code.

At the pinnacle of ethics governance are found the civil courts and other legal jurisdictions that affect the ethical practice of counselors. One of the primary mechanisms for this type of governance is through the use of malpractice suits in civil courts. In malpractice actions, one of the central points is to establish a violation of duty, requiring determining the standard of what constitutes "good professional practice" as applied to the matter at hand. This issue is difficult to determine because it is often ill defined and requires many types of considerations. It is not unusual that various expert witnesses would be called to testify regarding such practices. Additionally, there might be an attempt to establish a blatant violation of the general rules of the profession by reference to the profession's ethical standards (Thompson, 1990). Another standard of practice that might be applied would be consideration of whether the action or service in question was both within the scope of practice of the profession and within the individual's personal scope of practice. The profession of rehabilitation counseling has established its scope of practice, with which its practitioners must be familiar to appropriately and ethically establish their personal scopes of practice. Practitioners are ethically bound to limit their own scopes of practice to areas within the profession's scope in which they are personally competent to practice by virtue of appropriate types and levels of education, supervision, and professional experience (LaBuda, 1995).

It is through these six levels that the various professional governance entities interact to provide a network of mandatory and aspirational ethics functions. In their totality, an interactive system of research, educational and enforcement services shape and regulate the ethical practice of rehabilitation counselors. Taken together, these systems of knowledge, traditions, rules, and laws form the regulatory content, but they do not provide the practitioner with possibly the most crucial tool for ethical practice—knowledge and experience in application of a *decision-making process* that can be applied to this form and content.

ETHICAL DECISION-MAKING PROCESSES

The intent of an ethics code is to provide rehabilitation counselors with guidance for specific situations they experience in their practices. Authorities have long recognized, however, that ethics codes must be written in general enough terms that they apply across a wide range of practice settings. They also are reactive in nature; that is, they address situations that have already been part of the profession's experience (Kitchener, 1984;

Mabe & Rollin, 1986). As a result, even with the knowledge of the profession's code of ethics, rehabilitation counselors may find that they do not have sufficient guidance to resolve the dilemma in question. They may find that the particular situation with which they are faced is not addressed in their code, that their practice is governed by more than one code providing conflicting direction in the situation, or that conflicting provisions within any one code appear to apply to the situation. It is for that reason that rehabilitation counselors must be prepared to exercise their professional judgment in ethics responsibly. This type of occurrence is not so much a failure of ethical codes but rather a natural and appropriate juncture recognizing the importance and role of professional judgment. In other words, it is affirmation that one is involved in "practice of a profession," rather than "doing a job," however skilled. In order to exercise such judgment, the counselor must be prepared to recognize underlying ethical principles, conflicts between competing interests, and to apply appropriate ethical decision-making skills to resolve the dilemma and act in an ethical manner (Francouer, 1983; Kitchener, 1984; Tarvydas, 1987). Fortunately, the professional is assisted in this task by examination and refinement of his or her ordinary moral sense, as well as the availability of thoughtful models for the ethical decision making process. Many components of ethical decision-making involve teachable, learnable skills, to supplement the professional's developing intuitive professional judgment.

Several types of models exist that seek to explain and structure the process of ethical decision making. Some prominent examples view the ethics decision-making process as: professional self-exploration (Corey et al., 1993); a moral reasoning discourse (Kitchener, 1984); the result of a moral developmental process (VanHoose & Kottler, 1985); a multidimensional, integrative psychological process (Rest, 1984); and involving a hierarchy of four contextual levels that affect the process of decision making (Tarvydas & Cottone, 1991). Generally, ethical decision-making models can be thought of as having the characteristics of either *principle or virtue* ethics (Corey et al., 1993). *Principle* ethics focus on the objective, rational, cognitive aspects of the process. Practitioners who adhere to this perspective tend to view the application of universal, impartial ethical principles, rules, codes, and law as being the core elements of ethics. *Virtue* ethics considers the characteristics of the counselors themselves as the critical element for responsible practice. Thus, proponents of virtue-ethics approaches would tend to concern themselves more with counselors reflecting on and clarifying their moral and value positions. Additionally, they would examine other personal issues that might affect their ethical practice, such as unresolved emotional needs that might negatively affect their work with their clients. Preferred approaches to ethical decision making should include both aspects (Corey et al., 1993).

THE INTEGRATIVE DECISION-MAKING MODEL OF ETHICAL BEHAVIOR

In this book, the Integrative Decision-Making Model of Ethical Behavior (the Integrative Model) is introduced. This model integrates the most prominent principle and virtue aspects of several decision-making approaches and introduces some contextual considerations into the process. It emphasizes the constant process of interaction between the principle and virtue elements, as well as placing a reflective attitude at the heart of the process. The model also maintains a focus on the actual production of ethical behavior within a specified context, rather than prematurely terminating analysis by merely selecting the best ethical course of action. This approach respects the importance of setting and practice contextual factors that are crucial in rehabilitation counseling, in which the interdisciplinary and institutional influences have been very strong historically and currently.

Conceptual Origins of the Integrative Model

The Integrative Model builds on several well-known decision-making models widely used by professionals in the mental health and rehabilitation treatment communities. The work of Rest (1984) provides the Integrative Model with its core understanding of ethical decision making as a psychological process involving distinct cognitive–affective elements interacting in each component. Cognitions and emotions are seen as unavoidably intertwined at each component of the decision-making process and in the production of ethical behavior. Rest's (1984) model conceptualizes ethical decision making as more than a direct expression of moral or value traits, or stage in a moral-developmental process. He emphasizes considering the completion of ethical behavior as the necessary endpoint for consideration, rather than merely arriving at a cognitive decision or intent to do an ethical act. Therefore Rest's (1984) ethical decision-making components and many of his considerations are the foundation of the Integrative Model as presented here.

The work of Kitchener (1984) provides other core elements to the Integrative Model. She differentiates the useful distinction between the intuitive and critical–evaluative levels of ethical decision making, thus providing a forum in which to incorporate the richness and influence of the everyday personal and professional moral wisdom into the individual professional's process of ethical decision making. This personal and professional wisdom informs the first level of the process, the "intuitive" level. At that level both conscious and unconscious levels of awareness lead to decisions that are made calling into play the individual's existing morals, beliefs, and prior experiences. The experiences, morals, and beliefs that constitute our ordinary moral sense will also include prior professional learning and experiences. Kitchener notes that the intuitive level of process often is the professional's main decision-making tool when the situation is not perceived as one that is novel, unusual, or requiring some particular level of care. The intuitive level of analysis always constitutes the first platform of decision making, even when the practitioner recognizes the situation as requiring the more stringent level of analysis involved in the critical evaluative level of consideration. Thus, a person's ordinary moral sense is relevant to his or her ethical decision-making process; this fact reinforces the concerns raised by proponents of the virtue-ethics perspective.

If the ethical issues are not resolved at the intuitive level, the counselor progresses to Kitchener's (1984) critical–evaluative level of ethical analysis. This level involves three hierarchically arranged stages or tiers of examination to resolve the dilemma. At the first stage, the counselor would seek to determine if any laws or ethical rules exist that would provide a solution for the dilemma. If they do not exist, or provide conflicting dictates, the counselor would progress to the second tier by introducing consideration of how the core ethical principles apply to the situation. The benchmark work of Beauchamp and Childress (1983) identified autonomy, beneficence, nonmaleficence, and justice, as the ethical principles governing ethical behavior. Kitchener (1984) elevated fidelity to the status of the fifth ethical principle critical to the helping profession.

When the process of seeking guidance by recourse to the dictates of the ethical principles leaves continuing uncertainty as to the appropriate ethical course of action, counselors proceed to assessing the positions suggested by ethical theory. J. B. Patterson (1992) recommends that rehabilitation counselors be concerned with normative ethical theory and may benefit from considering the question of whether they would prefer their action to be decided based on a general or universal law. Kitchener (1984) suggested applying the "good reasons" approach in which the counselor attempts to make a decision based on what the counselor would wish for himself or herself, or someone dear to them. Another standard she suggests would be to take the action that results in the least amount of avoidable harm.

The final conceptual influence on the Integrative Model is the four-level model of ethical practice introduced by Tarvydas and Cottone (1991). This approach introduces an extended consideration of the contextual forces acting on ethical practice beyond the singular focus on the individual practitioner in relationship to the individual client. The four levels are hierarchical, moving to increasingly broader levels of social contexts within which ethical practice is influenced. The relationships among the domains are seen as interactive in nature. Peak ethical efficiency and lowest levels of ethical stress are reached when each level holds compatible values and standards, or endorses a mutually acceptable mechanism for the ethical dilemma's resolution. The most microlevel in the hierarchy is the traditionally central clinical counseling core, in which the counselor–client relationship is the focus. The second level is that of the clinical multidisciplinary team interaction. At this point, practitioner-to-practitioner dynamics are considered. Often team relationships and leadership, collaboration skills, and the interplay of the differing ethical codes and traditions becomes important to the process. At the next level the institutional or agency context and its constraints enter into the process. Dictates of agency policy, practitioner–supervisory style and practices, and staffing patterns are examples of factors that might have an influence. Additionally corporate or administrative operations, such as institutional goals, marketing strategies, and corporate-oversight processes may play a role. At the final macrolevel of impact the effects of overall societal resources and public policy have their considerations. Social concern for scarce health care resources, the movement to managed care, and the privatization of rehabilitation care are examples of broad themes and policies that relate to and may affect ethical practices at the practitioner level. Societal values or values related to such areas as independence and self-sufficiency, work and productivity, physical appearance, and other types of behavior do influence the work of rehabilitation counselors extensively (Gatens-Robinson & Rubin, 1995).

Themes/Attitudes in the Integrative Model

In addition to the specific elements or steps of the Integrative Model, there are four underlying *themes or attitudes* that are necessary to enact the potential of the model successfully. These attitudes involve mindfully attending to the tasks of: (1) maintaining a stance of *reflection* concerning one's own awareness of personal issues, values, and decision-making skills, as well as extending effort to understanding those of all others concerned with the situation, and their relationship to you; (2) addressing the *balance* between various issues, persons, and perspectives within the process; (3) maintaining an appropriate level of attention to the *context(s)* of the situation in question, allowing awareness of the counselor–client, treatment team, organizational, and societal implications of the ethical elements; and (4) seeking to use a process of *collaboration* with all rightful parties to the decision, but most especially the client.

By considering these background attitudes of balance, reflection, context, and collaboration, rehabilitation counselors engage in a more thorough process that will better preserve the integrity and dignity of all parties involved. This will be the case even when outcomes are not perceived to be equally positive for all participants in the process, as is often true in a serious dilemma when such attitudes can be particularly meaningful. Reflection is the overriding attitude of importance throughout the enactment of the specific elements of stages and components that constitute the steps of the Integrative Model. Many complex decision-making processes easily become overwhelming, either in their innate complexity, or in the real-life press of the speed or intensity or events. In the current approach, the practitioner is urged always to "Stop and think!" at each point in the process. The order of operations is not absolute, nor more important than being reflective and invested in a calm, dignified, respectful, and thorough analysis of the situation. It is not until we recognize that we are involved in the process and appreciate its critical aspects that we can call forth other resources to assist the process and persons within it. Such an attitude of reflection will serve the rehabilitation counselor well at all stages of this process.

Elements of the Integrative Model

The specific elements that comprise that actual operations within the Integrative Model include four main *stages* with several *components*

Table 5.1. The Integrative Model for Ethical Behavior In Rehabilitation Counseling

Stage I. Interpreting the Situation through Awareness and Fact-finding

Component 1.	Enhance sensitivity and awareness
Component 2.	Reflect to determine whether dilemma or issue is involved
Component 3.	Determine the major stakeholders and their ethical claims in the situation
Component 4.	Engage in the fact-finding process

Stage II. Formulating an Ethical Decision

Component 1.	Review the problem or dilemma
Component 2.	Determine what ethical codes, laws, ethical principles, and institutional policies and procedures exist that apply to the dilemma
Component 3.	Generate possible and probable courses of action
Component 4.	Consider potential positive and negative consequences for each course of action
Component 5.	Select the best ethical course of action

Stage III. Selecting an Action by Weighing Competing, Nonmoral Values

Component 1.	Engage in reflective recognition and analysis of personal competing values
Component 2.	Consider contextual influences on values selection at the collegial, team, institutional, and societal levels

Stage IV. Planning and Executing the Selected Course of Action

Component 1.	Figure out a reasonable sequence of concrete actions to be taken
Component 2.	Anticipate and work out personal and contextual barriers to effective execution of the plan of action, and effective countermeasures for them
Component 3.	Carry out and evaluate the course of action as planned

constituting the steps to be taken within each stage. As previously stated, the concepts summarized below are drawn in the main from the work of Rest (1984), Kitchener (1984), and Tarvydas and Cottone (1991). The specific elements are presented in Table 5.1.

Stage I. Interpreting the situation through awareness and fact-finding

At this stage the primary task of the counselor is to be sensitive and aware of the needs and welfare of the people around the counselor, and the ethical implications of these situations. This level of awareness allows the counselor to imagine and investigate the effects of the situation on the parties involved and the possible effects of various actions and conditions on them. This research and awareness must also include emotional as well as cognitive and fact-based considerations. There are four components that constitute the counselor's operations within this stage. *Component One* involves enhancing one's sensitivity and awareness. *Component Two* requires the counselor to reflect on what is known of the situation to determine whether a dilemma or issue seems to be involved. Not every situation with ethical overtones rises to the level of becoming an ethical dilemma. Rubin, Wilson, Fischer, and Vaughn (1991, p. 79) set four characteristics that a situation must meet before is considered to be an ethical dilemma:

1. A choice must be made between two courses of action.
2. There are significant consequences for taking either course of action.
3. Each of the two courses of action can be supported by one or more ethical principles.
4. The ethical principles supporting the unchosen course of action will be compromised.

In *Component Three* the counselor does an inventory to determine the persons who are major stakeholders in the outcome of the situation in question. It is important to reflect on any parties who will be affected and what their exact relationship is ethically and legally to the person at the center of the issue, the client. It is useful to imaging dropping a rock into a pond. The point of impact is where the central figure, the client, makes the impact. However, he or she is surrounded by persons at varying levels of closeness to him or her, such as parents, partners of intimate relationships, a spouse, children, employer, friends, and neighbors. They radiate out from the client in decreasing levels of intimacy and responsibility to the client. The ethical claims on the counselor's level of duty is not uniform. Almost all codes of ethics in counseling make it clear that the client is the person to whom the first duty is owed, but there are others who the counselor has lesser, but important levels of duty to consider. It is always important to determine whether any surrogate decision makers for the client exist such as a guardian or person with power of attorney, so that this person may be brought into the central circle of duty early on in the process. It is useful to be sensitive and proactive in working through situations in which the legal relationships do not coincide with the social and emotional bonds between the client and other persons involved in the dilemma. The final element in Stage I is *Component Four* in which the counselor undertakes an extensive fact-finding investigative process of such a scope as is appropriate to the situation.

Stage II. Formulating an ethical decision

This aspect of the process is that stage which is most widely known by professionals, and for many may erroneously be thought of as constituting its entirety. The central task in this stage is to identify which of the possible ethical courses of action appears to come closest to the moral ideal in the specific situation under consideration (Rest, 1984). Many decision-making models in other areas of counseling can be applied as a general template at this stage, but the following components are drawn from the work of VanHoose and Kottler (1985). In Component Two there is the addition of Kitchener's (1984) attention to ethical codes, laws, and ethical principles; and Tarvydas and Cottone's concern for the team and organizational context in the examination of institutional policies and procedures, which remind the counselor of other useful areas for consideration.

Component One suggests that the counselor should review the problem or dilemma to be sure that the most current and comprehensive understanding of it is used to analyze the dilemma. *Component Two*, as stated above, directs the counselor to research the standards of law and practice applicable to the situation. *Component Three* initiates the process of formally envisioning and generating possible and probable courses of action. As with all decision-making processes, it is important at this step not to prematurely truncate this exploratory process by prematurely censoring the possibilities, or succumbing to the sense of being overwhelmed or limited in options. *Component Four* is the logical outgrowth of determining courses of actions to consider in that potential positive and negative consequences are identified and assessed in light of the risks, as well as the material and personal resources available. Finally, the best ethical course of action is determined in *Component Five*.

Stage III. Selecting an action by weighing competing, nonmoral values

Many people would think that the ethical decision-making process is concluded at the end of Stage II. This impression is very limited in its realization of the many additional forces that may affect the counselor and result in the counselor not actually executing the ethical course of action selected at that point. *Component One* of Stage III interjects a period of reflection and active processing of the decision of what the counselor actually intends to do in view of competing, nonmoral values (Rest, 1984). It is important that counselors allow themselves to become aware of the strength and attractiveness of other values they hold that may influence whether or not they will discharge their ethical obligations. If they are self-aware, they may more effectively and honestly compensate for their conflicted impulses at this point. Counselors may have strong needs for acceptance by peers or supervisors, prestige, influence, avoidance of controversy, or financial success. These value orientations may come into conflict with the course of action that is necessary to proceed in an ethical manner, and must be reconciled with the ethical requirements if the client is to be ethically served. On the other hand, the counselor may place a high value on being moral or ethical, to be accepted as a respected professional with high ethical standards, or value the esteem of colleagues who place a high value on ethical professional behavior. Those forces should enhance the tendency to select ethical behavioral options. Therefore, the importance of selecting and maintaining ethically sensitized and positive professional and personal values should be recognized as critical to full professional functioning, as *Component Two* would suggest.

In Component Two the counselor systematically inventories the contextual influences on his or her choice at the collegial, team, institutional, and societal levels. Although this is not a simple process of weighing out forces, it should serve as an inventory of forces that are either dysfunctional or constructive for selecting the ethical course over other types of values present in these other interactions. The counselor may also use this type of information to think strategically about the forces he or she will need to overcome to provide ethical service in the situation under consideration. Beyond the immediate situation, it is important to recognize that the counselor should intentionally control his or her exposure to contexts that consistently reinforce values that run counter to the dictates of good ethical practices. This problem might result in terminating or curtailing certain relationships, changing employ-ment, or selecting another aspect of rehabilitation counseling service to provide.

Stage IV. Planning and executing the selected course of action

Rest (1984) described the essential tasks of this stage as planning to implement and then actually executing what one plans to do. This opera-tion includes *Component One* in which the counselor figures a reasonable sequence of concrete actions to be taken. In *Component Two* the task is to anticipate and work out all personal and contextual barriers to effectively execute the plan of action. It is very useful to consider and prepare spe-cific countermeasures for barriers that may reasonably be anticipated to arise. It is in this regard that the earlier attention to other stakeholders and their concerns may suggest problems and/or allies to the process. Additionally, earlier consideration of the contextual influences in Stage III assist the counselor in this type of strategic planning. *Component Three* is the final step in the linear aspect of this model in that it provides for the execution and evaluation of the course of action as planned. Rest (1984) notes that the actual behavioral execution of ethics is often not a simple task, frequently drawing heavily on the personal, emotional qual-ities, and professional and interpersonal skills of the counselor. He men-tions such qualities as firmness of resolve, ego strength, and social assertiveness. To this list could be added countless skills such as persis-tence, tact, time management, team collaboration, and conflict-resolution skills. Considerations are limited only by the characteristics and require-ments of the counselor and specific situation involved.

SUMMARY

Rehabilitation counseling continues to grow in stature and visibility as a profession. As a result, contemporary rehabilitation counselors should anticipate the need to demonstrate high levels of competency in the ethical aspects of their practices. The profession as a whole has provided substantial tools to inform this process; including ethical standards of practice, mechanisms to educate and govern the practice of these ethical standards, and knowledge and wisdom for individual counselors embodied within models of ethical decision making and behavior. With responsible utilization of these sizable assets for ethical practice, rehabilitation counseling should continue its leadership position in the counselor professionalization movement.

CHAPTER 6

Qualified Providers of Rehabilitation Counseling Services

Michael J. Leahy

A mong the various professionals (e.g., physiatrist, psychologists, social workers, medical case managers) who may provide services to individuals with disabilities during their individual rehabilitation process, the rehabilitation counselor represents a unique professional who can play a central role in the extramedical phase of the rehabilitation process for individuals with both acquired and congenital disabilities (G. N. Wright, 1980). Rehabilitation counseling emerged as a full-time occupation over 75 years ago. Unlike the beginnings of other counseling specialties and health-related occupations, rehabilitation counseling was mandated through federal legislation with the passage of the Smith–Fess Act in 1920, which established the public or state–federal rehabilitation program in this country. In the years following this land-mark legislation, rehabilitation counseling practice in the public and private sectors evolved and expanded to provide an extensive array of vocational and independent living services to an ever-increasing adult population of persons with a wide range of physical and mental disabilities (Leahy & Szymanski, 1995).

Although the occupational status of rehabilitation counseling was established in the 1920s, it was not until the mid 1950s, with the passage of the 1954 Vocational Rehabilitation Act Amendments, that the discipline embarked on a series of significant ongoing developments (e.g., preservice education, professional associations, code of ethics, regulation of practice) that have led over time to the professionalization of practice in rehabilitation counseling in this country, and to some extent internationally. Although initially a very heterogeneous group of practitioners in terms of educational background and professional competencies, rehabilitation counselors today, as a result of the professionalization process of the past 40 years, represent a group of professionals with a much higher degree of commonalty in relation to preservice preparation, practice, and professional identity than at any previous time in our professional history.

The purpose of this chapter is to review those elements of the profession that serve to both uniquely identify and provide the foundation for rehabilitation counseling practice in today's health and human services environment. Particular attention will be devoted to the scope and research-based foundation of practice, and the definition of qualified providers. In addition, preservice and continuing education, regulation of professional practice (certification and licensure), and the professional organizations in rehabilitation counseling will be reviewed.

SCOPE OF PRACTICE

Rehabilitation counseling has been described as a process in which the counselor works collaboratively with the client to understand existing problems, barriers, and potentials in order to facilitate the client's effective use of personal and environmental resources for career, personal, social, and community adjustment following disability (Jaques, 1970). In carrying out this multifaceted process, rehabilitation counselors must be prepared to assist individuals in adapting to the environment, assist environments in accommodating the needs of the individual, and work toward the full participation of individuals in all aspects of society, with a particular focus on career aspirations (Szymanski, 1985).

Over the years the fundamental role of the rehabilitation counselor has evolved (Jaques, 1970; Rubin & Roessler, 1995; G. N. Wright, 1980), with the subsequent functions and required knowledge and skill competencies of the rehabilitation counselor expanding as well. Regardless of their employment setting and client population, however, most rehabilitation counselors (a) assess client needs, (b) work with the client to develop goals and individualized plans to meet identified needs, and (c) provide or arrange for the therapeutic services and interventions (e.g., psychological, medical, social, behavioral) needed by the client, including job placement and follow-up services. Throughout this individualized process, counseling skills are considered essential components of all activities. It is the specialized knowledge of disabilities and of environmental factors that interact with disabilities, as well as the range of knowledge and skills required in addition to counseling that serves to differentiate the rehabilitation counselor from social workers, other types of counselors (e.g., mental health counselors, school counselors, career counselors), and other rehabilitation practitioners (e.g., vocational evaluators, job-placement specialists) in today's service delivery environments (Jenkins, Patterson & Szymanski, 1992; Leahy & Szymanski, 1995).

Utilizing a long-standing tradition in rehabilitation counseling research of studying the role and functions of qualified practitioners, in 1994 an official scope-of-practice statement was developed and adopted by the major professional, accreditation, and credentialing organizations in rehabilitation counseling. This statement, which is consistent with available empirical research, was required to more explicitly identify the scope of practice of the rehabilitation counselor to the public, consumers of services, related professional groups, and regulatory bodies. The statement, which was originally constructed by members of the Examination and Research Committee of the Commission on Rehabilitation Counselor Certification (CRCC), also contains major assumptions and underlying values associated with the scope of practice for rehabilitation counselors. The statement was formally adopted in 1994 and 1995 by the following organizations: the American Rehabilitation Counseling Association (ARCA), National Rehabilitation Counseling Association (NRCA), Alliance for Rehabilitation Counseling (ARC), National Council on Rehabilitation Education (NCRE), Commission on Rehabilitation Counselor Certification (CRCC), and the Council on Rehabilitation Education (CORE). The official scope-of-practice statement for rehabilitation counseling reads as follows.

> Rehabilitation counseling is a systematic process which assists persons with physical, mental, developmental, cognitive, and emotional disabilities to achieve their personal, career, and independent living goals in the most integrated setting possible through the application of the counseling process. The counseling process involves communication, goal setting, and beneficial growth or change through self-advocacy,

psychological, vocational, social, and behavioral interventions. The specific techniques and modalities utilized within this rehabilitation counseling process may include, but are not limited to:

assessment and appraisal;

diagnosis and treatment planning;

career (vocational) counseling;

individual and group counseling treatment interventions focused on facilitating adjustments to the medical and psychosocial impact of disability;

case management, referral, and service coordination;

program evaluation and research;

interventions to remove environmental, employment and attitudinal barriers;

consultation services among multiple parties and regulatory systems;

job analysis, job development, and placement services, including assistance with employment and job accommodations;

and the provision of consultation about, and access to, rehabilitation technology. (CRCC, 1994, pp. 1–2).

RESEARCH-BASED FOUNDATION OF PRACTICE

Underlying the practice of any profession or professional specialty area is the delineation of specific knowledge and skill requirements for effective service delivery. Job analysis, role and function, professional competency, critical incident, and knowledge-validation research are all terms that describe a process whereby the professional practice of rehabilitation counseling has been systematically studied to identify and describe important functions and tasks or knowledge and skills associated with the effective delivery of services to individuals with disabilities.

Over the past 40 years, an extensive body of knowledge has been acquired through these various research methods that has empirically identified the specific competencies and job functions important to the practice of rehabilitation counseling (e.g., Berven, 1979; Emener & Rubin, 1980; Harrison & Lee, 1979; Jaques, 1959; Leahy, Shapson & Wright, 1987; Leahy, Szymanski & Linkowski, 1993; Muthard & Salomone, 1969; Rubin et al., 1984; Wright & Fraser, 1975). This long-standing emphasis in rehabilitation counseling on the development and ongoing refinement of a research-based foundation in relation to practice and the required knowledge and skills has served to distinguish rehabilitation counseling from other counseling specialties that also seek to define and validate the scope of professional practice. These research efforts have also provided the profession with evidence of construct validity of rehabilitation counseling knowledge and skill areas (Szymanski, Linkowski, Leahy, Diamond, & Thoreson, 1993).

Although role and function approaches generally provide an empirically derived description of the functions and tasks associated with the role, the knowledge required to perform these functions is more indirectly assessed and inferred on the basis of the described functions and tasks. Roessler and Rubin (1992) in their review of recent major studies (Emener & Rubin, 1980; Leahy et al., 1987; Rubin et al., 1984) concluded that rehabilitation counselors have a diverse role requiring many skills if they are to effectively assist individuals with disabilities improve the quality of their lives. On review of the various studies they also concluded that the role of the rehabilitation counselor can be fundamentally described as encompassing the following functions or job task areas: (a) assessment, (b) affective counseling, (c) vocational counseling, (d) case management, and (e) job placement.

Conversely, knowledge validation and professional-competency approaches provide an empirically derived description of the knowledge and skills associated with a particular role, but the actual functions and tasks are more indirectly assessed and inferred on the basis of the knowledge and skills needed by an individual in order to practice. Recent research by Leahy et al. (1993) provided empirical support that the following 10 knowledge domains represent the core knowledge and skill requirements of rehabilitation counselors: (1) vocational counseling and consultation; (2) medical and psychological aspects of disability; (3) individual and group counseling; (4) program evaluation and research; (5) case management and service coordination; (6) family, gender, and multicultural issues; (7) foundations of rehabilitation; (8) workers' compensation; (9) environmental and attitudinal barriers; and (10) assessment. A complete listing of the knowledge domains and subdomains from the ongoing CRCC/CORE Knowledge Validation Study is provided in Table 6.1.

In terms of research utilization and application these empirically derived descriptions of the rehabilitation counselors role, function, and required knowledge and skill competencies have assisted the profession in a number of important ways. First, they have helped define the professional identity of the rehabilitation counselor by empirically defining the

Table 6.1. Knowledge Domains and Subdomains from the CORE/CRCC Knowledge Validation Study

Knowledge Domain/Subdomain

Vocational counseling and consultation services
    Planning for vocational rehabilitation services
    Vocational implications of various disabilities
    Physical/functional capacities of individual
    Occupational and labor market information
    Job-placement strategies
    Client job-seeking skills development
    Employer practices affecting return to work
    Job analysis
    Client job retention skill development
    Job modification and restructuring techniques
    Job and employer development
    Theories of career development and work adjustment
    Follow-up and postemployment services
    Accommodation and rehabilitation engineering
    Supported employment services and strategies
    Employer-based disability prevention and management
    Computer applications and technology
    Services to employer organizations

Medical and psychological aspects of disability
    Medical aspects and implications
    Medical terminology
    Psychosocial and cultural impact of disability
    Appropriate medical intervention resources

Individual and group counseling
    Individual counseling practices and interventions
    Individual counseling theories
    Behavior and personality theory
    Human growth and potential
    Family counseling theories
    Group counseling practices and interventions
    Group counseling theories

Program evaluation and research
    Evaluation procedures for assessing effective services
    Rehabilitation research literature
    Basic research methods
    Design of research projects and needs assessments

Case management and service coordination
    Case management process
    Community resources and services
    Services availability for a variety of populations
    Financial resources for rehabilitation services
    Rehabilitation services in diverse settings
    Planning for independent-living services
    Organizational structure of the public rehabilitation program
    Organizational structure of nonprofit service delivery system

Family, gender, and multicultural issues
    Societal issues, trends, and developments
    Psychosocial and cultural impact on the family
    Multicultural counseling issues
    Gender issues
    Family counseling practices

Foundations of rehabilitation counseling
    Ethical standards for rehabilitation counselors
    Laws affecting individuals with disabilities
    Rehabilitation terminology and concepts
    Philosophical foundations of rehabilitation
    History of rehabilitation

Workers' compensation
    Workers' compensation law and practices
    Expert testimony
    Organizational structure of the private-for-profit system

Environmental and attitudinal barriers
    Attitudinal barriers for individuals with disabilities
    Environmental barriers for individuals with disabilities

Assessment
    Interpretation of assessment results
    Test and evaluation techniques for assessment

uniqueness of the profession and by providing evidence in support of the construct validity of its knowledge base. Second, the descriptions have been extensively used in the development of preservice educational curricula in order to provide graduate training in areas of knowledge and skill critical to the practice of rehabilitation counseling across major employment settings. Third, the long-standing emphasis on a research-based foundation to practice has greatly contributed to the rehabilitation counseling profession's leadership role in the establishment and ongoing refinement of graduate educational program accreditation, through the Council on Rehabilitation Education, and individual practitioner certification, through the Commission on Rehabilitation Counselor Certification. Finally, this body of knowledge has also been useful in identifying both the common professional ground (shared competency areas) and the uniqueness of rehabilitation counseling among related rehabilitation disciplines (e.g., vocational evaluators, job-placement specialists) and other counseling specialties (e.g., career counselors, school counselors, mental health counselors). This process of further definition in the area of occupational competence is a normal sequence in the professionalization process for any occupation seeking public recognition.

QUALIFIED PROVIDERS

According to the professional associations (ARCA, NRCA, and ARC), qualified providers of rehabilitation counseling services are those professionals who have completed graduate degree training in rehabilitation counseling or a closely related degree program (e.g., counseling) at the masters level, have attained national certification as a Certified Rehabilitation Counselor (CRC) and have acquired the appropriate state licensure (e.g., Licensed Professional Counselor) in those states that require this level of credential for counseling practice. As an integral aspect of this professional identity, under this definition, qualified providers, are required to practice rehabilitation counseling within the guidelines and standards of the Code of Ethics for Rehabilitation Counselors and maintain ongoing professional development through relevant continuing education in order to maintain and upgrade their knowledge and skills related to practice. In addition to these professional requirements and responsibilities qualified providers are expected to be a member of a professional organization and contribute through professional advocacy to the advancement of the profession.

In recent years there has been a series of studies conducted to investigate the relationship between rehabilitation counselor education and service delivery outcomes that has provided consistent support for the position that rehabilitation counselors, as qualified providers, need to obtain preservice training at the graduate level in rehabilitation counseling or a closely related field prior to practice. Studies of the New York (Szymanski & Parker, 1989), Wisconsin (Szymanski, 1991), Maryland (Szymanski & Danek, 1992), and Arkansas (Cook & Bolton, 1992) state vocational rehabilitation agencies demonstrated that counselors with master's degrees in rehabilitation counseling achieved better outcomes with clients with severe disabilities than did rehabilitation counselors with unrelated master's or bachelor's degrees. In another group of studies involving rehabilitation counselors from a variety of employment settings, preservice education was linked to the rehabilitation counselors perceived (self-assessed) level of competency. Shapson, Wright, and Leahy (1987), and Szymanski, Leahy, and Linkowski (1993) demonstrated that counselors with master's degrees in rehabilitation counseling perceived themselves to be more competent or better prepared in critical knowledge and skill areas of rehabilitation counseling than did counselors with unrelated preservice preparation (Leahy & Szymanski, 1995).

Over the years, particularly the past 20, there has been a growing expectation among members of the profession, employers, and regulatory bodies that rehabilitation counselors who provide services to people with disabilities have the appropriate preservice education and credentials (certification and licensure) as identified above. Even today, however, there are individuals practicing as rehabilitation counselors in both the public and private rehabilitation sectors in this country who do not have this type of preservice preparation or appropriate credentials. Although this heterogeneity in professional background was once thought of as a natural consequence of a quickly expanding field, in more recent years the practice of hiring individuals without appropriate professional training and credentials has been heavily criticized by professional, educational, and regulatory bodies in rehabilitation counseling. According to Rothman (1987), one of the key characteristics of any profession is regulation of practice. Individuals who practice rehabilitation counseling outside of the profession are not accountable to or included in such regulation of practice, however, and are therefore not required to adhere to the profession's Code of Ethics or accepted standards of practice. Although this situation has improved over the years, it is still unacceptable. It is clear, however, that in the years to come the trend toward professionalization and particularly the movement toward state licensure and certification in this country will make it less likely that an individual will be able to practice as a rehabilitation counselor without appropriate training and credentials.

SPECIALIZATION AND RELATED PROVIDERS

Today, a majority of rehabilitation counselors practice in the public, private, and nonprofit rehabilitation sectors. More recently, however, rehabilitation counselors have begun to practice in independent-living centers, employee-assistance programs, hospitals and clinics, mental health organizations, public-school transition programs, and employer-based disability prevention and management programs. Although setting-based factors may affect the relative emphasis or importance of various rehabilitation counselor functions or may introduce new specialized knowledge requirements for the rehabilitation counselor, there remains a great deal of commonality in the role and function among rehabilitation counselors regardless of employment setting (Leahy et al., 1987, 1993). One aspect that is often affected by these various settings is the specific job title used by the rehabilitation counselor. Although the rehabilitation counselor job title is used in the majority of settings, one can also find the use of the title rehabilitation consultant or case manager among today's practicing rehabilitation counselors. In addition, as one advances up the career ladder within these various settings, rehabilitation counselors can assume supervisory, management, and administrative roles within these various organizations.

Although the majority of rehabilitation counselors are viewed as generalists, another aspect of variation among practicing rehabilitation counselors is the degree to which they specialize their practice. One particularly useful model for viewing this issue was developed by DiMichael (1967), who suggested a two-way classification of horizontal and vertical specialization in rehabilitation counseling. In DiMichael's model, horizontal specialization refers to rehabilitation counselors who restrict or specialize their practice with a particular disability group (e.g., deaf, blind, head injury, substance abuse) that requires a significant amount of specialized knowledge or skill, specific to the type of disability. Vertical specialization, on the other hand, occurs when rehabilitation counselors attend to only one function in the rehabilitation process (e.g., assessment or job placement) in their work with clients. Vocational evaluators and job-placement specialists are examples of vertical specialists in this model.

The previous section on qualified providers does not imply that only rehabilitation counselors should provide rehabilitation services for persons with disabilities. In fact, there are numerous other related work roles that contribute to the rehabilitation process and complement the role and services provided by the rehabilitation counselor. In addition to vocational evaluators and job-placement specialists, who can assist the rehabilitation counselor and client at critical stages in the rehabilitation process (assessment and job placement), other supportive resources could include physicians and physiatrists, physical and occupational therapists, psychologists, work-adjustment trainers, job coaches, and various vocational training personnel. Often times a very critical aspect of the rehabilitation counselor's role is the coordination of services provided by these various professionals within the context of a multidisciplinary team approach to effectively address the multifaceted needs of the client in the rehabilitation process.

PRESERVICE AND CONTINUING EDUCATION

Throughout this chapter the importance of appropriate preservice education in rehabilitation counseling has been emphasized. By the 1940s three universities (New York, Ohio State, and Wayne State) had developed graduate training programs in rehabilitation counseling (Jenkins et al., 1992). In 1954, with the passage of the Vocational Rehabilitation Amendments, federal grant support was provided for the first time to universities and colleges to develop graduate preservice training programs to prepare rehabilitation counselors for employment in the public and private nonprofit rehabilitation sectors. This federal training support, which continues to this day, accelerated the design and development of graduate training in rehabilitation counseling in this country and can be viewed as the beginning of the professionalization process for the formal discipline of rehabilitation counseling (Leahy & Szymanski, 1995).

During this initial period of program development, a conference report by Hall and Warren (1956), which documented the findings of a comprehensive workshop sponsored by the National Rehabilitation Association (NRA) and the National Vocational Guidance Association [now the American Counseling Association (ACA)], provided the initial guidelines for curriculum planning by the new, federally funded rehabilitation counselor education programs (G. N. Wright, 1980). In the years that followed, empirical research in the form of role and function and professional-competency studies (covered earlier in this chapter) helped guide curriculum redesign efforts to ensure that critical knowledge and skill areas needed in the field were reflected in the preservice training content.

As rehabilitation counselor education programs expanded in colleges and universities there was a need to devise a mechanism to standardize and accredit these training programs. In 1972 the Council on Rehabilitation Education was established as the national accreditation body for rehabilitation counselor education programs "to promote the effective delivery of rehabilitation services to individuals with disabilities by promoting and fostering continuing review and improvement of master's degree level programs" (CORE, 1991, p. 2). Research done at the University of Wisconsin laid the foundation for a multistakeholder program-evaluation process that was recognized in 1975 by the National Commission on Accrediting, a predecessor of the Council on Postsecondary Accreditation (COPA) that is still in use today (Linkowski & Szymanski, 1993). Today there are over 80 accredited master's-degree educational programs in rehabilitation counseling. As the oldest and most established accreditation body among the counseling professions, the CORE process remains firmly grounded in research. The knowledge standards (see Table 6.1) against which program curricula are measured are constantly validated though an ongoing, joint research project with the Commission on Rehabilitation Counselor Certification (Szymanski et al., 1993).

Following graduate-level preservice education, practicing rehabilitation counselors need to continue their professional development to maintain and upgrade knowledge and skills associated with the delivery of rehabilitation counseling services to persons with disabilities. For example, Certified Rehabilitation Counselors are required to obtain a minimum of 100 hours of relevant continuing education during their 5-year certification period. With the rapid pace of change in the field and the continual dissemination of new knowledge and expanded skills associated with practice, the rehabilitation counselor needs to be aware of the continuing educational opportunities available. Although there are numerous organizations and groups that provide this type of training, the primary sources and sponsors of continuing education for the rehabilitation counselor are the professional organizations (e.g., ARCA, NRCA), the Regional Rehabilitation Continuing Educational Programs (RRCEPs), Research and Training Centers (R&Ts), and university-based continuing-education programs.

REGULATION OF PRACTICE AND CREDENTIALING

Regulation of practice through professional certification and licensure are important characteristics of professions (Rothman, 1987). Rehabilitation counseling has been widely recognized as the leading counseling specialty in the development and pioneering of credentialing mechanisms through national certification and educational program accreditation, which serve as the cornerstones of the general counseling professionalization system (Tarvydas & Leahy, 1993). However, it has also been widely observed that the order of credentialing development in rehabilitation counseling is atypical of the expected order of progression seen in other, more established professions, such as medicine and law. The more classic evolution of credentials, according to Matkin (1983), has been for the profession to initially achieve state licensure, and then move to develop national specialty certifications or endorsements regulated by the professional organizations. In rehabilitation counseling, national certification was established first and then followed by a long period of legislative advocacy, in which other counseling specialty groups took the lead role along with rehabilitation counselors to establish state counselor licensure laws in individual states (Tarvydas & Leahy, 1993).

In our field, the CRC credentialing process is the oldest, and most established certification process in the counseling and rehabilitation professions. The purpose of certification is to ensure that the professionals engaged in rehabilitation counseling are of good moral character and possess at least an acceptable minimum level of knowledge, as determined by the Commission, with regard to the practice of their profession. The existence of such standards is considered to be in the best interests of consumers of rehabilitation counseling services and the general public. From a historical perspective, the CRC credentialing program was an outgrowth of the professional concerns of the ARCA and the NRCA.

Since the inception of the credential and the subsequent development of the CRCC in 1973, over 23,000 professionals have participated in the certification process. Today there are over 14,000 CRCs practicing in the

United States and several foreign countries (Leahy & Holt, 1993). Certification standards and examination content for the CRC have been empirically validated through ongoing research efforts throughout the 22-year history of the Commission, and are currently regularly examined as part of the ongoing CORE/CRCC Knowledge Validation Study, which is housed at the CRCC offices in Chicago. These standards represent the level of education, experience, and knowledge competencies (see Table 6.1) required of rehabilitation counselors to provide services to individuals with disabilities (Leahy & Szymanski, 1995).

In terms of regulation of practice, the most powerful credential is licensure. As differentiated from voluntary national certification, licensure regulates the practice of a profession through specific state legislation. Beginning in 1976, with the passage of the first counselor licensure bill in Virginia, there has been a long struggle by advocates of the counselor-licensure movement to enact legislation on a state-by-state basis to protect the title and regulate the practice of counseling. During the past 20 years over 40 states have enacted counselor-licensure legislation. The trend has been toward the passage of general-practice legislation (which covers various counseling specialty groups), which is consistent with the recommendations of the American Counseling Association's (ACA) Licensure Committee in its model legislation for licensed professional counselors (Bloom et al., 1990; Glosoff, Benshoff, Hosie, & Maki, 1995). Reflecting this trend, the most commonly used title in counselor licensure bills has been that of the Licensed Professional Counselor (LPC).

Counselor-licensure legislation is intended to regulate both the use of the terms by which the statute officially refers to professional counselors as well as to protect the practice of professional counseling as set forth in its definition and scope-of-practice provisions. This combination of title and practice bill is the most stringent form of credentialing and would prohibit anyone from practicing counseling unless fully qualified regardless of formal title. Title-only legislation on the other hand, which has been passed in 24 of the states, prohibits persons from using the specific titles restricted in the bill to those who have met the specified qualifications established by the bill and have achieved licensure. It does not, however, restrict persons from providing counseling services if their job titles avoid restricted language. Most title-only legislation was passed to avoid powerful lobbying efforts that would have been mounted to defeat the more restrictive title and practice bills. Clearly this type of legislation was seen as a first stage by counselor-licensure advocates in the overall drive toward eventual regulation of practice through future revisions of the initial legislation (Tarvydas & Leahy, 1993).

Although there are presently three states that have passed licensure laws specifically covering the rehabilitation counselor (Texas, Louisiana, and Massachusetts), the majority of states have enacted general-practice legislation covering all counselors. The professional associations in rehabilitation counseling (ARCA, NRCA, and the Alliance for Rehabilitation Counseling) have taken the position to strongly advocate for the inclusion of rehabilitation counselors within general counselor state licensure whenever possible. With this in mind, the Licensed Professional Counselor designation, combined with certification as a CRC would represent the appropriate credentials for rehabilitation counselors working with individuals with disabilities, in states with general-practice legislation.

PROFESSIONAL ORGANIZATIONS

According to Rothman (1987), professional organizations, provide a forum for the exchange of information and ideas among professionals, reflect the philosophical bases of a profession, and as political entities, are concerned with the organization of the profession and relations with external groups. In rehabilitation counseling, professional associations also provide an organizational home for individuals with similar professional identities, interests, and backgrounds who are committed to the further development and refinement of the profession.

Throughout the modern history of rehabilitation counseling there have been two divergent models of the profession that have served to define the professional organizations of the rehabilitation counselor. One model postulates that rehabilitation counseling should be viewed as a separate and autonomous profession, organizationally aligned with other related rehabilitation disciplines. The other model views the rehabilitation counseling profession as a specialty area of general counseling, organizationally aligned with other related counseling groups. These early beliefs are presently reflected in the profession's two major professional organizations, which also represent rehabilitation counseling's dual emphasis in counseling and rehabilitation.

The American Rehabilitation Counseling Association was founded in 1958 as a professional division of the American Personnel and Guidance

Association (now the American Counseling Association). The National Rehabilitation Counseling Association, was also founded in 1958 as a professional division of the National Rehabilitation Association. The presence of these two organizations, with similar missions and constituencies, has been the topic of much discussion and debate over the years. The perplexing aspect of these discussions is that depending on individual perspective, one can rationalize the efficacy of either organizational model. In fact, the argument can be made that formal organizational relationships with both the counseling and rehabilitation communities has over time served to strengthen, align, and confirm our dual orientations as rehabilitation counselors and has provided the profession with a very unique identity and heritage (Tarvydas & Leahy, 1993).

Throughout the years, there have been serious discussions of organizational merger (see Rasch, 1979; Reagles, 1981) and systems of collaboration (G. N. Wright, 1982) to repair the fragmentation and professional and public confusion created by the existence of two such organizations representing rehabilitation counseling (Leahy & Szymanski, 1995). To address these concerns, in 1993 the ARCA and NRCA boards created the Alliance for Rehabilitation Counseling (ARC) as a formal collaborative structure to marshal the strengths of both organizations into a unified professional policy and strategic-planning voice for rehabilitation counseling, while at the same time respecting the autonomy, heritage, and value of each of the individual organizations.

Although still in the early stages of this formal relationship, these two professional organizations have already coordinated their respective strategic-planning efforts, and developed and approved joint policy statements on impending federal legislation, counselor licensure, and scope of practice. In addition, they have developed joint committees, which will meet under the auspices of the Alliance in the areas of licensure, third-party reimbursement, and standards of practice, and have agreed to co-sponsor a comprehensive annual professional development conference. The Alliance for Rehabilitation Counseling appears to have been a major step forward for the profession in developing comprehensive and coordinated professional advocacy efforts at the national level and providing a mechanism under which all rehabilitation counselors in this country can unite as we continue down the path of professionalization in the years to come.

CHAPTER 7

Consumer: Individual and Families

Al Condeluci and Janet M. Williams

I n the course of our lives we play many roles. We are friends, neighbors, citizens, sons, daughters, husbands, wives, students, teachers, and the like. Indeed, when you think of the elements of a successful life, one could argue that it is the ability to master roles that leads to a fulfilling life. Of course, these roles are played within the context of the greater culture and subculture in which we hold membership.

The context of our individual roles within a family also take on significance as a family entity. We may interact on behalf of our entire family or as a family on behalf of an individual member. The context changes depending on the situation. Any constellation of roles can occur within a culture.

One may define culture as a network of people drawn together by common cause or celebration. Indeed, all of us are members of a variety of cultures (or subcultures) in the course of our lives. Most of us are also members of a spiritual culture where we practice a certain form of theology in an effort to nurture our spirits or souls.

We also belong to work, social, intellectual, and interest-oriented groups in which we share common focus with other people and are linked by the roles sanctioned by that culture. These are the settings of our lives and the way we find importance, esteem, and meaning in our existence. We feel good about ourselves when we are able to master or be accepted in the role success we exhibit.

As we enter a system often described as "human services" we enter a culture unto itself. Services evolve and roles change. Consumers, families, and rehabilitationists have begun an almost awkward dance to renegotiate who leads and who follows, which is clearly linked to who decides.

ROLES WITHIN REHABILITATION

The notion of role success has been linked to rehabilitation in a number of ways. One theorist, Wolf Wolfensberger (1983), initiated the concept of social-role valorization as the key to normalizing the relationships for people with developmental disabilities. Wolfensberger defined social-role valorization as the attainment of social roles as a means to enhancing ones value in the society. He postulated that the more people with disabilities are exposed and permitted to play viable social roles the more easily they would be assimilated into the mainstream.

Social-role valorization is an opportunity for consumers to see themselves within the greater context of a society rather than within a context of a human-service system. Families began to be told where their members fit rather than what was wrong with them. Hence, rehabilitation looked outward to the community for opportunities for inclusion.

Others, before and after Wolfensberger, have attested to the importance of role success within the context of society. Goffman (1959), for instance, wrote about the way people present themselves within the culture. He articulated the notion of the masks people wear within the roles they play. These masks allow us to navigate between roles in an effort to achieve life success.

Some years later, in thinking about social acceptance, the concept of community bridge building was initiated (Mount, 1989). This notion continued the thesis that generic social roles were a more viable route to friendships and relationships than the traditional skill-building programs offered by most human-service agencies. The idea of relationships is a critical one in human services today. That is, people become known more for the relationships they develop than for how they perform or function.

Mount and others argued that if the rehabilitationist focused on assets, capacities, gifts, and talents of people rather than to attempting to change their deficits, more progress could be made in mainstreaming people back to the community through commensurate cultural groups. This notion is somewhat novel because the traditional tenor of rehabilitation was to attend to what people could not do or did not do well.

Consumers were finally told you are okay just the way you are. Families were told to get on with life as it is and rehabilitationists were told to quit trying to fix people. This revolutionary change in roles evolved over time.

It is useful to examine the history of rehabilitation to further understand the evolution that started by saying people must be "fixed" to one that states that people are "consumers." The fix-it end of the spectrum begins with the medical model.

A LOOK AT THE MEDICAL MODEL

The primary driving force of the medical model is the influence of science and the prominence of the sick role. Indeed, Talcott Parsons (1951) wrote about the sick role in the mid-1900s identifying the ways medicine can be limiting. As a scientific model, the medical paradigm is one of precision and predictability. It starts with the notion that people are sick, ill, deficient, or defective. Given the knowledge of science, agents of this model endeavor to identify and then isolate the reasons for the deficiency, this identification develops from what is perceived to be wrong with the person. Indeed, the labels and diagnosis offered by medical agents are often descriptors of the deficiency. For example, the label of "cerebral palsy" literally means that the defective cerebral cortex is cause for the palsy or shaking exhibited by people with this condition.

Once labeled, and clearly defined through deficiency, the medical model attempts to isolate the problem and offer a treatment plan to rescind, or lessen the effects of the condition. In fact, it is hoped that the treatment plan will fully "cure" the problem. The goal is to fix, heal, or change the labeled person to be "normal" or typical to some defined standard. Once this occurs, the individual will then easily fit into the community. All three constituencies are often in agreement about the need to be "fixed" early on.

Another key feature of the medical model is the dominance of certified and sanctioned experts who hold publicly acknowledged certification. The more severe or stigmatic the condition, the more fully certified the expert must be. Along with the individually credentialed professionals, often the facilities too must be certified and meet some external test. For consumers and families it may be comforting to know that experts are available and in charge.

Because the medical model is scientific in nature it operates from the notion of cause and effect. That is, as the paradigm prompts a study and analysis of the ailment; it is drawn to make predictions about what to expect. This predictability can cause the medical agents to begin to see the labeled person as a separate set of dysfunctional parts that alter the individual wholeness.

All of these elements lead to a type of devaluation in which the labeled person is seen as sick, deficient, and incapable of making good decisions. Further, as the elements of their ailment are scientific, the patient does not have the background, understanding, or credential to make knowledge-able decisions for themselves. All of these factors distance the labeled person from the role of consumer. As a person begins to feel alienated he or she may begin to ask more questions, and begin to be labelled as "inap-propriate" for wanting to know.

Given this perspective, it is easy to see how people, who are histori-cally devalued and not in command of the medical nuances, are easily left out of the decision-making process. In fact, for most of us, devalued or not, the medical model is often one that is not to be challenged. Most of us are taught at an early age that the doctor is not to be challenged. Only recently have some people challenged the physicians perspective, or sought a second opinion.

THE FAMILY AND THE MEDICAL MODEL

The message of the medical model puts different pressures on families. Initially, a family may be forced to make life-and-death decisions for which they usually are not prepared. Naturally, they want to protect their fam-ily member from further harm. It is traditionally thought that being sur-rounded by technology and professionals means one is "protected." So, logically, families want their loved one to stay in this protective environment.

This protective reaction is reinforced over and over as the person begins to question the orientation dictated by the medical model. The con-sumer and family begin to realize that funding is often tied directly to deficits and problems, and not to the dignity of risk or the right to be wrong. People are tested, assessed, and evaluated to find out what is wrong with them so funding can be established to fix the person just right. Further, the all-encompassing structure of many medically based programs leads to the assumption that a person cannot function outside of the program structure. Meanwhile, the person may be working hard and want more independence, but the system, driven by the medical model, tells him or her not to take risks because the person is not yet competent, or will be without money and resources.

Under these circumstances families have been described as overprotective, unrealistic and in denial. This deficit-and-problem approach to labeling families is in line with defining behaviors as medical problems to be fixed. How often do you hear some well-intentioned rehabilitationist declare, "If only the family would. . . ." Seldom is attention given to the needs of families as being rightly concerned about further harm to the person, questioning why this happened to him or her, wanting the person to be different, or not being able to immediately grasp the enormity of life changes.

CULTURE AND ROLES

In *Interdependence* (Cordelvg, 1991) and *Beyond Difference* (Cordelvg, 1995) the notions of roles, culture, deficits and capacities are further explored by Cordeluci. If we want people included in jobs, neighborhoods, churches, and the like, we must think about culture and relationships and how the roles we play offer a route to inclusion. This means that the more we know about roles, the more we can understand/include. In this context, people are welcomed not for the functional things they might do, but for the roles they play within the culture and the similar interests that they have with others.

This concept is consistent to the typical norms of society. That is, most of us are not necessarily accepted into groups or associations because we are independent in our activities of daily living. Rather, we are accepted because we share an interest and passion in the topic at hand. We become known in these cultures because we share similar roles.

When one thinks about how similarities can bond different people, consider the television series, "Cheers." As most of us know, the "Cheers" bar became a dynamic venue for a diverse group of people to come together for a common exchange; to socialize. Although the characters were vastly different in what they did or what they wanted from life, at

"Cheers" they had a social similarity. Week in and week out, numerous stories wove around this diverse group as they dealt with a variety of situations. The group situations typify the bonding power of common roles that we play with others, and how these roles can override the difference we might have as people.

This type of thinking is a significant paradigm shift from the historical sense of rehabilitation. For many years, and consistent with the medical model, we have assumed that the route to community acceptance was through functional-skill competency. Using the "Cheers" example, traditional rehabilitation would want to make the characters in "Cheers" more functional and typical as a way to better be accepted in that venue.

Now it seems clear that although focusing on differences might be beneficial at times, this is not the best approach for the characters of "Cheers" to be included in the larger exchange of the social venue. In the same vein, the approach is not the best way for inclusion of people who happen to have disabilities and are interested in being a part of the greater culture. Rather, if we begin to think about role competence and overall cultural interests, the realities of community become more apparent.

THE ROLE OF CONSUMER

Of the many roles we play, one of the most interesting and complex is that of consumer. All of us, in many ways are consumers of goods, services, and products. The more we know about various goods, services, and products the more successful we will be in our decision making. In this context consumerism in rehabilitation means two important things. *One is how the person with a disability comes to be a better consumer in general. The other is in considering the person with a disability as a consumer of our rehabilitation services.*

Although both of these themes are independent, they are also tied together. That is, as the individual becomes more astute as a general consumer, he or she will also become more adept at analyzing and evaluating how professionals who act as their agents are performing.

Nowhere is this concept of consumerism more powerfully presented than in the independent-living movement initiated by people with disabilities in the early 1960s. As most rehabilitationists know, the independent-living movement was launched from the context of civil rights.

Much as racial discrimination was the focus of civil rights, the aspect of consumer control was (and is) the cornerstone of the independent-living movement (Shapiro, 1993).

These rights mean that individuals who use rehabilitation services should control how services are delivered and, at times, who delivers the service. This credo has led to the creation of centers for independent living (CIL), agencies dedicated to the consumer-control concept. A bona fide CIL is a center where the majority of staff and board are individuals with disabilities. The momentum of the CILs and the independent-living movement have resulted in key changes in formal aspects of rehabilitation. First with the Rehabilitation Act Amendments of 1973 and then again in 1978 when the Act was amended to further articulate independent living as a bona fide rehabilitation goal. The passage of the Americans with Disabilities Act created a legal basis for consumerism and declared that disability is within the natural context of the human endeavor. All these measures have had consumer control as a key element.

CONSUMERISM DEFINED

To better understand the basics of consumerism it is important to first examine definitions and social interpretations. Although one may consult dictionaries, it is important to explore these concepts with people from various locations around the country to enhance perspective. Clearly people know their own realities best, and, to this extent, are the best purveyors of information for professionals who seek to know more.

> *Consumer* 1. A person or thing that consumes. 2. A person or organization that uses a commodity or service. 3. An organism, usually an animal that feeds on plants or other animals (Random House, 1987).

> *Consumer* 1. One who or which consumes. 2. One who uses up an article of exchangeable value; one of the buying public (Funk & Wagnall, 1984).

> *Consumer* 1. One that consumes, especially one that acquires goods or services for direct use or ownership rather than for resale or use in production or manufacturing (American Dictionary, 1992).

All of these definitions imply a gathering of goods or services for some enhancement or accomplishment. They suggest that the consumer is able to articulate and differentiate between similar goods or services so as to make a decision that is best for their interest. So consumers are decision makers with specific interests in decisions. In most regards this means being a customer of products.

CONSUMER AS CUSTOMER

Another key aspect of consumerism is to consider a customer perspective. The popularity of the word "customer" as a descriptor of people with disabilities involved in human services is particularly intriguing. To some extent, the title seems too naive, as most people with disabilities in traditional human services are far from true customers. In these situations it seems as if the use of the word is more of a diluted sense of the term. That is, the rehabilitation system will describe people as customers, but it is really a misuse of the word's intent. Wolfensberger (1972) discussed ways that human-service systems can overuse, or misuse terms like consumer, customer, client, and the like. He articulated how human services have come to detoxify concepts as well. He shares that in earlier times people were punished by being relegated to dungeons. As society became more enlightened, we called these places a "time-out room." Now we refer to those isolated places as "client lounges." The bottom line, however, is that they still represent isolation and punishment. Perhaps "customer" is a similarly detoxified notion.

Regardless of the efficacy of the term, customer as a descriptor does have a powerful consumer base. In the classic sense the customer is one who chooses a product or service and indeed, usually has a litany of options. As a customer, the consumer of any type of product, as long as he or she has money to pay for that product, is truly in control.

However, the economic description of customer hardly plays in human services. In many cases people with disabilities and their families have very little impact on the way and means of rehabilitation services. There are many reasons for this, but the most prominent seems to be the perception that the individual with a disability does not truly understand the medical or psychological aspects of their situation. Again, this is a result of the medical models influence on rehabilitation. Like it or not, rehabilitation is originally the child of medicine, and the medical model makes consumerism and the customer perspective difficult to achieve.

DEVALUATION AND CONSUMERISM

Historically, devalued people have typically been relegated to a lower status as consumers. Some companies simply do not want the business of groups perceived to be less valuable. As an advocate, encountering experiences of such consumer devaluation is common. While promoting the ADA (Americans with Disabilities Act) to some local business people the case was made concerning the economic viability of people with disabilities as real consumers. It was suggested that the ADA and its emphasis on architectural and attitudinal accessibility was good business in that people with disabilities would be more active consumers of their services and products. Over and above the moral issue of equal access, the emphasis was that such activities were just good business. Later, during a break, two business people in the session were overheard to indicate that for the cost they anticipated for ADA accessibility, there would probably not be commensurate business. Further, the restaurateur of the duo thought that having people with serious disabilities in his eatery would deter other customers. He said, "Who would want to eat sitting near someone in a wheelchair?"

We hope these kinds of attitudes represent a minority perspective, but they are still harbored by some. This type of "spread" of devaluation from one type of situation to a vital social role is important for us to ponder. First we need to inspect the parochial attitudes of human service professionals to the consumer role that people with disabilities might play within our own organizations. Are people with disabilities and their families truly seen as viable consumers? Next we need to understand and address the devaluation of the consumer role that might be felt in the greater community.

In his writings, Goffman (1961, 1963) reflects on the sociological ramifications of stigma. He explored the basic concept of deviance juxtaposition in which the negatives of deviance can spread to others who are positioned together. In some ways this notion of putting devalued people together, however, is actually used as a methodology for rehabilitation treatment. In some states the criminal-justice system allows first-time offenders to "work off" their offense by doing volunteer community-service work. Often this work is done with people who have disabilities. In reality, this deviance juxtaposition keeps both groups devalued.

METHODS TO ENHANCE CONSUMER PARTICIPATION

Given the importance of consumerism in rehabilitation today, many organizations are exploring ways and means to enhance consumer participation. These efforts vary, but the most important ingredient is sincerity in wanting to have people served be more active in the daily operation of the organization. Some ideas to consider include:

• Consumer preparation classes: Probably the most basic idea, and one offered by many organizations that support people with disabilities, are classes on consumerism and decision making taught by other consumers. This kind of exposure can assist people who have limited experiences or those who need some compensatory strategies to develop decision-making skills.

• Service advisory councils: Advisory groups of consumers of products have long been used as a quality-assurance mechanism by many organizations. These councils will meet on a regular basis to review, evaluate, or critique services offered. In some cases council can have veto or approval power.

• Consumer/board participation: The ultimate authority for most human-service agencies rests with a board of directors. This chartered group develops policy and assures that the organization moves toward its agenda. Many organizations have developed policy or guidelines that call for a portion of their board to be representative of the constituency served by the organization. That is, agencies that serve minority groups, or special-interest groups will attempt to have like people on the board. Indeed, centers for independent living mandate that at least 51% of the board of directors be people with disabilities. These types of mandates, however, have been criticized recently by concerns that quotas are not the best route to the spirit of full participation. Nonetheless, having people who receive service from the organization on the board does tend to keep sensitivities sharp and the organization focused on it objectives.

• Staff positions: Another way to develop consumerism and to keep the organization on task is to have the agency hire people that it has served, where feasible. Nothing develops consumer skills better than the chance to be a direct consumer, and often this takes financial resources.

• Focus groups: In strategic planning, organizations have often used focus groups to help test assumptions and focus external factors. A focus group is often comprised of constituents, consumers, or stakeholders who have opportunities to interact with key agency representatives. Focus groups are excellent ways for consumers to enhance their independence skills.

• **Hiring/firing sign-offs:** In situations in which staff play a supportive or assisting role, consumer participation in hirings or firings offers another possibility for real consumer involvement. It is amazing how responsible people can be when they have this type of "consumer power."

• **Voucher options:** Perhaps one of the most direct means of consumer participation is to provide people full access to programs through vouchers or direct cash grants. In its purest form, people can take a voucher (or money) and shop for the service that best suits them. Food stamps are probably the best known voucher program. These programs make food coupons available to eligible people and then allow them to shop around for the best deals. Another example of vouchers is the Section 8 housing program offered through the U.S. Department of Housing and Urban Development (HUD). Like food stamps, the Section 8 program makes a certificate available to eligible individuals who then access private housing that is best suited for them.

THE FAMILY AS A CONSUMER

In many regards, when an individual becomes a consumer of rehabilitation services, this becomes a family affair. After injury, illness, or birth wherein a person now has a disability, the family is usually the first consumer. This is especially true with congenital birth defects or traumatic injuries. In these cases the individual with the disability is incapacitated or unable to play a direct role. The family, however, is usually serving as the voice and key decision maker for the individual about the needed services.

This focus on the family as consumer offers an interesting point for examination. Often the family is comprised of a number of players, each with individual concerns and perspectives. In these cases confusion or disagreement can be a problem. Some family members may want one course of action and others yet another option. In these situations, organizational professionals must assess and clarify who are the major constituents. In some regards the situation might dictate that the family is the primary consumer as the individual with the disability is not yet in a position to make decisions for him or herself.

This conflict in consumers is well known in mental health and

head-injury rehabilitation services. In some situations, the individual
with the disability wants one thing from the agency and the family quite
another. The individual may want full control and the family wants the
individual protected. As we understand the competing influences the
family has with the medical model and community-oriented approaches,
this conflict is understandable. Experience has revealed many of these
types of standoffs. In some of these cases the solutions came only after
legal action.

Another juncture at which consumer conflicts between users of services and their families occurs is revealed when people reach the adult
years. This period is challenging for any parent–child relationship, but in
situations in which the person has a disability the family may be more apt
to treat the individual in a childlike way. Again, families receive their
messages from the medical model and a society that often views people
with disabilities as childlike and incapable. Simple decisions on life-style
choices, to more complex issues, such as marriage, having children, and
the like, can seriously compromise the reality of consumerism.

In situations where families have disagreed with the decision of their
adult son or daughter there is no easy answer. Some considerations might
include:

- Educate: Reflect with the family on why they might want to protect
their child. Gain the family's trust and introduce them to other families
and consumers who may have felt that way at one time and have since
changed their perspective. If the professional can let the families educate
one another beneficial results often occur.
- Mediate: In this approach, the agency does not take sides, but merely provides the venue whereby the parties come to explore their points of
contention. Here the agency might assure that the individual is treated like
an adult, but focus on the reality of the impact of the decision.
- Find a mediator: In some cases, a mediator may help the dispute
reach resolution. In this area one may identifiy other family members
who serve as a mediator. In other cases, professional mediators might be
engaged.
- Offer a middle ground: As with most disputes, emotional issues have
a tendency to clutter the discussions, if a middle or common ground can
be found, often both sides can find reason to agree and move on.

SUMMARY

Social roles are critical to life success. Rehabilitation has come to understand this principle and embrace it within the rehabilitation framework. A key function of using social roles as a stepping stone to community inclusion is to better understand the roles we play and how these roles can be enhanced.

This chapter has attempted to explore the general notion of roles in rehabilitation and focuses on the critical role that people play as consumers. Indeed, there are many roles we play in daily life and all of them merit review, but the role of consumer is of particular interest in rehabilitation.

The consumer role is critical for a number of reasons. One reason is that as the cornerstone of the disability rights/independent-living movement, consumer control has become a paramount issue. People with disabilities, the movement contends, know their situation best and given the appropriate resources will make the best decisions as to their needs. This role and responsibility is an integral part of the Rehabilitation Act Amendments and the Americans with Disabilities Act.

Consumer control, however, has been compromised in those situations in which people cannot make the best decisions for themselves. In these cases, others, parents, advocates, or relatives have stepped in to assume this responsibility. In many situations, medical or clinical specialists have assumed a decision-making role concerning the needs of the person. This medical-model influence unfortunately still dominates many human-service agencies today.

CHAPTER 8

Cultural Pluralism: Contexts of Practice

Carl Flowers, Charlotte Griffin-Dixon, and Beatriz Treviño

The profession of rehabilitation counseling has undergone various changes since its inception in the early 1900s. The services it provides and the people it serves has expanded considerably. Amid all the transformations in the profession, however, one concept has remained constant—the philosophy (DiMichael, 1969; B. A. Wright, 1983) and practice (Jenkins, Patterson, & Szymanski, 1992) of diversity. That is, the rehabilitation profession is diverse and practices pluralism as a system. Rehabilitation professionals, consumers of disability services, and the various aspects of service delivery are all intertwined. Although various facets of the rehabilitation process are addressed in greater detail elsewhere in this volume, the issues and considerations associated with providing appropriate rehabilitation services to ethnic and cultural minorities with disabilities are the focus of this chapter.

This chapter is not designed to provide readers with menus of "do's and dont's" to serving persons with disabilities from various ethnic and cultural backgrounds. It does, however, provide the following discussion for rehabilitation practice: (a) ethnic minorities, (b) cultural minorities, (c) minorities with disabilities, (d) rehabilitation counseling professionals, (e) diversity nomenclature, and (f) culturally skilled counselors.

ETHNIC MINORITIES

Demographic projections of the next several decades suggest that minority group members will comprise approximately one-third of the U.S. population (U.S. Bureau of the Census, 1991). Additionally, as the growth rate of minority populations increase, the number of minority individuals with disabilities will also increase (Campbell, 1991). Consequently, the need to address issues relevant to the provision of rehabilitation counseling and services for minorities with disabilities becomes of paramount importance.

Four ethnic groups comprise nearly 33% of the population of the United States (U.S. Bureau of the Census, 1991). Census data also indicates a significant rate of increase among African Americans (13.5%), Asian Americans/Pacific Islanders (107.8%), Native Americans (37.9%), and Hispanic/Latino Americans (53%) between 1980 and 1990. Non-Hispanic whites, on the other hand, had the lowest growth increase (6%) during the same period. As evidence that diversity within the United States is growing, demographers estimate that by the year 2020 the white non-Hispanic population will peak in size then steadily decrease, whereas minority populations will steadily increase (U.S. Bureau of the Census, 1986). Furthermore, by the year 2050 minorities and non-Hispanic whites are expected to be almost evenly divided (*Time,* 1993). Additional demographic information, the history of casteism on each of the four largest minority groups follows.

African Americans

African Americans constitute the largest minority racial group, representing 12.1% of the U.S. population or 29.9 million people (U.S. Bureau of the Census, 1991). It is estimated that the growth rate among African Americans will increase nearly 2% over the next 20 years, compared to the less than 1% anticipated growth among whites. By 2050 it is estimated that the African American population will have doubled and will exceed 60 million.

According to national data, 31% of African Americans live below the poverty level, have lower average family incomes and lower levels of education than their white counterparts, and rank among the lowest, as a racial and ethnic group, in terms of health status (U.S. Bureau of the Census, 1990). Research indicates that nearly 20.8% of all working-age

(15–64) African Americans report having a disability, and 12.7% report having a severe disability (U.S. Bureau of the Census, 1993).

Asian Americans

Asian Americans, as an ethnic group, are the fastest growing minority population in this country, having increased from 3.5 million in 1980 to 7.27 million in 1990 (U.S. Bureau of the Census, 1991). This 107% increase is not only dramatic, but twice the next largest percentage increase among Hispanics/Latinos, during the same period. Japanese, Chinese, and Filipinos constitute the largest groups of Asian Americans in the United States. Although usually grouped together, Asian Americans are made up of persons from several Southeastern countries, including Cambodians, Laotians, Vietnamese, as well as immigrants from China and Japan. Additionally, demographic references to Asian Americans usually include individuals from the Pacific Islands (i.e., Samoa).

Asian Americans are traditionally referred to as the "model minority," due in part to the perception of their higher educational attainment (i.e., 73% of persons over age 25 are high-school graduates), lower participation in juvenile crime (U.S. Bureau of the Census, 1991), and lowest reported incidence of disability (9.6%) and severe disability (4.5%) (U.S. Bureau of the Census, 1993). However, poverty is still prevalent, particularly among subgroups (i.e., Chinese, 13.1%) of this population.

Hispanic/Latino Americans

Hispanics/Latinos are the youngest and second fastest growing ethnic minority group in the country (García, 1991). Based on the 1990 census data, Hispanics/Latinos comprise 9% of the U.S. population or 22.35 million people. The term "Hispanic" is a generic title used by the U.S. government to describe all people of Spanish origin and descent. Hispanic and Latino are often used interchangeably, however, the preference for Latino is growing among this population (Gonzalez, 1991). For purposes of this discussion the preferred term Latino will be used throughout this chapter to describe all people of Spanish origin and descent. Latinos are divided into five subgroups: Mexican origin (64%), Puerto Rican origin (10.5%), Cuban origin (4.9%), Central and South American origin (13.7%), and Other Hispanic (6.9%) (U.S. Bureau of the Census, 1991). The census figure does not include the estimated 5 million persons of Mexican origin who are not legal citizens. Four states with the largest Latino population in the U.S. are California (7.7 million), Texas (4.3 million), New York (2.2 million), and Florida (1.6 million) (U.S. Bureau of the Census, 1993).

Latinos have the highest immigration rate (Gonzalez, 1991) of any ethnic group with varying levels of acculturation (Keefe & Padilla, 1987) and an affinity for the Spanish language (de la Garza, Dean, Bonjean, Romo, & Alvarez, 1985; Sue & Sue, 1990). Latinos have low levels of educational attainment (Perez & Salazar, 1993; U.S. Bureau of the Census, 1991) and high educational needs (Cummins, 1984, 1986; Cummins & Swain, 1986) that lead to limited occupational opportunities (Chapa & Valencia, 1993; Morales & Bonilla, 1991). Over 25% of Latinos, mostly of Puerto Rican and Mexican origin, live below the poverty level. Furthermore, working-age (15–64) Latinos experience a high incidence of health problems that lead to disability (16.9%) and severe disability (9.1%) (U.S. Bureau of the Census, 1993).

American Indians/Native Americans

American Indians, Eskimos, or Aleuts are the smallest ethnic minority group in the U.S. In 1990 American Indians numbered at 1.9 million people, or about 0.8% of the U.S. population (U.S. Bureau of the Census, 1991). American Indians are mostly rural people with over one-half living outside of metropolitan areas. The Bureau of Indian Affairs (BIA) has designated 278 reservations and other trust lands referred to by Native Americans as "Indian Country" (Snipp & Summers, 1992). Over one-third of the American Indians reside in designated lands. The remainder reside in urban areas such as Los Angeles, San Francisco, Seattle, Oklahoma City, Chicago, and Minneapolis.

Before the *War on Poverty*, American Indians had the highest poverty, lowest educational attainment, and most limited employment opportunities (Snipp, 1989) of any minority group. By the 1980s those who had become more educated and had better employment opportunities raised their income levels above poverty. However, American Indians who resided in the reservations still had a considerable amount of poverty. U.S. census (1993) data indicate that American Indians, Eskimos, or Aleuts report the highest rate of disability (26.9%) and a comparable rate of severe disability (11.7%) to African Americans and Latinos with the working-age (15–64) group.

Castification Profile

The castification process of minorities can be best understood through the lens of history, but before the process can be understood the term must be defined. "Castification is fundamentally an institutionalized way of exploiting one social group (ethnic, racial, low-income, or other minority group), thus reducing this group to the status of a lower caste that cannot enjoy the same rights and obligations possessed by the other groups." (Trueba, 1993, p. 30). African Americans, Asian Americans, Latinos, and American Indians share the castification experience (see e.g., Acuña, 1988; Leong, 1995; Takaki, 1989; Trueba, Rodriguez, Zou, & Cintron, 1993). For example, African American ancestry traces back to the times of indentured servitude and slavery. American Indians, on the other hand, were already occupying America, but were pushed off their land and placed in reservations. Latinos trace their roots to the Mexican Revolution (Mexico won its independence from Spain) and the Treaty of Guadalupe Hidalgo that ended the Mexican–American War (Mexico lost half of its territory—Texas, California, New Mexico, Nevada, and parts of Colorado, Arizona, and Utah—to the United States). Asian Americans were allowed to enter the U.S. to work in the mines, on the farms, and then in railroad construction. When cheaper labor was found, race riots broke out and Anglo Americans called for their expulsion from the United States, leading to the Chinese Exclusion Act of 1882.

Given that population groups do not function in a social vacuum, minorities in particular are vulnerable to social, cultural, and political influences (Gonzalez, 1991). Ethnic minorities in the U.S. display several distinct characteristics that put them "at risk" of being excluded from equality and opportunity in the social, political, and economic arena: high rates of immigration and reproduction, low levels of education, high rates of urbanization, unemployment and underemployment, high levels of poverty (Garcìa, 1993), and high incidence of disability (U.S. Bureau of the Census, 1993). Much of the isolation and segregation that dominated then still exists today. A history that cannot be denied or ignored is what shapes our present challenges.

Cultural Minorities

The Civil Rights Movement inspired other minority groups, such as cultural minorities, to articulate their demands for equitable treatment in society (Rittenhouse, Johnson, Overton, Freeman, & Jaussi, 1991).

Cultural groups, such as people with disabilities, specifically the deaf culture, lesbians and gay men, will be discussed, albeit many other such groups exist.

Deaf Culture

A census of the deaf population in the United States indicates that over 13 million people reported having a significant hearing loss and almost 2 million were unable to distinguish speech (Schein & Delk, 1974). The hearing community has accepted deafness to mean the inability to hear. The deaf population has gone beyond the physical or audiological perspective to a cultural definition, however.

> Deaf people are accomplishing something of extreme importance today. They are redefining deafness. They are rejecting the old "clinical pathological model" and replacing it with the "cultural model." They are rejecting the view that deafness is a disability, and insisting instead that deaf people are a community which is culturally distinct. (Glikman, 1984, p. 25)

In defining American Deaf Culture, Padden (1980, 1988) provides a more subjective definition closely linked to ethnic identity.

> A culture is a set of learned behavior of a group of people who have their own language, values, rules for behavior, and traditions. A person may be born into a culture. . . . Or, a person may grow up in one culture and later learn the language, values, and practices of a different culture and become "enculturated" into that culture. (Padden, 1980, p. 92)

Hall (1991) conducted an ethnographic study of a Deaf club and found that everything from etiquette and conversational rules to sharing Deaf history and mentoring younger members were identified functions of the club. In fact, one deaf participant indicated that the club was "like a second home" something that hearing people did not have. Studies on multiple minority statuses (i.e., ethnic identity and deafness) indicate that individuals have a stronger bond with the Deaf cultural group (Page, 1993; Rittenhouse, Johnson, Overton, Freeman, & Jaussi, 1991).

Lesbians and Gay Men

Lesbians and gay men are now often perceived as a quasi-ethnic, or a cultural minority group that is struggling for civil rights (Altman, 1982; Herek, 1991; Murray 1979). Lesbians and gay men remain largely outside the law in all but four states (Wisconsin, Massachusetts, Hawaii, and Connecticut) where discrimination on the basis of sexual orientation is not prohibited in employment, housing, or services (Herek, 1992). Cultural heterosexism dominates in the United States and any nonheterosexual form of behavior, identity, relationship, or community is denigrated (Herek, 1990). Consequently, concealment of homosexuality is rooted in fear of ostracism, taunts, violence, discrimination, harassment, and the loss of occupational opportunity and advancement (Kitzinger, 1991).

Gays and lesbians have been increasingly visible since WWII and the 1969 Stonewall rebellion (Herek & Berrill, 1992). In *coming out* they have challenged long-standing stereotypes and created an unprecedented community infrastructure that has helped them foster significant political and social gains (Bérubé, 1990; D'Emilio, 1983). They also made themselves more vulnerable to hate crimes, however. For example, since the AIDS epidemic began tens of thousands of gay or bisexual men have died, and AIDS has been used to rationalize prejudice, discrimination, and violence against gay men and lesbians (Herek & Berrill, 1992).

Minorities with Disabilities

Minorities with disabilities comprise the majority of the 48.9 million persons counted as having a disability and the 24.1 million as having a severe disability (U.S. Bureau of the Census, December 1993). Furthermore, minorities with disabilities are at risk of becoming increasingly unemployed or underemployed without further education and training. Rehabilitation service delivery systems can begin to help by understanding their health and social services' utilization patterns and identifying cultural considerations for effective practice.

Utilization Patterns

The underutilization of rehabilitation services by minorities with disabilities has been discussed by numerous researchers (Belgrave & Walker, 1991; Pedersen, 1982; Sue & Sue, 1990). By the same token, several studies have examined various potential barriers to utilization of health care and social services (Bruhn & Fuentes, 1977; Burma, 1970; Estrada, Treviño, & Ray, 1990; de la Garza et al., 1985). Barriers exist both on the part of the consumers and the service delivery systems. Barriers associated with consumers include, but are not limited to, language and cultural differences, lack of transportation, geographic inaccessibility, financial constraints, and isolation from the mainstream culture. Barriers associated with systems are as broad as the widespread, but ineffective use of traditional counseling techniques when dealing with minority groups (Pedersen, 1985, 1991; Smith & Vasquez, 1985). In fact, Nwachuku and Ivey (1991) contend that the most prominent counseling theories begin with traditional theoretical assumptions that are culturally biased and therefore cannot be adopted in multicultural and cross-cultural approaches.

Cultural Considerations

"Culture is an enormously powerful determinant of what we think, how we behave and what we believe" (Shephard, 1989, p. 7). Cultural considerations for effective practice include, but are not limited to, language, ethnicity, values, and life-styles. Language is the most fundamental cultural consideration. Although English is the most commonly used language in this country, it has been observed that by the year 2000 Spanish will be as commonly used as English. Institutions that provide services to Spanish-speaking consumers will need to communicate with the consumers' native language or use interpreter services (Leal-Idrogo, 1995; Smart & Smart, 1995). Likewise, African American consumers who use "Black language" may be misunderstood in counseling sessions or during vocational evaluations (Alston & McCowan, 1994; Smith, 1973). American Indians, on the other hand, have over 300 languages and dialects with the most common today being Cherokee, Navaho, and Teton Sioux (La Framboise, 1988). Similar challenges are encountered with Asian Americans.

Ethnicity, values, and life-style may also be affected by cultural traits, such as interaction styles, nonassertive attitudes, self-blaming attitudes, low self-concept, differing concepts of time, interdependence with family members, and a host of other traits. Several researchers have identified specific cultural considerations for minority groups (e.g., Corey, 1991; Hong, 1993; Ong, 1994; Sue & Sue, 1990). The reader is cautioned not to assume, however, that all minorities follow these cultural traits.

Rehabilitation Counseling Professionals

Rehabilitation professionals who take the cavalier approach that "business as usual" is the standard model of services provision is doing an injustice to minorities with disabilities and the profession as a whole. For example, several researchers have indicated that the "business as usual" approach to service delivery has resulted in inconsistencies in the quantity and quality of services offered to minorities with disabilities (Dziekan & Okacha, 1993; Herbert & Chatman, 1988; Herbert & Martinez, 1992; Santiago, 1988; Sheppard, Bunton, Menifee, & Rocha, 1995; Walker, Turner, Haile-Michael, Vincent, & Miles, 1995; Wheaton, 1995; T. J. Wright, 1988, 1993).

Sensitivity to the unique needs, based on cultural differences, of consumers is a requisite for serving consumers from diverse backgrounds and cultures. Cultural awareness and sensitivity among counselors also includes respect for the differing values, classes, language factors, and unique experiences that consumers bring to the counseling relationship. Culturally sensitive counselors working with minorities with disabilities must be cognizant of and prepare to use different approaches, as opposed to assuming that one approach can or should be generalized for use with all consumers.

Another important issue is the need for counselors to be aware of their own biases, and their possible impact on the consumer relationship. For example, when counselors make assumptions that consumer behavior is normal based on their personal experiences, the end result is the expectation of consumer assimilation and, ultimately, counselor stereotyping.

Diversity Nomenclature

Rehabilitation counseling professionals are recognizing the importance of clearly defining and understanding the meanings of terms used with ethnic and cultural minorities. Various terms appear frequently in the rehabilitation literature to describe minorities in service delivery systems. Following is a brief list of the most widely used terms and their definitions. The reader is cautioned to note that there is no consensus among social scientists on any one of the definitions. Segall (1984) indicates that consensus is not absolutely necessary to advance knowledge, however. Therefore, the definitions selected are the most practical ones for the purpose of our work.

Acculturation

Redfield, Linton, and Herskovits (1936) began defining the process of acculturation with the American Indian cultures. They state: "acculturation comprehends those phenomena which result when groups of individuals having different cultures come into continuous first-hand contact with subsequent changes in the original cultural patterns of either or both groups" (p. 149). Their definition remains generally accepted today.

 ## Assimilation

Keefe and Padilla (1987) refer to assimilation as the social, economic, and political integration of an immigrant or ethnic minority into mainstream society. Furthermore, in order for assimilation to occur, the minority group member must have acculturated to some extent and must be accepted by the dominant group. The social aspects of assimilation include primary (i.e., family members, friends) and secondary (i.e., work, school, social agencies) relations. Economic assimilation is the process whereby ethnic minorities are provided equal opportunity in competing for education, income, and occupational status. Political assimilation is the elimination of any bias for ethnic political action.

 ## Culture

Triandis et al. (1980) are quite explicit about the psychologically relevant elements that constitute culture. Triandis et al. refers to both physical and subjective cultures. Physical culture refers to objects such as roads, buildings, and tools, whereas subjective culture includes elements such as social norms, roles, beliefs, and values. Subjective cultures can include a wide range of topics, such as familial roles, communication patterns, affective life-styles, individualism, collectivism, spirituality, and religiosity, which become amendable to measurement.

 ## Ethnicity

Ethnicity is used to characterize groups in terms of nationality, culture, or language. However, individual ethnic identification is different in that the knowledge and practice of cultural traits is not necessary to identify with a certain group. For example, one might be more knowledgeable about one ethnic group, yet at the same time prefer another group (Keefe & Padilla, 1987).

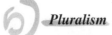

Pluralism

Keefe and Padilla (1987) describe pluralism as the cultural, social, and structural ways in which ethnic groups are maintained as distinct groups within a single political state. More specifically; pluralism as a social condition is that state of affairs in which several distinct ethnic, religious and racial communities live side by side, willing to affirm each other's dignity, ready to benefit from each other's experience, and quick to acknowledge each other's contributions to the common welfare.

> Pluralism is different from the contemporary concept of *diversity* in which individuals from various groups are merely present, just as it differs for the idea of *integration* in which individuals are asked, explicitly or implicitly, to abandon their cultural identity in order to merge into the majority community. (Brown University, 1986, p. ix)

The plural society is one that reaches a state of peaceful coexistence; violence may occur, but is considered destructive to the plural system.

Race

Zuckerman (1990) poses several problems with using race to explain group differences. For example, race generally defines physical characteristics (i.e., skin color, facial features) that are common to a geographically isolated population. Latinos, for instance, are often referred to as a racial minority group, but who can be White, African American, Asian, American Indian, or any combination thereof. For rehabilitation counselors it is more important to understand the relationship between identified biological factors and chronic health problems. That is, African Americans are at higher risk of hypertension than Anglo–Americans (Anderson, 1989), and Latinos have the highest incidence of diabetes (*National Hispanic Reporter,* 1992).

Stereotyping

Terborg (1977) described stereotyping and control as taking on both descriptive and prescriptive beliefs. Descriptive beliefs tell how most people in a group supposedly behave, what they allegedly prefer, and where their competence lies. For example, women are good secretaries, but poor welders, or African Americans are good athletes, but poor scholars.

Prescriptive beliefs are much more controlling, in that they purportedly tell how certain groups *should* think, feel, and behave. For instance, women should be nice, or Asian Americans should be good at math. In short, stereotypes control people and reinforce one group's or individual's power over another.

Cross-cultural Counseling

Das (1995) defines cross-cultural counseling as the practice of counseling American minorities who are seen as culturally different.

Cultural Awareness

Betz and Fitzgerald (1995) describe cultural awareness as an opportunity for counselors to examine the biases and limitations of their culture, learn about other cultures, and be open to continued learning.

Multicultural Counseling

Vontress (1988) had described multicultural counseling as the situation in which the counselor and the client are culturally different because of socialization acquired in distinct cultural, subcultural, racioethnic, or socioeconomic environments.

CULTURALLY SKILLED COUNSELOR

The process associated with counselors becoming culturally skilled may be described as a journey. Sue and Sue (1990) observe that becoming a culturally skilled and sensitive counselor is "an active process, that is ongoing" which "never reaches an end point" (p. 166). This section provides readers with a summary of sensitivity skills needed to effectively serve minorities with disabilities. Attainment of cultural sensitivity involves a minimum of five actions: (1) movement from being culturally unaware to being aware and sensitive of his/her own cultural heritage and to valuing and respecting differences; (2) counselor awareness of his/her own values and biases and how those biases may affect culturally diverse persons with disabilities; (3) developing and increasing the comfort level with differences that exist between themselves and persons being served, in terms of race and beliefs; (4) sensitivity to circumstances (i.e., personal biases and stages of ethnic identity) that may dictate the referral of a culturally diverse individual with a disability to a member of his/her own race/culture; and (5) acknowledgment and awareness of his/her own beliefs, attitudes, and feelings (Sue, 1992).

SUMMARY

Counselors working with minorities with disabilities should, at a minimum, be aware of treatment issues relevant to diverse groups. In the absence of such awareness, counselors are likely to continue perpetuating biased behaviors, using proven ineffective counseling models, and conducting themselves in a business-as-usual fashion. Conversely, rehabilitation counselors who focus on awareness, understanding, and appreciation of differences among minorities and other culturally diverse persons with disabilities take the business-as-unusual approach. As a result, counselors are more likely to experience success in establishing a trusting relationship with consumers. Sensitivity, based on cultural differences, and attention to the unique needs of consumers is a requisite for serving consumers from diverse backgrounds and cultures. Cultural awareness and sensitivity among counselors includes respect for the differing values, classes, language factors, and unique experiences that consumers bring to the counseling session. Culturally sensitive counselors working with minorities with disabilities must be cognizant of the need for and be prepared to use different approaches, as opposed to assuming that one approach can be generalized for all clients.

PART 2

Practice

CHAPTER 9

Public and Private Rehabilitation Counseling Practices

Ralph E. Matkin

A nnual reported figures approximate that rehabilitation counselors help 49 million Americans with disabilities live independent, productive lives (Mariani, 1995). These specialized counselors accomplish this by combining counseling skills with knowledge of mental, physical, and developmental disabilities in relation with information about work adjustment, the current labor market, projected employment trends, job development, and job placement. All of these factors generally are exercised by rehabilitation counselors to assist their clients in selecting, obtaining, and retaining viable jobs. The setting in which rehabilitation counselors practice, however, plays an important role in the nature and scope of the activities they perform, and the knowledge and skills required on the job.

This chapter offers a comparative perspective of activities, knowledge, skills, and other personal traits required by these specialized counselors working in selected sites in public and private sectors.

EXPANDED EMPLOYMENT OPPORTUNITIES

From their occupational origins as vocational rehabilitation workers assisting disabled World War I veterans reassimilate to productive civilian lives, to their rise as a professional group of postgraduate-trained rehabilitation counselors working with all ages and types of clients with disabilities, these specialized counselors were employed principally in publicly funded state–federal rehabilitation agencies (from 1918) and private nonprofit sheltered workshop facilities (from 1954) until the mid-1980s (Bitter, 1979; Obermann, 1965; Rubin & Roessler, 1995). Beginning in the mid-1970s, however, increasing numbers of rehabilitation counselors began seeking career outlets in the private (for profit) business sector (Matkin & Riggar, 1986).

Expansion into private-sector employment can be attributed to several significant factors. First, state workers' compensation statutes began incorporating mandatory provisions as early as 1975 for vocational rehabilitation services to be offered to eligible injured workers. Traditional rehabilitation agencies in the public sector, however, were unable to respond initially in a timely manner to these new service mandates directed at the insurance industry. This service vacuum in California, for example, virtually spawned a private rehabilitation industry overnight. Second, the competitive nature of business and industry facilitated a rapid expansion by private rehabilitation firms and practitioners into other insurance-based disability systems and practices in addition to workers' compensation. Among these were personal injury claims from automobile accidents, railroad disability insurance, longshore and harbor workers' compensation, occupational health and safety, employee assistance programs, and a variety of legal suits involving such issues as wrongful termination of employment and lost wage calculations.

A third contributing factor to the rise in private-sector rehabilitation involved the changing nature of the clients served by public rehabilitation agencies, caseload size, and the extent to which services were provided directly by counselors in the state–federal system. When vocational rehabilitation services became available to civilians in 1920 through the Smith–Fess Act, workers' compensation statutes already existed that offered medical services for federal employees and most privately employed workers in 42 states (Matkin, 1985; G. N. Wright, 1980). Vocational services for these clients were intended to be provided through the growing system of public rehabilitation agencies. The predominant clientele served by the public rehabilitation sector until the mid-1970s, therefore, consisted of working-age people who reasonably could be expected to return to gainful employment. The characteristics and numbers of people served by rehabilitation agencies in the public sector, however, changed dramatically when legislation expanded its definition of eligible conditions to include developmental disabilities.

Beginning with the 1973 Rehabilitation Act, and subsequently mandated by its 1978 amendments, highest priority for services was extended to clients with the most severe disabling conditions to include those acquired early in life or at birth. Although the benefits of rehabilitation services now could be provided to virtually all citizens with disabilities, rehabilitation counselors in public agencies were confronted with increasing client caseloads to manage and an increasing average duration per case because the most severe disabling conditions required more services and longer periods of care. These events led to greater numbers of client referrals to external providers for longer term treatment and specialized rehabilitation services.

Compounding these events was the fact that funding allocations to public rehabilitation agencies were not keeping pace with the increasing costs required to serve clients with the most severe disabilities. Furthermore, the historic "return on investment" revenues generated through taxes paid by competitively employed, vocationally rehabilitated clients were declining significantly because jobs were not as readily attainable for many clients with severe disabilities compared to those who had incurred a disability after reaching working age.

STATE–FEDERAL REHABILITATION AGENCIES

Job Duties

Rehabilitation counselors have been employed in a state–federal agency system that was created by Congress in 1917. The Smith–Hughes Act established a public program in vocational education that provided a basis for a system of vocational rehabilitation. The following year, disabled veterans were included through the passage of the Smith–Sears Veterans Rehabilitation Act of 1918 (Bitter, 1979). Although the nature of eligible disabling conditions and the scope of rehabilitative services have been expanded and redefined by public laws since that time, the occupational functions of rehabilitation counselors in the public sector generally have remained the same. The *Dictionary of Occupational Titles* (DOT) (U.S. Department of Labor, 1991, p. 52), for example, identifies seven broad categories of tasks:

1. Interviews and evaluates handicapped applicants, and confers with medical and professional personnel to determine type and degree of handicap, eligibility for service, and feasibility of vocational rehabilitation.
2. Accepts or recommends acceptance of suitable candidates.
3. Determines suitable job or business consistent with applicant's desires, aptitudes, and physical, mental, and emotional limitations.
4. Plans and arranges for applicant to study or train for job.
5. Assists applicant with personal adjustment throughout rehabilitation program.
6. Aids applicant in obtaining medical and social services during training.
7. Promotes and develops job openings and places qualified applicant in employment.

In addition to the specialized counselor occupation described above, the *DOT* identifies a "vocational rehabilitation consultant," which includes tasks that also may be performed by state–federal rehabilitation agency counselors who have been promoted to supervisor or administrator levels (U.S. Department of Labor, 1991, p. 75). These activities include:

1. Develops and coordinates implementation of vocational rehabilitation programs.
2. Consults with members of local communities and personnel of rehabilitation facilities, such as sheltered workshops and skills training centers, to identify need for new programs or modification of existing programs.
3. Collects and analyzes data to define problems and develops proposals for programs to provide needed services, utilizing knowledge of vocational rehabilitation theory and practice, program funding sources, and government regulations.
4. Provides staff training, negotiates contracts for equipment and supplies, and performs related functions to implement program changes.
5. Monitors program operations and recommends additional measures to ensure programs meet defined needs.

These occupational descriptions suggest that the role of rehabilitation counselors in the state–federal agency system is multifaceted. The current position stresses that their job requires expertise in counseling, coordinating, and consulting functions (Hershenson, 1990). In their counseling function, rehabilitation counselors assist clients to examine/reexamine and reconstitute their self-concepts, personal goals, and vocational goals. Coordinating skills are needed to select and monitor an array of physical, social, and vocational services that clients require to achieve their rehabilitation goals. Consulting functions are needed by rehabilitation counselors when working with the client's family, service providers, and employers (Rubin & Roessler, 1995).

Personal Characteristics

Rehabilitation counselors must possess an above-average ability to learn and understand theoretical and technical materials, and to communicate orally and in writing to perform their job duties (EUREKA, 1996). The *DOT* classifies the required skills of this occupation among the highest with respect to working with data and people. Data is defined as, "information, knowledge, and conceptions, related to data, people, or things, obtained by observation, investigation, interpretation, visualization, and mental creation. Data are intangible and include numbers, words, symbols, ideas, concepts, and oral verbalizations" (U.S. Department of Labor, 1991, p. 1005). Rehabilitation counselors are expected to be able to coordinate, analyze, compile, compute, copy, and compare data in their job activities [Occupational Access System (OASYS)-Job Match, 1996].

The people skills of rehabilitation counselors include "dealing with individuals in terms of their total personality in order to advise, counsel, or guide them with regard to problems that may be resolved by legal, scientific, clinical, spiritual, or other professional principles" (U.S. Department of Labor, 1991, p. 1006). These activities require abilities to mentor, negotiate, instruct, supervise, divert, persuade, speak, serve, and take or provide instructions (OASYS–Job Match, 1996). The work situations rehabilitation counselors encounter in the state–federal agency system demand personal temperaments that are attuned to directing, controlling, or planning activities of others, moving from one task to another using different skills, seeing details accurately, making decisions that affect others using data and facts, taking responsibility for one's decisions, and reaching conclusions based on a combination of objective and subjective criteria (EUREKA, 1996; OASYS–Job Match, 1996; U.S. Department of Labor, 1991).

DEPARTMENT OF VETERAN AFFAIRS

Job Duties

Federal employment of rehabilitation counselors is governed by the qualification standards and policies of the U.S. Office of Personnel Management (OPM) (1990), which is part of the Executive Branch of government. OPM is responsible for developing and issuing minimum standards to determine applicants' qualifications for General Schedule (GS) positions at pay grades GS-1 through GS-15. The standards and requirements found in OPM's Handbook must be met by all appointees to positions in competitive service and placement. Furthermore, federal executive branch agencies are responsible for applying the appropriate standards in individual personnel actions and developing selective factors, when needed, to supplement the Handbook (OPM, 1990).

In 1992, 588 personnel classified by OPM as vocational rehabilitation specialists (GS-1715) were employed in four federal agencies: Department of Health and Human Services, Department of Interior, Department of Labor, and the Department of Veterans Affairs (VA) [Federal Occupational Career Information System (FOCIS), 1992]. Of that total, 400 were employed in 81 VA medical centers and regional offices (FOCIS, 1992) throughout the country.

The OPM Handbook (1990) identifies three broad categories of specialized experiences required by vocational rehabilitation specialists:

1. Work that required obtaining and applying occupational information for the handicapped, knowledge of the interrelationships of the involved professional and specialist services, and skill in employing the methodology and techniques of counseling to motivate and encourage individuals served by the program.
2. Experience which demonstrated knowledge of the vocational rehabilitation problems characteristic of the disabled, including familiarity with available resources and skill in identifying, evaluating, and making effective use of such resources to serve disabled individuals; or of the disadvantaged, including knowledge of adjustment problems of the educationally or culturally disadvantaged, familiarity with available adult education and training resources, and ability to recognize problem areas needing special attention.

3. Experience in vocational guidance or teaching in a recognized vocational rehabilitation program or school; developmental or supervisory work in programs of vocational rehabilitation or training programs for the disadvantaged; or personnel or employment placement work that provided extensive knowledge of the training and adjustment requirements necessary to place persons having disabilities or social adjustment problems. (June 1991, p. 36)

Using these work-experience requirements, these specialists deal with the vocational rehabilitation problems of people with physical or emotional disabilities, or other individuals served by the VA whose backgrounds and lack of job skills impair their employability. The work generally performed by vocational rehabilitation specialists involves counseling, planning training programs, job placement into gainful employment, and supervising clients while they are in training and during their adjustment to employment (FOCIS, 1992).

Personal Characteristics

The entry-level pay grade of a federally employed vocational rehabilitation specialist is GS-5, which requires four academic years above high school leading to a bachelor's degree or a bachelor's degree (OPM, 1990). Full professional counseling knowledge, however, is not required despite the nature of the work described above (FOCIS, 1992). On the other hand, this position generally is filled by those with a master's degree (GS-9) or higher (GS-11). The work situations that vocational rehabilitation specialists encounter, especially in VA medical centers, demand personal temperaments that are attuned to working as part of a medical team, planning activities of others, moving from one task to another using different skills, making decisions that affect others using data and facts, and reaching conclusions based on a combination of objective and subjective criteria.

PRIVATE SECTOR REHABILITATION

The phrase "private rehabilitation sector" generally has been associated or frequently used as synonymous with a "for-profit" work setting. For the purpose of this chapter, however, the private sector includes rehabilitation counselors working as employees of rehabilitation firms, as private practitioners, and as employees of private nonprofit rehabilitation workshops and facilities. Each of these settings relies on revenue generated through services contracted with third-party funding sources or individuals seeking services for themselves. The respective profit or nonprofit business status of these settings affects the distribution and use of their net profits.

JOB DUTIES

Employees of rehabilitation firms

Over 38% of practicing Certified Rehabilitation Counselors (CRC) are employed by private for-profit rehabilitation firms (Matkin, Bauer, & Nickles, 1993). The occupational duties of these counselors have been studied extensively since 1981. The majority of the investigations were conducted to identify and establish a content-valid examination for national certification of insurance rehabilitation specialists which has been renamed subsequently as the certification of disability management specialists. The duties performed by the vast majority of rehabilitation counselors in the private sector focus on five categories: (1) case management and human disabilities, (2) job development and vocational assessment, (3) rehabilitation services and care, (4) disability legislation, and (5) forensic rehabilitation (Matkin, 1995).

Case management and human disability activities comprise approximately 20% of the work time in the private rehabilitation sector. This area requires knowledge of the nature of disabling conditions, coping mechanisms, and personality and motivation dynamics found among clients. Job development and vocational assessment activities compose nearly 30% of the job; counselors need to be knowledgeable about methods used to assess vocational capability, they must analyze labor markets, conduct job analyses, and place clients in training and employment. Rehabilitation services and care activities account for approximately 20% of a counselor's work. These activities require knowledge of methods for determining the range of available client services in a community (including medical, psychiatric, or psychological services), the availability of transportation, counselors must also analyze the need for posthospital care and determine a client's need for assistive devices.

Knowledge of disability legislation comprises approximately 15% of a counselor's duties. An essential ingredient of successful practice in the private sector is keeping abreast of laws and regulations that affect service delivery and making timely adjustments when necessary. Rehabilitation counselors are required to possess a working knowledge of key disability legislation, such as workers' compensation, Americans with Disability Act, legal residency requirements of their clients, and the interrelationships between labor unions and employment practices. Finally, nearly 15% of a rehabilitation counselor's time in the private sector is consumed by forensic application. This area requires a working knowledge of the manner in which courtrooms, hearings, and depositions are conducted; the role of expert witnesses; methods of legal inquiry/questioning; the difference between fact and opinion; the purpose and use of hypothetical questions in testimony; and methods used to establish or undermine a witness' credibility (Matkin, 1995).

Private Practitioners

Over 7% of all practicing CRCs reported themselves as working primarily in private practice (Matkin et al., 1993). What remains unclear from this information, however, is whether these counselors are sole proprietors with fewer than six employees or owners or co-owners of private companies or corporations with more than five employees. Presuming they are sole proprietors, it may be reasonable to assume that these rehabilitation counselors perform a combination of administrative and direct-service duties. Generally speaking, the direct services of private practitioners are those performed by their privately employed counterparts mentioned. On the other hand, administrative management tasks must be performed routinely to maintain the business practice.

The duties of any small business owner include planning, organizing, directing, diverting, monitoring, evaluating, and managing activities of the operation. In order to maintain the viability of their practice, these rehabilitation counselors must be able to administer fiscal operations to include preparation of payroll and tax forms, negotiate business contracts, market their services, establish and coordinate services, plan public relation strategies, represent the practice at community or business meetings, purchase needed equipment and supplies, and hire and fire employees (OASYS–Job Match, 1996).

Employees of Nonprofit Rehabilitation Workshops and Facilities.

Nearly 15% of practicing CRCs are employed in nonprofit rehabilitation facilities composed of privately operated (over 11%) and state–federally operated (slightly more than 3%) sheltered workshops and facilities (Matkin et al., 1993). Work activities of rehabilitation counselors employed by the privately managed facilities typically emphasize performing vocational evaluation, work-adjustment training, job modification, job development and employer negotiation to provide opportunities to people with disabling conditions, job placement, job coaching, independent-living-skills training, and case management (Rubin et al., 1984; Rubin & Roessler, 1995).

Personal Characteristics

Working in private practice or as an employee of a for-profit rehabilitation firm represents perhaps the most demanding situations of all settings in the field. Not only are the knowledge and skills associated with the previously mentioned work sites required, but rehabilitation counselors must also adjust to a higher degree of legal scrutiny, when the preponderance of services they offer are performed (e.g., workers' compensation, personal injury, wrongful employment termination). Additionally, private-sector rehabilitation counselors, particularly those in private practice, are confronted frequently and routinely with cost issues such as level of business income versus expenses (generating sufficient billable hours), acquiring and maintaining the highest practitioner credentials available in the field, and remaining abreast of current standards and practices recommended in their fields of expertise. On the other hand, rehabilitation counselors in private nonprofit facilities may be requested to develop and implement activities to market services to nontraditional funding sources for direct referrals (e.g., insurance companies, private rehabilitation firms, private practitioners, private industry councils, schools). All of these activities demand personal temperaments that involve high degrees of perseverance, creativity, tolerance for stress, planning activities of others, moving from one task to another using different skills, making decisions that affect others, and reaching conclusions based on data and facts.

PERSONALITY FACTORS

The preponderance of occupational research on rehabilitation counselors has concentrated on identifying their work roles and functions, skills and competencies, and training needs in various employment settings. The handful of studies that focus on personality characteristics of rehabilitation counselors have investigated a limited range of variables, such as empathy, genuineness, job satisfaction, respect, warmth, "case manager" versus "therapist" personality comparisons, and working styles. Although Kunce and Cope (1987) noted that rehabilitation counselors with different personality patterns may be equally successful in their occupation choice, these authors cautioned that problems may arise when specific job responsibilities are not compatible with unique sets of personality characteristics.

According to John Holland (1973), "people search for environments that will let them exercise their skills and abilities to express their attitudes and values" (p. 4). This seems to imply that for every vocation, only particular personality types or trait groups are available to interact congruently with specific work situations (Agada, 1984). These relationships are depicted clearly in Holland's (1985a, 1985b) hexagonal presentation of **R**ealistic, **I**nvestigative, **A**rtistic, **S**ocial, **E**nterprising, and **C**onventional types. The following results were obtained from a national random sample of 20% of all practicing CRCs (Matkin & Bauer, 1993; Matkin et al., 1993).

Counselors working in state–federal rehabilitation agencies appear to have high social interests, responsible for and in control of their actions, have an expectation of status or prestige from their occupation, and have artistic (creative) tendencies. Vocational rehabilitation specialists employed in VA medical centers or general hospitals can be described as having a need for self-control, being responsible for and interested in helping others, having a preference for therapeutic and teaching roles, and having an expectation of occupational status and prestige derived from the medical surrounding in which they work. CRCs who are in private practice have high expectations of personal and professional achievement, occupational status, and creative expression. They tend to be self-confident and self-reliant with multiple interests. Furthermore, they enjoy using their analytic abilities, seeking opportunities for personal development, and acting independently and autonomously. CRCs employed by private for-profit rehabilitation firms tend to view themselves as responsible for and in control of their actions, with an inclination for using scientific, research, and evaluative abilities. Finally, counselors employed in private nonprofit rehabilitation facilities tend to rely on scientific, research, or mathematical abilities. They tend to value highly opportunities that lead to personal development, personal achievement, and that use their abilities to the fullest.

CHAPTER 10

Professional Practice: Assessment

Norman L. Berven

A ssessment is basic to virtually all functions performed in rehabilitation counseling practice. The scope of assessment is broad, extending well beyond the description of individuals, their functioning, and needs, to include: (a) the identification of problems experienced by individuals seeking assistance and the analysis, definition, and redefinition of those problems in a manner in which they can be more readily resolved; (b) the development of vocational and other life goals and objectives, and the identification of barriers that must be overcome in order to achieve them; and (c) the identification of strategies to resolve problems and to achieve the goals and objectives established, and the organization of those strategies into comprehensive service plans (see Vocational Evaluation and Work Adjustment, 1975). Assessment occurs at many different levels in rehabilitation counseling practice. At a more global level, assessment forms the basis for the overall service plans guiding the rehabilitation counseling process with a particular individual; at a more specific level, assessment forms the basis for the identification of appropriate strategies to follow in response to an unexpected crisis; and, at an even more specific level, assessment at a particular moment in time forms the basis for determining an appropriate verbal response or action to take at that moment that will be consistent with the individual's needs and will produce the intended response or outcome.

Many diverse methods are used in assessment, extending well beyond the psychological, educational, and vocational tests that are typically associated with assessment. Also included are interviews, direct observations, job tryouts, and medical examinations, among a variety of other methods. In addition, not only is assessment directed at understanding individuals and their characteristics but also at the situational contexts that surround individuals and substantially influence their functioning and potential.

The purpose of this chapter is to discuss the assessment process and contemporary assessment practices in rehabilitation counseling, including assessment methods used, the synthesis and interpretation of assessment information, and the types of decisions and determinations for which assessment is commonly used. In addition, current trends and future developments in assessment are briefly discussed.

ASSESSMENT PRACTICES

In the rehabilitation process the roles of consumers or individuals served in relation to rehabilitation counselors or other service providers can be conceptualized along a continuum of control over decision making. At one extreme, the more traditional service-delivery model, the rehabilitation counselor maintains control of the process and serves as the primary decision maker in service delivery. Midway along the continuum the rehabilitation counselor and consumer function as a team, assuming joint control and collaborating in the decisions to be made. At the other extreme the consumer assumes control as the primary decision maker, and the rehabilitation counselor serves as a consultant, providing information and opinions to the consumer to facilitate his or her independent decision making. A move along the continuum toward greater consumer control of the rehabilitation process has been advocated by many as moving away from a medical model of service delivery toward an approach that is less paternalistic toward people with disabilities and more empowering (e.g., Holmes, 1993; Nosek, 1992).

Assessment is often associated with control of the decision-making and service–delivery processes by the rehabilitation counselor rather than the consumer. Whether service delivery and treatment decisions are to be made by the professional, the consumer, or by the two in collaboration, assessment provides the information base for those decisions, and the rehabilitation counselor has special expertise to bring to the process in developing that information base. To the extent that consumers assume greater control over decision making, consumers needs to be involved as active participants in the assessment process, and the information that is accumulated needs to be communicated to consumers in a form that can be effectively used by them to facilitate their own decision making.

Assessment begins at the time in the rehabilitation process when the first information is received by a rehabilitation counselor about an individual to be served, perhaps through a phone call from the individual or a written or verbal referral from another professional, sometimes accompanied by previous treatment or service records. From the time that this initial information is obtained, the rehabilitation counselor begins to form impressions about the individual and his or her needs, as well as goals that might be appropriate and services or intervention strategies that might be indicated. As additional information is accumulated, it is interpreted and synthesized with the information previously obtained to develop an increasingly sophisticated and complex understanding of the individual and his or her needs, which can be used to predict how the individual might behave in different situations or respond to different intervention strategies. These predictions, in turn, facilitate the decisions to be made in treatment and service delivery.

BASIC CONCEPTS

Cronbach (1990) has distinguished between indicators of "maximum" performance and indicators of "typical" performance, and this distinction can be useful in understanding the purposes of various assessment methods in rehabilitation counseling (Berven, 1980; Maki, McCracken, Pape, & Scofield, 1979). Indicators of maximum performance are used to predict the behavior of an individual when performing at his or her best, for example, in training or employment, and may be further categorized into indicators of ability or aptitude and indicators of current skills or achievement. Indicators of ability or aptitude assist in the determination of potential to develop skills if given appropriate opportunities through training or other experiences, whereas indicators of current skills or achievement can assist in determining current mastery of skills. For example, a measure of mathematical aptitude might be used to determine one's potential to learn math skills, whereas a measure of mathematical achievement might be used to determine whether an individual already possesses the math skills required for a particular type of employment or training (e.g., carpentry) or whether some further training in math might be required. Indicators of typical performance are used to determine how an individual might typically behave in various situations and may be further divided into indicators of interests, facilitating predictions about likely satisfaction in different work and life situations, and indicators of personality characteristics.

With all assessment methods it is important to consider reliability and validity of the scores or other information provided. Reliability refers to "the degree to which scores are free from errors of measurement" (American Educational Research Association, American Psychological Association, & National Council on Measurement in Education, 1985, p. 19) or, alternatively, "the consistency of scores obtained by the same persons when reexamined on different occasions . . . or under other variable conditions" (Anastasi, 1988, p. 109). Validity refers to "*what* the test measures and *how* well it does so. It tells us what can be inferred from test scores" (Cronbach, 1990, p. 139). As an example, the reliability and validity of a bathroom scale might be assessed by having an individual step onto and off the scale, each time recording the weight registered; reliability of the scale as an assessment device would be reflected by the extent to which the scale is consistent in registering the same weight on each occasion, and validity would be reflected in the extent to which the weight registered provided an accurate indication of the individual's true weight. The reliability and validity of any assessment procedure are largely responsible for determining its value as an assessment method.

Standardization is another concept that is important in understanding the variety of "standardized" or "norm-referenced" assessment devices that are commonly used in rehabilitation counseling practice. A standardized assessment procedure is a test or other assessment device that has been administered to one or more large groups of individuals, identified as the standardization or normative sample, according to carefully specified procedures. When the device is then used in assessment, it is administered according to the same standardized procedures, and the individual's performance can then be compared to the standardization or normative samples in interpreting the scores. However, the comparison of performance to standardization or normative samples can be made *only if* the standardized procedures have been strictly followed, and the presence of limitations associated with disability may render standardized administration procedures impossible, and the accommodations required will serve to complicate the interpretation of scores and other performance measures (e.g., see Berven, 1980; Nester, 1993; Sherman & Robinson, 1982; Willingham et al., 1988). In addition, the presence of functional limitations can influence the meaning or inferences to be drawn from test scores in other important ways (e.g., see Berven, 1980).

ASSESSMENT METHODS

A wide variety of assessment information is typically used in the rehabilitation process. The information obtained includes scores and other quantitative data from standardized tests and related instruments, as well as qualitative data obtained through such methods as interviews or direct observations. Sources of assessment information include the individual him or herself, other people who have known or have worked with the individual, and physicians and other professionals who may be called on to conduct examinations or evaluations of current functioning or potential. Although assessment is heavily concentrated in the initial stages of the rehabilitation process, it continues throughout the entire process. Some of the methods utilized are the same as those used in other counseling and human service specialties and settings, whereas others have been specifically developed to meet the needs of people with disabilities in rehabilitation settings.

Interviews

As in other counseling and rehabilitation specialties and in other human-service professions, the interview is probably the most widely used assessment method. It is often the first point of contact between a rehabilitation counselor and an individual seeking assistance and serves to initiate assessment. The interview provides a rich source of self-reported information, as well as an opportunity to observe the individual. Observations may include interpersonal skills, thought processes, affect, deficits in memory, and follow-through on plans and commitments after the conclusion of an interview. Unlike standardized tests, the interview is not restricted to prespecified questions and directions of inquiry, with the counselor able to move the information-gathering process in whatever directions seem to be most productive as the interview unfolds.

There are many potential sources of error in information obtained through interviews (see Kaplan & Saccuzzo, 1993). These sources of error include subjectivity on the part of the counselor in interpreting statements and observations during the interview; intentional or unintentional distortions in information reported by the individual; the manner in which questions are asked by the counselor that can influence the responses obtained (e.g., leading, closed-ended questions that can substantially influence the answers given); and the relationship established between the counselor and the individual that can influence openness in responding. In addition, observations made during interviews may be situation specific and may not generalize to other situations in which predictions regarding the behavior of the individual need to be made. Although reliability and validity issues are often not considered in the use of interviews and have not been extensively addressed through research, it would seem likely that information obtained through interviews may be highly inconsistent, and the information and observations obtained may not be particularly useful in making good inferences and predictions about future behavior in other types of situations.

The usefulness of the interview as an assessment method can be enhanced through awareness of the potential sources of error in information obtained through interviews and by continuing vigilance in attempting to counter those sources of error. Evidence exists that the reliability and validity of information obtained from interviews can be enhanced through the use of more highly standardized interview procedures (e.g., see Baker & Spier, 1990, who discuss the merits of standardization of employment selection interviews). Such standardization, if carried too far, however, can reduce some of the advantages of interviews, particularly their flexibility and individualization. Some standardized interview protocols have been developed specifically for use in rehabilitation settings, including the Preliminary Diagnostic Questionnaire (Moriarty, Walls, & McLaughlin, 1987), the Vocational Decision-Making Interview (Czerlinsky, Jensen, & Pell, 1987), and the Employability Maturity Interview (Morelock, Roessler, & Bolton, 1987). In addition, attempts have been made to comprehensively identify important questions and lines of inquiry for initial interviews in rehabilitation settings (e.g., Esser, 1980; Roessler & Rubin, 1992; Rubin & Roessler, 1995).

Standardized Tests and Inventories

Standardized psychological and vocational tests and inventories include a wide variety of paper-and-pencil, apparatus, and computer-administered devices. With the exception of interviews, standardized tests and inventories are probably the next most widely used of all assessment methods. Tests of maximum performance include achievement tests and batteries, particularly those focusing on academic skills such as reading and mathematics, and aptitude tests and batteries, focusing on intelligence and other cognitive and neuropsychological abilities and a wide variety of vocational aptitudes, including clerical and mechanical aptitudes and dexterity. Tests of typical performance include vocational inventories, that focus on vocational interests, attitudes, and values, which may be used to predict likely satisfaction in different occupations and vocational situations and, consequently, the likelihood of persisting in those occupations, as well as personality inventories and related measures, designed to measure a wide variety of emotions, motives, values, beliefs, attitudes, and related characteristics in order to contribute to understandings of individuals that will help predict how they will likely behave in different situations.

Literally thousands of tests and inventories have been developed, many available through a number of different commercial publishers and distributors, and textbooks on testing and assessment typically focus primarily on these types of instruments. Reviews of available tests and inventories are provided through a number of sources; best known is the *Mental Measurements Yearbook* (Kramer & Conoley, 1992), which reviews the most widely used instruments and is also available in electronic form on CD–ROM (Kramer & Conoley, 1993). Of all assessment methods, reliability and validity tend to be most extensively documented for standardized tests and inventories; however, the reliability and validity of even the best tests and inventories tend to be more limited than commonly believed, and a great deal of caution is necessary in interpretation of scores and other performance measures (see Berven, 1980).

Simulations of Work and Living Tasks

Simulations of tasks actually performed in specific occupations or clusters of occupations are known as work samples, which have been widely used in rehabilitation counseling practice. In a similar manner, physical functioning and independent-living tasks may also be simulated as a method of assessing physical capacities and self-care and independent-living skills. Traditionally, the term work sample has been used to refer to a simulation of the tasks in a particular occupation, thus having a direct, one-to-one correspondence with that occupation. For example, a work sample could be developed to simulate an entry-level occupation that individuals who enter a particular training program may often pursue, and performance on the work sample may then indicate potential to pursue the training and, ultimately, the occupation. Alternatively, work samples are often conceptualized and used as performance aptitude tests, assessing a cluster of aptitudes important for performance in many different occupations, and inferences may be drawn from scores and other performance indicators regarding potential for all occupations requiring that cluster of aptitudes.

Work samples, like tests, are typically standardized and are administered to individuals served under those same standardized conditions, with scores then being compared to norm groups or to industrial standards established through engineering studies. In addition to assessment of potential, the completion of a variety of work samples can provide individuals with opportunities for career exploration, trying out a variety of occupational tasks in a short period of time in order to explore potential interests in a less abstract manner than provided through traditional interest inventories. A number of commercially available work sample and related vocational assessment systems are commonly used, and Brown, McDaniel, Couch, and McClanahan (1994) have provided reviews of a number of the available systems. According to Brown et al., evidence regarding reliability and validity of many of the available systems is limited and sometimes totally nonexistent, and considerable caution is thus warranted in drawing inferences from scores and performance observed.

Simulated and Real Environments

In contrast to work samples, which involve the simulation of tasks in a particular occupation, entire work environments may also be simulated. Similarly, a kitchen or entire apartment may be simulated in a hospital rehabilitation unit to assess independent-living skills, potential, and behaviors. Historically, work environments have been simulated in sheltered employment settings in order to assess work behaviors and potential for employment and to identify behaviors to target for intervention in order to facilitate employability. Although such applications of situational assessment are still practiced, contemporary thought has questioned the validity of such assessments because of the contrived nature of the simulated environments, varying in many important ways from real work environments, and these differences can dramatically influence the behaviors observed.

Observations of individuals functioning in real work or living environments, such as job tryouts, can be viewed as the most definitive of all assessment approaches in determining potential, skills, and behavior related to functioning in that specific environment or other similar environments. For example, individuals may be placed in the same environment in which they previously worked prior to the onset of a disability, or in a new occupation and work environment being considered for the future; accommodations can be implemented, training can be provided in vivo, and observations can be made to assess both maximum performance (i.e., aptitudes, skills, and behaviors in relation to the demands of that work environment) and typical performance (e.g., attitudes and interests in pursuing that particular type of occupation in that particular type of environment). Similarly, an individual recovering in an inpatient rehabilitation unit from the recent onset of a physical disability can be observed during short stays in the home environment to assess independent living skills and to determine needs for further training in activities of daily living, aids and appliances that might improve independent-living skills, and the accommodations that might be required in the home environment.

Behavioral observations of individuals in simulated and real environments, as well as in other assessment situations (e.g., work samples and interviews), can be facilitated through the use of systematic behavioral assessment methods and a variety of rating scales (see Galassi & Perot, 1992; Silva, 1993). Many rating scales commonly used in rehabilitation settings are homemade scales that are loosely constructed with little or no reliability or validity data available. Several scales are available through commercial publishers, however, and reviews of available rating scales have been provided (e.g., Esser, 1975; Harrison, Garnett, & Watson, 1981; Power, 1991).

Functional Assessment

Functional assessment may be defined as any systematic approach to describing an individual's functioning in terms of skill (what an individual "can do"), current behavior (what an individual "does do"), or both (Brown, Gordon, & Diller, 1983). Functional assessment is typically conducted with the aid of scales, with the items representing comprehensive lists of areas of functioning, so that each can be comprehensively rated, evaluated, or described. Some scales produce summary scores and score profiles, whereas others rely on checklists and narrative descriptions of an individual's functioning in each area included in the scale. In most cases, multiple sources of information are integrated in the completion of functional assessment measures (e.g., interviews, client self-report, direct observation, and examinations, evaluations, and reports completed by other professionals); in fact, any of the assessment methods described above may contribute information relevant to functional assessment. A number of functional assessment measures are available for use in rehabilitation settings, and reviews and discussions of instruments have been provided (Crewe & Dijkers, 1995; Halpern & Fuhrer, 1984; Tenth Institute on Rehabilitation Issues, 1983). Functional assessment measures have been widely used in rehabilitation counseling practice, and their use will likely continue to grow.

INTERPRETATION AND SYNTHESIS OF ASSESSMENT INFORMATION

As information is gathered about an individual, the meaning of the various pieces of information must be determined, any inconsistencies with other available information must be resolved, and all of the information gathered must be organized and synthesized into an overall picture of the individual. This process of making sense of diverse bits of information in order to understand individuals and their needs is much like the process of research, which involves the discovery of the order underlying the phenomena under study (Sundberg & Tyler, 1962).

Interpretation of Assessment Information

Several authors have described the process of interpreting assessment information in which they identify different levels of interpretation, each characterized by different degrees of inference (Sundberg, 1977; Sundberg & Tyler, 1962). At the lowest level of inference, bits of assessment information can be viewed as samples of behavior in their own right, with full consideration given to the situational context in which the behaviors occurred. At the next higher level of inference, bits of information are interrelated in search of consistencies and generalizations. At the next higher level of inference, a hypothetical construct (e.g., depression, motivation, self-esteem) may be used to describe the essence of the consistencies or generalizations identified. When making such interpretations, it is important to remember that inferences are often far removed from the observations on which they are based and, consequently, interpretations must be made with caution, remaining tentative and open to change as new information emerges.

Organization of Information According to Assets, Limitations, and Preferences

In order to make sense of the myriad of information typically available in working with individuals in rehabilitation settings, it is important to organize the information in a way that will facilitate the assessment process. The information accumulated includes not only information about the individual, but also information about the environmental context surrounding the individual, including barriers to the improvement of quality of life and resources available. Relevant information may include such diverse elements as personal characteristics described in terms of hypothetical constructs (e.g., flat affect, positive self-esteem, perseverance in the face of obstacles to progress); credentials held by an individuals (e.g., a driver's license or a high school diploma); and resources available (e.g., social support, financial resources, stable living arrangements). All such information may have a great deal of relevance to the rehabilitation process in assisting individuals in finding their place in society and improving the quality of their lives.

One approach to making sense of the myriad of information typically available is to organize the information in a continuing process, as it is accumulated, according to assets, limitations, and preferences. Assets include the strengths of the individual and his or her surrounding situation that may facilitate the accomplishment of rehabilitation goals and thus may be relevant to rehabilitation planning, whereas limitations represent those characteristics that may serve as barriers. Preferences represent the individual's likes and dislikes, interests, and needs, which are significant in developing rehabilitation plans that will result in outcomes that will be satisfying to the individual. As assessment information is accumulated, interpreted, and organized, increasingly sophisticated statements can be formulated regarding assets, limitations, and preferences, which can facilitate rehabilitation planning.

Synthesis of Information into a Comprehensive Working Model of the Individual

A number of authors have described the process by which counselors and other professionals process information and conceptualize individuals with whom they work and their problems and needs (e.g., Goldman, 1971; McArthur, 1954; Pepinsky & Pepinsky, 1954; Strohmer, Shivy, & Chiodo, 1990). In general, effective clinicians systematically construct a "working model" or conceptualization of an individual and then use that working model as a basis for clinical or service decisions. The process of building the working model begins with *inductive* reasoning in which inferences are drawn about individual bits of information and apparent consistencies between them. To the extent that inconsistencies appear, inferences are revised in an attempt to resolve the inconsistencies, increasingly seeking broader inferences to incorporate more and more of the information available and continually building an increasingly sophisticated working model of the person. *Deductive* reasoning is then used to formulate and test hypotheses regarding the usefulness of the working model in accounting for already available information and for making future predictions. To the extent that hypotheses tested do not account for the information or do not result in accurate predictions, the model of the person is revised so as to account for the new information. In this manner a comprehensive working model or conceptualization of the individual is derived that can then be used to make predictions about the behavior and outcomes likely to be achieved by the individual in a wide variety of situations.

Potential Sources of Bias in Interpretation and Synthesis of Information

Tversky and Kahneman (1974) described three judgmental heuristics or cognitive processing strategies that are used in processing information and making judgments that lead to biased inferences, and Nezu and Nezu (1993), among others, have applied these heuristics to understanding sources of bias in clinical inferences. The *availability heuristic* is invoked when a previous experience that is readily called to mind exerts an undue influence on the inferences of a counselor; for example, a counselor may have recently attended a training program on alcohol and other drug abuse that may lead to a quick judgment or inference that an individual is abusing alcohol or other drugs, and the counselor may fail to consider other possible explanations for the behaviors observed. The *representativeness heuristic* is invoked when individuals who share one characteristic are also believed to more likely share another characteristic; for example, stereotypes about women, African Americans, or people with a particular type of disability may lead to inferences from behaviors observed that an individual is "depressed" or "unmotivated," again failing to give adequate consideration to other possible explanations or inferences. The *anchoring heuristic* is invoked when quick determinations are made about an individual on the basis of initial impressions, and these determinations are resistant to change, because any subsequent information that is inconsistent with those impressions will be ignored or discounted, whereas information that is consistent will be given more weight, resulting in a confirmatory bias. A number of authors have empirically examined and discussed these sources of bias in counseling and the importance of recognizing and avoiding them in making inferences in assessment (e.g., Morrow & Deidan, 1992; Turk & Salovey, 1985).

MAKING CLINICAL AND SERVICE DECISIONS AND DETERMINATIONS

The final phase of assessment involves the translation of information into any of a number of different clinical decisions and determinations that vary depending on the purposes of the assessment. The most common decisions and determinations in rehabilitation counseling practice include selection for service, establishment of vocational objectives, identification of needed interventions and formulation of case service plans, and disability determinations. In making all of these various decisions and determinations, the "working model" of the individual that has been developed through synthesis and reasoning is used to make predictions corresponding to the decisions and determinations to be made.

Selection for Service

Virtually all rehabilitation agencies, as well as other human-service programs, have criteria established for determining who will be served.
Some criteria may be relatively objective and easily determined, such as
the presence of a particular diagnosis or type of disability or the presence
of a prespecified level of financial need. Others rely on more subjective
determinations. Perhaps the most universally used criterion concerns the
perceived benefits that are likely to occur if treatment or services are provided and whether these likely benefits are sufficient to justify whatever
time, effort, and expense would be required to achieve those benefits. In
making such determinations, the working model of the individual is projected into the future to predict the likely outcomes of the rehabilitation
process if services were to be provided, the extent to which those outcomes would be considered "successful," and the costs that would be
associated with the services required to achieve those outcomes. These
determinations are highly subjective and are based in part on the experience of the rehabilitation counselor with other individuals judged to be
similar to the individual being assessed, and the outcomes achieved with
those individuals. A decision regarding selection for service then requires
that a value judgment be added to this determination concerning whether
it is "worthwhile" to proceed with the provision of treatment or service.

Establishing Career or Vocational Objectives

Career or vocational objectives are some of the most common goals
established in rehabilitation counseling practice, and the interventions
and services provided are then directed toward achieving those objectives.
To establish career or vocational objectives, the working model of the
individual is projected into work environments associated with different
occupations in order to predict likely functioning and, consequently, likely satisfactoriness and satisfaction (Lofquist & Dawis, 1969). To the
extent that assets, limitations, and preferences of the individual have been
comprehensively identified in developing the working model of the individual, the process will be facilitated as a suitable vocational objective
will capitalize on the assets of the individual, will minimize the impact of
limitations, and will be consistent with preferences. Assets and limitations must be considered in terms of any changes that are expected to
occur as a result of intervention and service. In addition, as the working

model of an individual is projected into a potential work environment and likely functioning is predicted, other assets or limitations may be identified that are specific to that particular environment. Information about the ability requirements and sources of satisfaction provided by different work environments can be found in printed sources of occupational information, as well as through job analyses and other direct observations of work environments. Finally, similar procedures can be used in establishing other types of life objectives and plans to be pursued, such as the identification of a suitable living arrangement that is consistent with an individual's assets, limitations, and preferences.

Treatment and Case Service Plans

The comprehensive listing of assets, limitations, and preferences of an individual provides the basis for developing treatment and case service plans, as problems or barriers that need to be targeted for intervention will be found among the limitations identified. In those instances in which a career or vocational objective is being pursued through the rehabilitation process, the working model of the individual is projected into work environments consistent with that objective, and the impact of the individual's limitations on functioning in those environments can then be predicted (employability determinations). Similarly, the impact of limitations identified can be determined on *obtaining* employment in that occupation (placeability determinations) and in functioning in whatever environments might be required in preparing for that occupation. Those limitations that are predicted to pose barriers to accomplishment of the objective are then targeted for intervention. Limitations targeted might include skill deficits (e.g., specific vocational skills, academic skills, social skills, independent travel skills, test-taking skills, and job-seeking skills), inconsistencies between typical behavior and environmental expectations (e.g., punctuality, mannerisms, and speed), lack of credentials (e.g., degrees, diplomas, and licenses), or a wide variety of other limitations that may pose barriers (e.g., limitations in self-confidence, social support networks, finances, and transportation).

For each limitation that is targeted for intervention, one or more treatment or intervention strategies or services must be identified. Possible interventions would include counseling or other strategies provided directly by the rehabilitation counselor, whereas other agencies or professionals would be called on to provide other interventions or services.

The technique of "brainstorming," which involves the identification of as many alternative intervention strategies as possible while temporarily suspending judgment about their appropriateness, can serve to stimulate creativity in identifying a comprehensive array of alternatives. Decisions regarding the interventions of choice can then be achieved by projecting the working model of the individual into the future to predict the likely outcomes of each alternative intervention, while also considering the practical costs associated with each alternative (e.g., monetary costs, time, and effort). Intervention strategies selected to address the barriers and problems identified are then organized into a comprehensive, integrated treatment or service plan that is then implemented.

Disability Determinations

Rehabilitation counselors are often called on to provide expert opinion regarding the vocational implications of disability in Social Security, workers' compensation, personal injury, and related proceedings. Lynch (1983) has conceptualized vocational expert opinion as including both employability and placeability opinions. Employability opinions require the identification of occupations that are compatible with an individual's residual capacities. Formulation of those opinions would involve procedures similar to those described in establishing vocational objectives, in which the working model of the individual is projected into work environments associated with different occupations to predict likely functioning. Placeability opinions concern the likelihood of actually obtaining employment in particular occupations, and are influenced by the opinions of individuals empowered with hiring decisions regarding the suitability of candidates for employment. To formulate placeability opinions, the working model of the individual is projected into the hiring process to predict the likelihood of a favorable hiring decision. In addition, the availability and competition for jobs in a geographically defined labor market must be determined.

The determinations required of rehabilitation counselors serving as vocational experts vary depending on the type of proceeding (Field & Sink, 1981; Rothstein, 1991). In Social Security proceedings determinations must be made as to whether or not an individual is prevented by disability from engaging in substantial and gainful activity in jobs that are available in significant numbers in the national economy. In workers' compensation and personal injury proceedings, a determination must be made regarding the loss of earning capacity resulting from a disability; this requires a comparison of earning in jobs available to the individual in the local labor market prior to the onset of the disability with earning from those available following onset. Field and Sink (1981) have described the Vocational Diagnosis and Assessment of Residual Employability (VDARE) system, which provides one step-by-step systematic procedure to facilitate such determinations.

FUTURE PERSPECTIVES

In recent years there has been an enormous growth in assessment devices available to rehabilitation counselors. The number and range of standardized tests and inventories available are particularly overwhelming; for example, a total of 3,009 commercially published instruments are referenced in *Tests in Print IV* (Murphy, Conoley, & Impara, 1994), and many other instruments not available through commercial publishers are also used in rehabilitation settings. The number of work sample and related assessment systems has also grown, with a total of 18 systems reviewed by Brown et al. (1994), in addition to 12 "job search software" systems. Finally, a wide variety of functional assessment measures, rating scales, and other assessment devices are available for use. It is anticipated that the numbers and variety of instruments and systems will continue to grow dramatically in the years ahead.

Rehabilitation counselors involved in conducting assessments that involve any of the various types of assessment devices will have a wide range of devices from which to choose, and identifying the available alternatives will continue to become increasingly difficult. By the same token, virtually all rehabilitation counselors involved in interpreting assessment reports from psychologists, vocational evaluators, and other professionals will be frequently confronted with scores and other performance measures on unfamiliar tests and systems. If counselors are to be effective consumers of such assessment information and avoid deferring completely to the judgment of professionals preparing assessment reports, they will need to maintain access to sources of information on new tests and systems and be diligent in consulting those sources of information when needed.

The application of computer technology in assessment is another trend that will certainly continue in future years. Bunderson, Inouye, and Olsen (1989) have discussed four generations of computer applications in assessment, and only the first generation, computerized conventional tests, has been applied extensively in rehabilitation counseling practice. More specifically, as discussed by Burkhead and Sampson (1985), the types of computer applications in assessment in rehabilitation settings include: standardized testing; structured interviews; vocational evaluation systems, including work samples; job matching systems, which may stand alone or be integrated with vocational evaluation systems; and assessment components of computer-assisted career guidance systems. Computers may be used to score responses to tests and other assessment devices, with answer sheets sent to a computer-scoring service or entered or scanned into a microcomputer for either computation and profiling of scores or the generation of narrative interpretive reports. Computers may also be used to administer assessment devices, in addition to the immediate scoring and reporting of results.

The second generation of computer applications discussed by Bunderson et al. (1989), which has not been widely used to date in rehabilitation settings but holds much promise for the future, is computerized adaptive testing (Embretson, 1992; Weiss, 1985; Weiss & Vale, 1987). Computerized adaptive testing involves the construction via computer of an individually tailored test for each person taking a particular test by over-sampling test items near the individual's level of the characteristic being tested (e.g., ability level), while excluding items that are either well above or well below that level (e.g., items that are too easy or too difficult). Anastasi (1992), among others, has suggested that adaptive testing is one of the most significant current trends in testing. One example of a computer-based adaptive test available for use in rehabilitation settings is the Differential Aptitude Tests: Computerized Adaptive Edition. The third and fourth generations of computer applications discussed by Bunderson et al., continuous measurement of dynamic changes and intelligent measurement, along with computerized adaptive testing, could serve to revolutionize assessment in rehabilitation counseling practice in the years ahead.

Despite the central role of assessment in rehabilitation counseling practice, the empirical basis for assessment in rehabilitation settings is often lacking (see Berven, 1994). For example, in a review of vocational evaluation systems commonly used in rehabilitation settings, Brown et al. (1994) found no evidence whatsoever regarding reliability and validity for 4 of the 18 systems reviewed, and they indicated that the available evidence for several of the other systems was either extremely limited or equivocal. Similarly, there is little empirical basis underlying the interview as an assessment tool, sources of bias that influence the judgments of rehabilitation counselors, and the processes by which they make clinical judgments and determinations. Given the importance of assessment to all aspects of rehabilitation counseling, the improvement of assessment methods and practices should be given a high priority if rehabilitation counselors are to effectively assist individuals with disabilities in maximizing quality of life.

CHAPTER 11

Counseling as a Recursive Dynamic: Process and Relationship, Meaning, and Empowerment

Lisa Lopez Levers

The contemporary practice of rehabilitation counseling has evolved extensively from its roots in the vocational education and vocational rehabilitation legislative mandates of the early 20th century. The field has seen a theoretical shift from a purely vocational emphasis in counseling to a focus on traditional person-centered therapy, then to psychosocial counseling, and most recently to more systemic- and ecologic-oriented approaches to counseling.

Rehabilitation counselors continue to work in traditional settings, for example, state vocational rehabilitation systems and rehabilitation hospitals, and the defining axis of rehabilitation counseling continues to be disability and related psychosocial issues. However, the scope-of-practice for rehabilitation counselors has broadened to include work in community mental health, substance abuse and chemical dependency, psychiatric rehabilitation, proprietary rehabilitation, and other clinical settings. Although some view rehabilitation counseling as having developed historically as an independent profession, others view contemporary rehabilitation counseling as one specialty area within a wider field of professional counseling. The controversy surrounding this issue remains unresolved (Leahy & Szymanski, 1995). For the purpose of this chapter, the focus presented here is on general professional counseling as it applies to the variety of settings in which rehabilitation counselors practice.

As the gateway to health care in the 21st century rapidly approaches, regardless of work settings or personal theoretical orientations toward counseling, rehabilitation counselors must be mindful of the emergence of managed care precepts—in both governmental and private arenas— aimed toward briefer, more strategic, outcome-oriented counseling techniques. It is a reasonable assumption, in the current economy of health care/health care economic climate, that a time-limited rather than time-unlimited counseling format is the norm for most counselors entering the rehabilitation services system.

This chapter is written with the understanding that the current set of service delivery systems is complex, if not confusing. Adapting to the professional services environment and adopting one's orientation to counseling are not easy matters, and therefore, this chapter is written with the new counselor and counselor trainee in mind. The information that follows assumes an introductory knowledge of beginning counseling theories, techniques, and professional issues or that the reader will have that introduction very soon. The material here is intended as a meaningful supplement to the foundational knowledge base of counseling and is presented in a way that anticipates eventual field work.

This chapter is aimed at moving the entering counseling student beyond the preliminary conceptualization of micro counseling skills as the basic building blocks of rehabilitation counseling to a consideration of how the counseling process and the relationship between client and counselor can serve to sequence counseling sessions in a way that (1) assists the client in deriving maximum meaning from his or her situation, (2) empowers the client toward desired outcomes, and (3) strategically addresses the time limitations currently imposed in most human-service settings. Because limited space is an important writing consideration here, just as limited time is an important consideration in providing counseling, a metaphor is borrowed from the literary composition field to help keep the message clear and succinct.

LEARNING TO WRITE AS A METAPHOR
FOR LEARNING TO COUNSEL

In the field of literary composition, instructors of basic composition spend much time helping students to learn the mechanics of effective writing in the hope that with much practice and skill development, the students will learn to use those tools in the creative and technical application of the craft. One important dimension of contemporary literary composition is the notion of *recursive writing*. *Recursive* is the adjectival form of the noun *recursion*. The word *recursion*, like its root *recur*, is derived from the Latin *recurrer*, which means to run back. In terms of writing, the implication is that the whole continually refers back to parts of itself. Some writing can be reasonably straightforward—or "linear"— in which a standard format is available for a standard content, the more or less recursive working out of the format having been done in the past. For cases in which the anticipated content is neither standard nor even known—except in the form of a fragmentary, elliptical intuition—the writing process takes on a complex, recursive dynamic in which the writer keeps going back, keeps recurring to a more or less vague sense of a developing intention in order to move forward and discover more of the developing meaning.

From a literary composition perspective, the implication is that effective writing is imbued with meaning, making tacit connections more evident to the reader. In order to accomplish its purpose, effective writing must be iterative or self-referent, generative, and it must invoke parallel structures. Therefore, for writing to be meaningful, that is, effective, it must be recursive.

Like effective writing, effective counseling must be recursive. In the same way that an effective writer first masters the use of the basic building blocks of language—how to construct a sentence, then a paragraph, then an essay—before the ability to write effectively evolves, the effective counselor must master the use of the basic technology of helping. The notion of recursion is a reminder that everything that happens within the counseling process with a particular client must loop back to the client's context, thus evoking greater insight through self-reflection. The effective counselor helps the client to make connections that are meaningful. The counseling process, as a recursive one, implies an interactive relationship that is also self-reflexive. In a parallel process, then, recursion also implies self-reflection on the part of the counselor, and extends even to the counselor's supervisor as well.

A TECHNOLOGY OF HELPING

Talk of a "technology of helping" may cause dissonance for some counselor trainees. Many students are attracted initially to the field of professional counseling because they view it as an art form, rather than as science. This dichotomy is problematic.

Survival in an academic environment ostensibly encourages this type of dichotomous thinking—*either/or* logic—rather than dialectical thinking. Effective counseling is, however, more often than not, a nonlinear process, thereby requiring that the practitioner be capable of thinking dialectically. Dichotomizing *art* and *science* creates an artificial distinction, one that leads to a more linear mode of thought and inquiry, and that, in relationship to counseling, has the potential to cause harm—and the most basic legal and ethical caveat in this field is to *do no harm*. The issue of potential harm is raised here, because by ignoring the scientific aspects of the profession, such as relevant theory and research, a counselor may not be prepared adequately for some of the client situations that he or she is sure to encounter eventually.

Although counseling certainly can be viewed in part as art, it is also science. Art and science are both essential aspects of the counseling process. Rollo May (1989) wrote brilliantly on *The Art of Counseling*. However, even the esteemed Dr. May, an early student of Alfred Adler, one of the earliest proponents of a major tenet of professional counseling —emphasizing human potential rather than focusing only on pathology— pointed to the importance of using basic technical skills and of understanding essential theories related to personality.

The technology of counseling includes all those basic listening and communication skills that beginning counseling students spend several academic terms learning. Most foundations of counseling texts emphasize such basic skills as attending, listening, empathy, and probing; and they elaborate on such basic counselor values as respect, understanding, warmth, genuineness, and client self-responsibility. These skills and values are the building blocks of counseling's technology, and the research that explores the efficacy of what counselors do and how they do it serves as the mortar that holds these blocks together. This counseling technology has its utility in providing counselors with a framework for helping clients to self-explore and to solve problems.

THE REST OF THE CHAPTER

Two fundamental elements have emerged from this discussion so far: the recursive process of counseling and the recursive relationship between client and counselor. These two elements combine to form a nexus with the constructs of meaning-making and empowerment, providing a dynamic structure for understanding how a client can move sequentially from the presenting problem to making a successful change. The focus of this chapter elaborates on understanding the importance of this structure, especially as it relates to an ecological consideration of the client's context.

COUNSELING AS A RECURSIVE DYNAMIC

The major theoretical approaches to professional counseling traditionally and categorically have included psychodynamic approaches, existential–humanistic approaches, and cognitive–behavioral approaches. In more recent years, discussions of the efficacy of more eclectic, systemic, and synergistic approaches have prevailed in the literature. In reviewing research literature related to comparable therapeutic gains across therapies, however, Horvath and Greenberg (1994) have stated that the results "suggest that different therapies produce comparable outcomes despite differences in premises, different assumptions about the etiology of human dysfunction, and different techniques" (p. 1). This of course raises questions about the specific elements of particular therapies and forces the question of commonality across counseling approaches.

Patterson and Welfel (1994) have hinted at such commonality by generically defining counseling as "an interactive process characterized by a unique relationship between counselor and client that leads to change in the client" (p.21). Counseling is typically defined in terms of process and relationship. This particular definition is offered here as a generic beginning point for the discussion of these two major elements, especially as it anticipates discussion of the client's meaning-making and client empowerment.

PROCESS

The counseling process can take the form of psychoeducation, therapy, habilitation, rehabilitation, recovery, healing, or some combination thereof. The determination of format selection must be guided by client need and client context.

The primary dimension of the recursive counseling process is self-knowledge—both of the client in his or her quest and the counselor in his or her helping strategy. By using selected counseling strategies, the counselor helps the client to construct new self-knowledge. By extension, self-knowledge recurs to self-reflection, which generates increased self-knowledge. This form of personal knowing (Polanyi, 1962) becomes heuristic—a process of self-discovery that predicates client action.

Action

The notion of a client taking action is central to the process of counseling. For example, a counselor may need to assertively challenge a client's irrational beliefs in order to assist the client in getting "unstuck" and taking action to make needed change. The client's needs and context must be assessed in relationship to taking action, however, and a full range of action-oriented strategies must be considered. The primacy of taking action is a notion that has cultural implications, and counselors working with clients representing diverse populations must consider carefully, respectfully, and even cautiously the action/change dimension of counseling.

Taking action does not always necessarily connote only overt observable behavior. Action can include less observable, more cognitively oriented frameworks. For example, the client may decide to do nothing or decide to confer with elders or significant others before making further decisions. There is a huge difference between intentionally deciding not to act and simply not acting without consideration of consequences.

Readiness to take action anticipates change. Change can take place at multiple levels, including cognitive reframing, emotional growth, increased insight, heightened awareness, spiritual progress, and so on.

Change

Counseling is a growth process, a problem-solving process, a self-reflexive process, that is, a process of change. Clients seek help with various concerns, dilemmas, crises, and problems, representing a continuum from normal developmental task issues, to unexpected crises, to extreme dysfunction. Personal transformation is possible and is enabled through the process of counseling. Such transformation is contingent on client readiness to take action and counselor facilitation of needed change as that change has been collaboratively determined by both client and counselor.

Regardless of the client's context and the counselor's theoretical orientation, the ensuing process is about change; and change, here, implies recursion. A typical outcome of the change process is an increased ability on the part of the client to manage or better manage the problem or concern that brought him or her to counseling. An essential outcome of the change process, if growth has really taken place, is that the client has gained a better understanding of his or her situation or life circumstance and has derived some meaning from addressing the issue that led him or her to engage in counseling.

Meaning

People seek meaning in their lives (May, 1973, 1991). Humans react to personal crises with a plethora of visceral and behavioral responses, but ultimately they attempt to derive meaning from even the most traumatic events (Frankl, 1985). Assisting people to find meaning in the face of personal crises leads to the discovery of proactive pathways of healing.

Carlsen (1988) proposed that "meaning-making" is a backbone of the counseling process. In her treatise on "meaning-making therapy," she referred to the "evolving definitions of meaning in an individual's life," stating that "meaning is interpreted as both a process and an ideal, as a structure and a sequence, as possibility and constraint, as an achievement and an intending, and as both noun and verb as it forms and reforms through the ongoing stages of adult life" (p. 5).

Meaning-making is recursive. In the cognitive framing of important client events, the counselor helps the client refer back to personal history and personal knowledge to derive meaning. Personal transformation is possible by helping the client to arrive at personal meaning-making, by taking action, and by making desired changes.

RELATIONSHIP

The relationship between client and counselor is punctuated by such counselor values as respect, warmth, understanding, genuineness or congruency, authenticity, and positive regard. Within the framework of these values, and by using situation-specific skills, the counselor establishes a relationship and forms a bond with the client. The successful counseling relationship is one that is collaborative in its partnership. Counselor and client form a partnership or alliance based on trust and formulated in the pursuit of a mutually agreed on client concern.

Working Alliance

An important dimension of the counseling relationship is the therapeutic alliance, a working alliance based on collaboration and partnership between the client and counselor. The counselor engages in a partnership with the client to resolve problems and eliminate barriers associated with disability, illness, or other psychosocial issues. The counselor and client also assess any client strengths or assets that may help to empower the client. The quality of the working alliance has been cited as a significant factor in successful client outcomes (Bordin, 1994; Brower & Nurius, 1993; Henry & Strupp, 1994; Horvath & Greenberg, 1994; Meier & Davis, 1993; Steenbarger, 1992).

Collaboration

The counseling relationship can be viewed as a partnership and collaboration as an instrumental aspect of the counseling partnership. The construct implies that client and counselor work together cooperatively to establish a counseling agenda that meets the client's needs and expectations. Although the construct is democratic in its underlying philosophy, it does not imply a relationship of absolute equality; there is always a power differential that must be acknowledged between the role of the counselor and the role of the client. To ignore the power dimension of the relationship in the name of collaboration is a mistake—an error in professional judgment that has the potential to lead to dual-role problems.

The prudent counselor proceeds with the partnership in a way that is respectful of the client yet realistically acknowledges the counselor's role as an employee of the service-providing agency or facility. This may seem to be a bit paradoxical to the new counselor, but there are important ethical considerations around this issue that relate to professional boundaries and that can be more fully examined within the context of a professional ethics course.

Person as a Multidimensional Being

An essential tenet of the counseling profession is maintaining a holistic view of the individual. One important aspect of such a holistic view is striving toward optimal balance in the various dimensions of one's being. All people operate in multiple dimensions, including the physical, cognitive, emotional, psychological, social, vocational, existential, and spiritual. The client requesting counseling services is far more complex than his or her presenting problem, disability, or diagnosis. Therefore, it is important to take full or holistic account of the client and his or her context.

Context

It is imperative that the counselor view the client within the client's contextual framework. This does not mean that any one counselor is capable of fully understanding all nuances of each and every client's context. However, the counselor can maintain a sensitivity to contextual issues and develop greater awareness of a particular client's context by asking for needed information rather than making assumptions.

Considering a client's context becomes a foreground/background issue. Nearly everyone has seen the white figure on black background used in building the Gestalt psychology theories circa 1910. When focusing on the white figure in the foreground, one sees a vase; however, when focusing on the black background, one sees two mirrored facial profiles. If a counselor only focuses on the individual client, the counselor misses important background or contextual information. A client's world view, value system, family members, relationships with significant others, and relationships within social units may be instrumental in mediating a successful counseling intervention. Taking such elements of client context into consideration brings the whole person into focus and can more easily facilitate the client's sense of empowerment.

Empowerment

The issue of empowerment is directly related to the client's ability to make positive changes within his or her context. The ability to change and to learn how to change is empowering. Egan offers the following ways of assisting client progress toward a greater sense of self-responsibility: "us[ing] a participatory rather than directive model of helping; help[ing] clients discover and use the power they have; accept[ing] helping as a natural, two-way influence process; becom[ing] a consultant to clients; and democratiz[ing] the helping process" (1994, pp. 60–61).

SEQUENCE OF SESSIONS

The individual sessions that comprise the counseling process for a particular client need to be sequential in terms of that client's development. In this sense, counseling can be conceptualized as a dialectical process. Although no rigid sequencing of sessions can (or should) be imposed, it is helpful to think of the whole counseling intervention as occurring in fluid stages.

Stages of Counseling

In the literature, the counseling process is typically characterized as consisting of three stages. Of course the stages are arbitrary, but the notion of step-wise progression is useful in terms of conceptualizing how the client moves from problem statement to successful change, and how the sessions can therefore be sequenced. It is also useful to think of the stages not as linear, but as fluid, interactive, and recursive.

The initial stage sets the tone for trust-building and serves to open the gateway to constructing an effective working alliance. The intermediary stage establishes and mediates goals, and client change is initiated. The final stage provides resolution to client concerns, problems, and/or dilemmas, and marks the extent to which progress and growth have been achieved as a result of the counseling process. Generally, stage one takes place in the first few sessions, if not in the first session, and stage three takes place in the last couple of sessions. It is stage two that is more elastic, because goals are negotiated and progress is mediated by new insights, increased awareness, and perhaps the necessity of reordering, redefining, or establishing new goals.

The length of the whole therapeutic intervention depends on the needs of the client, the type of setting in which the counseling takes place, and the extent to which external factors impose time limitations. The following list provides a categorical ordering of major counseling dynamics that occur throughout the sessions.

Stage I (initial session, often first several sessions)

- professional disclosure
- client role induction
- establishing trust
- data collection
- identifying problems—identifying purpose
- conceptualizing the case
- initiating the working alliance

Stage II (usually sessions 2 or 3 through acquisition of meaningful gain)

- developing the working alliance
- refining case conceptualization/diagnosing
- setting goals—marking purpose
- planning interventions
- meaning-making
- checking progress

Stage III (last one or several sessions)

- facilitating client-acquisition of therapeutic gain
- determining an end point
- planning termination
- potential referrals for additional or ongoing services
- termination

The above set of stage-determined dynamics is offered as a potentially useful map for conceptualizing a client's sequential development through the counseling process. There is some overlap from stage to stage, and the timing is, of course, flexible. For example, in a counseling setting with a 6-week intervention limit, the first stage probably would consist of session 1; with dynamics such as trust building, working alliance, and case conceptualization leading into session 2; the second stage would be approximated by sessions 2 through 5; and the third stage, beginning at the end of session 5 would lead through to session 6. One primary issue, that cannot be emphasized enough, is that this sequential progression through stages is always recursive.

CULTURE, COUNSELING AND THE 21ST CENTURY

Pedersen (1991) has referred to multicultural counseling as the fourth force in counseling. It is incumbent on rehabilitation counselor educators to ensure that a sensitivity to issues of diversity is infused throughout the curriculum, including issues related to race, ethnicity, gender, able-bodiedness, religion or spirituality, and sexual orientation. It is essential that skill training reflects culture-centered counseling (Pedersen, 1994; Pedersen & Ivey, 1993).

Sue and Sue (1990, p. 137) have pointed out that "world views are not only composed of our attitudes, values, opinions, and concepts, but also they may affect how we think, make decisions, behave, and define events." The importance of attending to culture and understanding variations in world view carries vast implications for counselors (Axelson, 1993).

Rehabilitation counseling must take place in an environment that reflects the diversity of the populations being served and that honors variations in world views. The counselor must be aware that rehabilitation services may operate on multiple axes in a multicultural context including any combination of issues related to race, ethnicity, gender, religion, sexual orientation, and disability. To a large extent, multicultural counseling includes systems of counseling that honor the primacy of the client's context by way of exploring that context. One such contextual consideration is to view the client from an ecological perspective.

AN ECOLOGICAL PERSPECTIVE

Clients come to the counseling relationship with personal histories and personal contexts that are parts of larger environments. It is essential to recognize, in assessing the individual client, that humans are social beings. People have mates or partners, families, friends, and other significant others in their lives. They affiliate with groups, organizations, churches, and so on, and work and recreate in various locations and capacities.

Individuals are a complex part of a larger culture, with perhaps many subcultural affiliations. Therefore, although it is important to understand intrapersonal dynamics, it is also important to understand interpersonal dynamics. It is important to assess the individual's systemic relationships as a way of understanding where and how the individual interfaces with his or her various environments. This type of ecological perspective supports the philosophical view that "considers a person's disability within the context of the whole person and in relationship to how the person interacts with the environment" (Levers & Maki, 1995, p. 133).

Adopting an ecological perspective enables the counselor to focus on the individual's needs within the person's context. It allows for an understanding of the spaces in which the client interfaces with other individuals, significant social units, and other systems. It permits a constructivist view that acknowledges areas of personal meaning. It endorses a holistic perspective that accounts for assets as well as liabilities, and tacit constructions of personal knowledge as well as more tangible forces that have an impact on the person. From an ecological perspective, the counselor can operate with an integrative approach, using the theories and techniques that have the best ecological fit. The counselor can also affirm the client in restoring, or indeed, creating greater balance in his or her life-style.

SUMMARY

This chapter has provided an overview of the professional practice of counseling as it applies to the many venues of rehabilitation counseling. Counseling has been examined as a recursive process that allows the client to move toward productive change and personal meaning-making. The effective counseling relationship has been identified as a working alliance that is predicated on a collaborative dynamic aimed at client empowerment.

By attending to the recursive dimension of the counseling process, the counselor can effectively facilitate the client's move through sequential stages of development related to the problem. Viewing professional counseling from an ecological perspective allows for a holistic view of the client and enables the counselor to use an integrative approach to problem resolution in a time-efficient manner. Viewing the practice of counseling as a recursive dynamic provides the rehabilitation counselor with a metaphoric style manual that assists in facilitating a process and developing a relationship aimed at client meaning-making and client empowerment.

CHAPTER 12

Professional Practice: Consultation

Ruth Torkelson Lynch, Rochelle Habeck, and Margaret Sebastian

T he rehabilitation counseling profession faces many new opportunities to expand services through the realm of consultation. Although the profession has developed a substantial portion of its identity from the state–federal vocational rehabilitation program and has been characterized by direct clinical service provision to individuals (e.g., counseling), it has become increasingly apparent that rehabilitation counseling skills and knowledge are also valuable resources for new settings and expanded applications. This chapter addresses the importance of this phenomenon to the rehabilitation counseling profession, provides a background regarding consultation theory and practice, supplies examples of consultation services by rehabilitation counselors, and discusses key skills, knowledge, ethical, and professional issues relevant to consultation practice.

The evolution of consultation opportunities for rehabilitation counseling can be viewed as a mark of achievement for the profession. Greater recognition of the value of rehabilitation counseling skills and knowledge in the broader labor market provides further stability for the future. Change into new arenas of practice has required some adjustments by the profession. Although distinctions have been made among these service delivery systems and "who pays the bill" (e.g., the government, a business, an individual client with a disability, or an insurance company), it is important to remember that many of the services provided are essentially the same. It is true that significant differences in perceived importance of knowledge domains have been found with respect to employment setting and job titles (Leahy, Szymanski, & Linkowski, 1993); but a common body of knowledge has also been identified that underlies the practice of rehabilitation counseling across employment settings (Szymanski, Linkowski, Leahy, Diamond, & Thoreson, 1993). The extensive body of empirical research about the competencies of rehabilitation counselors provides the profession with a basis for identifying the skills and services that are potentially available through consultation. In general terms, consultation can involve a combination of evaluation/assessment, problem solving, information synthesis, and plan development, which involves the core skills of rehabilitation counselors and can be provided to either groups (such as rehabilitation agencies, schools, and businesses) or individuals (such as other providers, consumers, or advocates). As in any other type of rehabilitation counseling practice, appropriate academic preparation, credentials, professionalism, skills, and ethics are of critical importance for consulting.

The growing demand for the application of our skills and services as consultants in new arenas should be viewed positively and optimistically. When diverse payors recognize the need for and the value of consultation provided by rehabilitation counselors, then the profession has made a very significant step in its evolution. Although services to enhance the lives of persons with disabilities one individual at a time will always be a primary contribution of rehabilitation counseling, consultation also provides the opportunity to impact the lives of persons with disabilities at organizational and policy levels.

CONSULTATION MODELS AND PROCESSES

Consultation within human services has developed primarily from (a) clinical models in medicine and mental health (Caplan, 1970) (i.e., diagnosis of a problem and prescription of treatment by a consultant with specific expertise), (b) behavioral psychology (e.g., Bergan, 1977), and (c) organizational applications (e.g., Lippitt & Lippitt, 1986). Current definitions of consultation vary depending on theoretical focus and discipline-specific perspectives. However, a synthesis of the purposes and targets of intervention used by human service professionals (Brown, Pryzwansky, & Schulte, 1995), which is based on previous models for mental health consultation (Brown, Wyne, Blackburn, & Powell, 1979; Morrill, Oetting, & Hurst, 1974), can provide an initial structure for a consultation model that applies to rehabilitation counseling. In the conceptualization offered by Brown et al. (1995), consultation is an *indirect service*, in contrast to direct interventions, which involve face-to-face contact with individuals or groups (e.g., teaching, supervision, counseling, and therapy), provided to a consultee (a group or individual requesting consultation). Consultation may be *formal*, requiring a contractual agreement and usually payment; or *informal*, taking place with a senior colleague, an expert on a topic, a peer, or a group of peers. Consultation also may be *inter-professional*, with someone outside of one's own professional domain (Clayton & Bonger, 1994) and it is frequently *interdisciplinary*, with rehabilitation counseling expertise being a specialized component of an interdisciplinary consulting team. The consultant may be *internal*, an employee of the consultee, or *external*. Although the consultant's relationship to the organization can influence the consultation experience, most of the theoretical principles and processes of consultation remain the same. Internal consultants have an established image that can help or hinder the process, they may have or be perceived to have vested interests in the presenting problems, and they cannot exit the system on termination of the consultation request (Kurpius & Fuqua, 1993). External consultants are more readily perceived as experts but they may lack some of the important background information available to an internal consultant.

Consultation can occur as *expert consultation*, in which the consultee contracts with the consultant to provide an intervention or a problem solution. In the expert mode, the consultant has responsibility for the design, implementation and ultimately the success of the intervention. Or consultation can occur as *process consultation*, an arrangement in which the consultant is actively working with the consultee to design and implement changes and success is the responsibility of the consultant and the consultee (Kurpius & Fuqua, 1993). Schein (1969, 1991) used the terms purchase-of-expertise model, doctor–patient model, and process-consultation model to draw distinctions between process and expert models. In reviewing these models, Rockwood (1993) proposed that the purchase-of-expertise model may be most effective when a problem is straightforward and expert information is needed; the doctor–patient model applies when the consultee knows that something is wrong but is unsure of the true problem or how to resolve it; and the process-consultation model (which involves the consultee throughout the diagnostic and problem-solving process) works best to reduce potential resistance to change and improve problem-solving ability for the future. Consultation activity is actually likely to shift in and out of the process-and-content modes to provide effective help.

The actual process of consultation, whether short or long term, individual or organizationwide, can be analyzed in terms of the following six stages, as described by Kurpius, Fuqua, and Rozecki (1993):

1. Preentry. This involves self-assessment by the consultant evaluating personal competencies relative to needs and articulating services related to those skills.
2. Entry, problem exploration, and contracting. In this step, the problem is explored by the consultee with the consultant to determine if a contract is necessary and feasible.
3. Information gathering, problem configuration, and goal setting. In this step, qualitative and quantitative data are gathered with valid and reliable measures involving appropriate consultee staff to define and/or confirm problems.
4. Solution searching and intervention selection.
5. Evaluation of intervention success with possible redefinition of the problem, if necessary.
6. Termination, which may include a debriefing and reflection about the process.

Consultation may focus on primary prevention (e.g., enhancing communication, decision making, or coping skills); secondary prevention (e.g., job-enrichment programs; remediation of learning difficulties); or tertiary prevention (e.g., reducing the impact of functional handicaps) with any of four target groups: individuals, groups, organizations, communities (Brown et al., 1995). This latter concept of four target groups is a key one for expanding rehabilitation counseling consultation because it extends the profession's traditional emphasis from clinical services for individuals to systemic interventions through services to groups and organizations. The importance of this larger focus for the profession and for resolving disability issues has been made clear in recent years.

The individual-oriented service model has been criticized for paying inadequate attention to the larger environment within the service process, failing to address factors that contribute to disability and others that can resolve it (Council of State Administrators of Vocational Rehabilitation,

1993; Habeck, Kress, Scully, & Kirchner, 1994; Olshesky, 1993; Stubbins, 1982; Vandergoot, 1993). An ecological or systems perspective takes into account the economic, political, architectural, and social organizational forces that impact the disability experience, and requires interventions that are designed for the appropriate level. This ecological perspective is embodied in the Americans with Disabilities Act (ADA) and the Rehabilitation Act as amended in 1992. Consultation strategies that are targeted toward organizations and groups provide rehabilitation counselors with an opportunity to facilitate public disability policy goals and influence change in other community, work, and school environments that affect many individuals with disabilities.

EXAMPLES OF CURRENT CONSULTATION PRACTICE

Three newer arenas of practice are presented below to illustrate the application of consultation models and processes in rehabilitation practice. Each of these examples may be applied to address a variety of impairments and disability problems.

Consultation in the Legal Arena

Legal definitions of disability (e.g., under Social Security, Workers' Compensation) reflect the importance of work in relation to adult functioning. The employability, placeability, earning loss, and earning capacity of an individual who has sustained physical, mental, or emotional limitations because of disease or injury is critical to determination of compensation and damage awards (e.g., personal injury litigation, workers' compensation). Vocational rehabilitation counselors with strong assessment and analysis skills have become valuable resources to the legal system as vocational experts capable of rendering opinions concerning the vocational and rehabilitation implications for specific cases.

The credibility of vocational opinions is related directly to the competence, training, and experience of the individual who conducted the analysis (Lynch, Lynch, & Beck, 1992). A consultant who is a vocational expert consultant is responsible for numerous steps that require thorough preparation and competency:

(a) critically reviewing supporting documentation (e.g., medical); (b) performing a vocational diagnostic interview; (c) noting critical work behaviors; (d) translating residual functioning capacity into vocationally relevant terminology; (e) locating, assessing, and integrating rehabilitation research relevant to the type of disability involved; (f) understanding vocational development theory, job requirements, and the world of work; (g) securing labor market and wage information; and (i) presenting logical and substantiable conclusions based on objective findings (Lynch et al., 1992, p. 88).

The vocational expert may be called on to present conclusions in written reports, in consultation meetings with referral sources, and in legal testimony (e.g., depositions, jury trials, before a hearing examiner). Because scrutiny of conclusions is integral to the legal process, consulting in the legal arena requires attention to detail, an understanding of the broad perspectives of how performance and life functioning are impacted by life events, and effective skills for communicating opinions. It is critical for consultants in the legal arena to be objective, concise, well-organized, and clear when providing an expert opinion.

Consultation in Business and Industry

As a result of rising health care costs and competitive economic conditions, many employers have become increasingly aware that disability is an important aspect of human resource and business management. Formerly, disability costs, such as workers' compensation and long-term disability, were simply ignored as "a cost of doing business." Insurance was recognized as a sufficient means of administering these benefits and handling financial risk. During the 1980s, innovative corporations and rehabilitation experts realized that the occurrence of disability and its costs and outcomes could be significantly influenced by assuming responsibility at the work site with the concepts and practices that have become known as disability management.

Akabas, Gates, and Galvin (1992) defined disability management as:

A workplace prevention and remediation strategy that seeks to prevent disability from occurring or, lacking that, to intervene early following the onset of disability, using coordinated, cost-conscious, quality rehabilitation service that reflects an organizational commitment to continued employment of those experiencing functional work limitations. (p. 2)

Effectively implemented, disability management is intended to achieve a win–win situation that addresses the common interests of employers and employees for maintaining a safe, productive, and profitable employment environment.

Although disability management programs traditionally have been thought of as employer-based, many insurance-based and provider-based disability management services have emerged to serve employer organizations. Service providers from a variety of professions now offer a wide range of services under the banner of disability management, from safety education and ergonomics through medical case management and return-to-work programs.

In addition to economic incentives, the Americans with Disabilities Act of 1990 (PL 101–336) added legislative requirements for employers to accommodate workers who become disabled and to enable their return to work. As Akabas et al. (1992) have pointed out, compliance with the ADA is a compatible goal to be achieved in an effective disability-management program. That is, having policies and practices in place that provide reasonable accommodation and avoid discriminatory practices unrelated to essential functions are just as necessary as components of a productive disability-management program as they are for assuring that new applicants for employment who have disabilities are considered within the spirit and the letter of the ADA.

Concurrent with these developments and in response to the crisis in health care costs, have been the phenomenal growth in the use of individual case management and the rise of managed health care. In particular, insurers and third-party administrators have turned increasingly toward the use of nurses and rehabilitation counselors for the provision of medical and vocational case management to guide and control the effective use of health care services and to achieve timely, appropriate return to work. These case management services are typically obtained through credentialed providers of disability case management services, either independent practitioners or organized networks of member providers in a managed care system. Insurers hire case managers as internal or contracted employees to directly deliver and control case management services within the claims management process of the insurance contract. Employers who are self-insured typically make arrangements for providers of these services through their benefits administrator, through external contracting, or by hiring case managers as internal employees. Regardless of the mechanism used to provide professional case management services, an effective disability-management program requires that general case management responsibilities for employees who have developed a potentially disabling injury or health impairment be assigned to someone internal to the company to facilitate coordinated activities within the workplace and with external parties that will result in timely and appropriate resolution.

In disability management program consultation, the employer organization is viewed as the client or consultee. An organization-level focus (i.e., professional services provided to a group rather than an individual) is therefore critical to disability management consultation. The individual who assists in the development, administration, and/or implementation of a corporate-based disability management program "must be critically aware of the context in which the . . . program will operate, as well as the changing internal and external forces that will influence the process and the outcomes" (Mitchell, 1995, p.1).

This organizational perspective is evident in corporate level program development, which is recommended to initiate a disability management process: (a) evaluate the present situation (needs assessment); (b) convene a coordinating committee; (c) establish policy and procedures; (d) provide a mechanism for case finding and early intervention; (e) appoint a case manager and develop ties with community agencies; (f) offer flexible employment options; and (g) provide training to key participants (Akabas et al., 1992). Mitchell (1995) also emphasizes the organization focus in delineating the critical steps that a consultant uses to develop a disability management program: (a) define the nature and scope of disability in the work force by collecting data and analyzing patterns of injury, illness, work disruption, work performance, and costs; (b) identify the competing internal and external self interests [force field analysis]; (c) specify the conditions needed for success on the part of all parties; (d) determine the program elements, policies, responsibilities, and incentives for performance, and the processes and mechanisms for coordination; (e) conduct staff development and supervisor training; (f) monitor and evaluate key indicators as the program is implemented; and (g) modify and adjust the program as needed.

Disability management consultation can be clarified using the organizational consultation models reviewed by Rockwood (1993). There are many specific technical expert services that can be offered in the workplace from either the"purchase-of-expertise" or "doctor–patient" models. Purchase of expertise for specific services within disability management (e.g., ADA compliance review, job description development with identification of essential functions, development of modified work assignments, individual case management) may be the type of consultation that requires minimal further professional development because these services are closely associated with core competencies of rehabilitation counselors (e.g., job placement, environmental barriers, assessment). However, one must be cautious not to market specific services that are narrow in scope (e.g., case management, return to work) in such a way that the buyer has expectations for the large-scale effects that can only be achieved in a disability management *systems* intervention (e.g., the "process consultation" model). The most significant outcomes of disability management occur at the employer–organizational level.

The role of the larger work environment in creating and resolving disability has become clear, as evidenced in ADA policy and disability-management research. Rehabilitation counselors who shift toward environmentally directed competencies can increase the scope and impact of their services. At the organizational level of disability management consultation, considerable content knowledge and advanced process skills are required (Habeck, Kress, Scully & Kirchner, 1994; Habeck & Munrowd, 1987). Therefore, advanced training in organizational and systems models, theories and techniques of consultation, general business knowledge, and their interface with advanced knowledge of the technical and clinical elements of disability management would be necessary for experienced practioners who wish to provide disability management at the organizational level.

Consultation in the Schools

Current educational reform efforts emphasize school restructuring and collaborative school environments that respond to the diverse needs of students, including students with disabilities. School environment accessibility and programming to transition students from school to work are examples of school restructuring efforts that directly effect students with disabilities. In these efforts within schools, a rehabilitation counselor may be a valuable consultant regarding such issues as the impact of disability, environmental access, and school-to-work transition.

In the provision of special education services to students with disabilities, rehabilitation counseling is considered a related service (House of Representatives Reports 101–544, 101–787, 1990a, 1990b). A primary focus of that service to schools is in facilitating the transition from school to working life, an outcome-oriented process encompassing a broad array of services and experiences that lead to employment (Will, 1984). Rehabilitation counselors become involved at the school level because transition is most effective when interdisciplinary and interagency collaboration and cooperation is emphasized and the process is started early (Hanley-Maxwell & Szymanski, 1992). The potential rehabilitation counseling functions for transition include, but are not limited to the following: career and psychosocial counseling, consultation regarding the vocational implications of disability and potential educational adaptations, job placement, job analysis, job modification and restructuring; coordination of job-support services, and promotion of transition to adult service agencies (Szymanski & King, 1989). These services could be provided by a rehabilitation counselor employed by the school or by a consulting rehabilitation counselor. The focus of consultation may be at the individual level (e.g., developing a transition plan for a specific student) or at the organizational level (e.g., facilitating transition program development for a school district).

Consultation skills play an important role when trying to implement school structure changes at an organizational level with a collaborative school team (West & Idol, 1993). Interactions may occur "(a) between any two or more individual professionals; (b) among members of a child-study team; (c) between parents of students and school professionals; (d) with community agencies and persons outside the school; (e) with persons responsible for special programs for the school; or (f) among school professionals responsible for specified tasks, such as behavior management and discipline" (West & Idol, 1993, p. 680). The consultant can function as a change agent by promoting team building and identifying model strategies that facilitate change (e.g., schoolwide commitment to transition).

School consultation frequently involves a triadic relationship (Kurpius & Fuqua, 1993) involving a consultee (e.g., school administration) and a client (e.g., student). The interventions and recommendations may be focused on organizational process or program development (e.g., development of a school-to-work transition program) or on individual students through expert interprofessional consultation (e.g., behavioral or career-development services for a specific student). A consultant may discover that the identified problem has resulted from a simple communication problem between the student and the consultee or that the problem requires outside agencies (e.g., community mental health, state rehabilitation agency) to be called in for assistance (V. Theilsen, personal communication, July 18, 1995).

Whether a counselor is internal or external to the school can affect the nature of practice. An internal consultant (i.e., a school employee) may have a valuable in-depth understanding of the school system but have difficulty being recognized as a resource or expert. External consultation may be more effective in addressing process consultation needs because the consultant is not perceived to have a vested interest in the presenting problems, is less likely to have personal relationships with staff and clients affected, and can effect the system on termination of the contract.

At the school's organizational level of the school, the consultant can facilitate vision, enhance staff skills, identify resources, encourage the development of incentives, and formulate an ongoing planning system (B. LeRoy, personal communication, July 24, 1995) using a five-step process:

1. Create a shared vision and get involved parties to understand and agree on what is trying to be accomplished; facilitate the process through a number of methods including consensus retreats, administrative roundtables with administrators from other districts, parent-awareness panels, and teacher exchange days between school districts.
2. Enhance school staff skills through inservice programs, teacher retreats, mentoring programs, and modeling by the consultant.
3. Identify previously untapped resources (such as ancillary staff, scheduling designs, and equipment appropriation).
4. Identify incentives (e.g., flex time, conference attendance, work time to do individual reading or special projects/research) that are reinforcing to the individuals who commit to the extra work that change often entails.
5. Summarize formative decisions, implement changes, and assess and evaluate continual progress and needs.

Consultation in the schools by rehabilitation counselors can be considered using the Schein (1969, 1991) purchase-of-expertise, doctor –patient or process-consultation models. Similar to disability management, purchase of expertise for specific services (e.g., planning for school-to-work transition, establishing a career development system) involves core rehabilitation counseling competencies such as case management, assessment, rehabilitation plan development. School system intervention (i.e., process consultation) will be most effective if the consultant has additional competencies in organizational and systems models (e.g., Beer & Spector, 1993; Cooper & O'Connor, 1993; Fuqua & Kurpius, 1993).

IMPLICATIONS FOR THE REHABILITATION COUNSELING PROFESSION

The marketplace is rapidly changing in health care and human service delivery with new terminology, policies, and practices (e.g., managed care, capitation, contracted/preferred providers) appearing at a rapid pace. These changes will continue to affect service delivery and require individual professionals as well as professional groups to assert their identities and market their expertise and skills in providing effective and cost-efficient services. Rehabilitation counselors must be able to recognize their skills and assert their expertise as a valuable resource in order to be identified as the most qualified providers for services such as assessment and vocational rehabilitation planning.

Rehabilitation counseling has a rich history of systematic research regarding critical knowledge areas, roles and functions, and professional competencies (e.g., Emener & Rubin, 1980; Jaques, 1959; Leahy, Shapson, & Wright, 1987; Muthard, & Salamone, 1969; Szymanski et. al., 1993; Wright & Fraser, 1975). Because consultation involves the sharing of professional knowledge and skills, practitioners should be encouraged to use the research findings about the profession as a framework for understanding and marketing present and future consultation services. The process of consultation provides an important medium for extending these services to new and broader arenas of need.

The primary knowledge domains of rehabilitation counseling identified by research and used in rehabilitation counseling certification and accreditation are: (a) vocational counseling and consultative services; (b) medical and psychosocial aspects of disability; (c) individual and group counseling; (d) program evaluation and research; (e) case management and service coordination; (f) family, gender, and multicultural issues; (g) foundations of rehabilitation ; (h) workers' compensation; (i) environmental and attitudinal barriers; and (j) assessment (Linkowski et al., 1993). Within the context of consultation, certain of these skills are particularly valuable as reimbursable consultative services. Comprehensive assessment, which integrates the physical/functional, vocational, and psychosocial implications of a disease or injury, is a service valued by individuals or groups who require a thorough summary of the impact of a disabling condition (e.g., legal arena) or a comprehensive plan (e.g., individual with a disability, insurance carrier). Case management and vocational rehabilitation planning are services that are valued in the context of achieving positive outcomes and containing costs. The consultation practice examples described enumerate further competencies of value in specific settings. Finally, there is considerable scrutiny by third-party payors and government agencies over the practices, outcomes, and efficiency of service delivery systems; therefore, skills in research methodology, program evaluation, and/or outcome analysis are also valuable consultative skills.

Finding consultation opportunities depends on the rehabilitation counselor recognizing and possessing specific skills that are valued and relevant. Therefore prior to identifying oneself as a consultant, a self-analysis of personal skills and qualifications is necessary to define current skills and identify needs for skill enhancement and new skill development. Jacobs (1995) suggests that both personal (e.g., skills, knowledge, time) and environmental resources (e.g., supplies, support services, equipment, space) be assessed. After the necessary additional skills to provide consultation have been acquired through continuing education and further experience, it is usually necessary to build a base of referral sources for consultation services. Rehabilitation professionals who have specific, recognized expertise (e.g., visible professional service, community involvement, publications) may be contacted directly to provide consultation. In other instances, a rehabilitation counselor may build on past experience and training to develop a network for consultation referrals. Competencies related to an appropriate knowledge base, specialized skills, and judgment (Brown, 1993), and professional ethics provide the crux of effective professional consultation and are essential for developing a future in consultation. Therefore, new professionals entering the field should see consultation as a future career development option following the crystallization of one's professional expertise and rehabilitation counseling identity.

The ultimate value of a consultant lies in the skill, ability, preparedness, and objectivity of the rehabilitation professional (Lynch et al., 1992). It is the responsibility of each consultant to identify, develop, and enhance personal competencies (e.g., through continuing education and experience) in order to provide effective consultation and represent the profession ethically and professionally. Enhanced training for new counselors as well as continuing education opportunities are integral for consultation activity. For example, extensive understanding of organizational systems (e.g., business, schools) and organizational development processes is necessary for consultation directed toward the organizations themselves. Rehabilitation counselors can thereby affect individuals functioning within larger systems (e.g., students with special needs, employees with disabilities). Our professional organizations and credentialling/accrediting bodies can provide leadership and marketing assistance to enhance consultation opportunities in the future. Consultation provides valuable career opportunities for qualified, experienced rehabilitation counselors and it offers expanded opportunities to share valuable skills, knowledge, and expertise. Rehabilitation counselors have a great deal to offer as consultants.

CHAPTER 13

Professional Practice: Placement

Robert Stensrud, Michael Millington, and Dennis Gilbride

lacement has been identified consistently as one of the fundamental functions of rehabilitation counselors in both public (Berven, 1979; Muthard & Salomone, 1969; Parker & Szymanski, 1992; Rubin et al., 1984; Sink & Porter, 1978) and private for-profit organizations (Collignon, Barker, & Vencill, 1992; Gilbride, 1993; Lynch & Martin, 1982). Because of its central role in the practice of rehabilitation counseling, placement is an important part of the knowledge base for professional development. The practice of placement generally includes the following activities: contacting and developing ongoing relationships with employers; educating consumers regarding job seeking, resume writing, interviewing, and job selection; collaborating with consumers and employers to make workplace accommodations; and following consumers to ensure satisfaction with their placement. This chapter discusses the history of placement, its role in the rehabilitation process, current issues relevant to the profession, and future directions requiring study.

THE IMPACT OF LEGISLATION ON PLACEMENT

The initial delivery of placement services to people with disabilities can be traced to two pieces of legislation: the Smith-Hughes Act of 1917 (P.L.

64–347) and Soldier Rehabilitation Act of 1918 (P.L. 65–178). These Acts, which supported vocational education and rehabilitation, provided the legislative foundation for today's state–federal partnership. Early legislation mandated vocational education, vocational guidance, occupational adjustment, and placement services. The goal of services was employment: All services had to clearly relate to a feasible vocational goal and an employment outcome.

There were clear social needs responsible for this vocational focus. Dislocated workers were traveling from rural areas to cities without the necessary skills to enter the labor force. Many wounded veterans survived, returning with significant disabilities that limited their employment options. The legislation was not intended to correct some societal wrong or please a vocal interest group. It was intended to use the available human resources efficiently and move the nation into the mainstream of the industrial revolution.

Vocational rehabilitation (VR) service providers formed a professional association, the National Civilian Rehabilitation Conference (now the National Rehabilitation Association), in 1924. Shortly after that, an interest group called the National Vocational Guidance Association was formed within the American Personnel and Guidance Association (now the American Counseling Association). It was not until 1954, with passage of the Vocational Rehabilitation Act Amendments (P.L. 83–565), that these employees were recognized as professional rehabilitation counselors. This Act provided money for training rehabilitation professionals, including counselors. It also supported research and demonstration projects to develop and extend new knowledge. Despite years of developing a professional association and additional years working as rehabilitation providers, it took the 1954 Act to provide the foundation for the profession of vocational rehabilitation counseling.

Shortly after passage of the 1954 Act, debate over the professional role of rehabilitation counselors entered the professional literature. C. H. Patterson (1957, 1966, 1967) argued that professional rehabilitation counselors should provide psychological counseling, whereas less professional rehabilitation coordinators should provide, among other things, placement services. This distinction had little effect on the actual practice of vocational rehabilitation counseling in the public sector. Studies of how VR counselors spent their time suggested they were generalists rather than specialists (Muthard & Salomone, 1969) and performed all the functions C. H. Patterson recommended for counselors and coordinators.

But, as well as professionalizing counselors, the Act professionalized the activity of counseling. After the Act, face-to-face counseling assumed a more important role than other activities until services directly related to placement consumed only a fraction of counselors' time (Vandergoot, 1987; Zadney & James, 1977). Placement is recognized by practitioners as one of the most important areas of competency, but counseling is considered the most important skill (Wright, Leahy, & Shapson, 1987). This leaves rehabilitation counseling and placement, as presently practiced, as separate skill domains.

The Act of 1954 also promoted the expansion of nonprofit rehabilitation facilities as community-based centers for work-adjustment training. During the 1950s and 1960s, these facilities provided services to people with severe disabilities, especially people with developmental and psychiatric disabilities. Facilities were more apt than public agencies to employ specialists for specific tasks. Starr (1982) suggested that this was because they followed a hospital-type organizational structure for service delivery and employed people in more diverse positions. Although public vocational rehabilitation counselors worked as generalists providing all things to all people, facility personnel worked within more tightly defined job descriptions providing only specialized services.

In terms of overall personnel, vocational rehabilitation in both the public and private nonprofit sectors grew tremendously through the 1950s and 1960s. Funding increased, the types of disabilities approved for services increased, and the number of rehabilitation professionals subsequently increased. A growing economy provided more jobs than there were applicants, so the idea of equal employment was widely accepted. People with disabilities came for services, counseling and training were provided, and people found jobs. The one place this was not the case was in facilities where the majority of consumers had severe disabilities. For these people, placement was more difficult. This may be why the movement for placement specialization originated among facility personnel.

On October 9, 1963, Robert Eddy, the manager of handicapped placement services for Goodwill Industries of Chicago, brought together several people who worked as job-placement specialists to form a professional association. Participants in this meeting agreed that placement specialists and the services they provided would be better served by creating a professional division within the National Rehabilitation Association (NRA). This meeting resulted in the formation of the Job Placement Division (JPD) of NRA and recognition of job placement as a specialized profession (Tooman, 1986). The group elected an ad hoc committee that worked to make the division official within the NRA. The division held its first organizational meeting on November 10, 1964, at the NRA Annual Conference in Philadelphia. The first president of JPD was Louis Ortale, who worked for the state Vocational Rehabilitation agency in Des Moines, Iowa.

JPD sought to enhance professionalism through several means. Members were recruited and the role of the division was clarified. JPD established conferences and training programs, including the Louis Ortale Memorial Lecture at the annual NRA conference (he died in 1967 when he was immediate past-president). The forerunner of the *Journal of Job Placement* began as an intradivisional communication device. Finally, the division sought to establish standards and competencies for placement professionals.

The initial professional competencies and standards were proposed by William Usdane, who was employed by the Rehabilitation Services Administration, during his presentation at the fourth Louis Ortale Memorial Lecture in 1973. The lecture included a statement of scope of practice that said placement professionals should be given responsibility for: job development, job solicitation, economic job forecasting, labor market information, job engineering, job placement, and postjob adjustment. From description of the role of placement professionals, the National Rehabilitation Job Placement/Job Development Institute at Drake University was developed to design the competencies for a master's degree based on Usdane's lecture. Howard Traxler, who was director of that program, gave the Ortale Lecture in 1978, laying out competencies and a training agenda for graduate degree programs in placement and rehabilitation counseling.

These competencies remained central to the role of job-placement specialists in public and nonprofit rehabilitation agencies through the 1970s and 1980s. Rehabilitation counselor education programs, still driven by federal funding to prepare people for public-sector jobs, included these competencies in their program requirements, but did not emphasize them. Placement was important, there just were not many people doing it. The people who were supposed to do it put a higher value on providing counseling (Emener & Rubin, 1980; Neely, 1974).

In 1992 consumers sent a new message in the form of the Rehabilitation Act of 1973 as Amended (P.L. 102–569). The consumer involvement mandated by the 1973 Act was important, but employment outcomes needed to be reemphasized. With the 1992 reauthorization, the initial focus of vocational rehabilitation—employment—had returned to the central position it held at the beginning of the century. Employment remained the fundamental purpose of disability services, but consumers' expectations had changed over 70 years. Consumers expected to be actively involved in a rehabilitation process that assisted them in achieving their own personal and career goals. They also expected a high standard of quality in the services and outcomes they received from vocational rehabilitation.

PRIVATE REHABILITATION

Placement as a cluster of professional activities evolved in a sector of the workforce that until recently was separate from public and nonprofit vocational rehabilitation. This other sector is the private for-profit sector that serves industrially injured workers. The increasing cost of medical care and workers' compensation insurance gave rise to private (insurance) rehabilitation in the mid-1970s. Growick (1993) stated that rehabilitation and workers' compensation were "made for each other" because both viewed return to work for people with disabilities (albeit for different reasons) as their primary goal.

Because private for-profit rehabilitation needed to meet the needs of *both* employers and people with disabilities, it traditionally focused more on employment and return to work than did public rehabilitation (Collignon, Barker, & Vencill, 1992; Gilbride, 1993; Gilbride, Connolly & Stensrud, 1990; Matkin, 1983b, 1987). During the late 1970s and early 1980s, there was a movement toward state-legislated rehabilitation as states viewed private rehabilitation as a cost-effective way to help injured workers return to work.

In recent years, however, there has been a major reduction in mandatory rehabilitation services for people with work-related injuries (Lui, 1993). Spiraling costs of workers' compensation insurance provided impetus for many state legislatures to repeal the mandatory rehabilitation provisions of their workers' compensation systems (e.g. Colorado, Kansas, Minnesota) or to dramatically constrain the provision of rehabilitation services (e.g. California). At least part of this backlash was a result of private rehabilitation providers' inadequate documentation of their effectiveness in returning injured workers to employment (California

Workers' Compensation Institute, 1991; Washburn, 1992). The continued use of rehabilitation in nonmandatory states and the limited extant empirical data suggest, however, that appropriate rehabilitation services often are successful at putting injured workers back on the job while saving employers money (Collignon et al., 1992; Growick 1993).

Private for-profit rehabilitation, like private nonprofit rehabilitation, held placement as a central component of the service delivery system. Structurally, for-profit rehabilitation was more like public rehabilitation in that a single counselor managed a single case (but much smaller total case load) from beginning to end. In the case of for-profit rehabilitation, however, payment mechanisms made employment outcomes more critical than in public rehabilitation and careful documenting of activities less important (Growick, 1993).

Public rehabilitation agencies provided involvement-oriented counseling to people with disabilities but offered few placement services. Private nonprofit rehabilitation agencies provided a specific focus on placement services primarily to people with severe disabilities but low compensation limited the professionalization of the industry. Private for-profit rehabilitation companies focused on placement but the intense outcome orientation resulted in limited documentation of effectiveness. Each sector evolved somewhat separately and with its own strengths and weaknesses. The question became: How do we attain the focus of private nonprofit rehabilitation, the documentation capabilities of public rehabilitation, and the outcome orientation of private for-profit rehabilitation? No one asked this question because until recently there were few incentives to do so.

CURRENT TRENDS

In the mid-1990s, federal budget deficits, concern over the size and influence of the federal government, and questions about the effectiveness of the state–federal Vocational Rehabilitation program (General Accounting Office, 1993), led to a general rethinking regarding the manner in which public vocational rehabilitation services were delivered. Although the Rehabilitation Act amendments of 1992 (P.L. 102-569) again underscored the centrality of employment outcomes and Rehabilitation Services Administration (RSA) directives discussed "quality placements," many consumer groups and policy-makers remained skeptical. Their input to state plans and federal legislation focused on having these concerns addressed by rehabilitation providers. In response, new service delivery models such as "block grants" and "one-stop shopping" for employment services were explored.

The current policy debate over block grants and one-stop shopping reflects three current policy themes: states' rights (devolution), market forces (vouchers), and workforce development areas (service integration). From the beginning of civilian rehabilitation, tension existed between states and the federal government regarding roles and responsibilities for assisting people with disabilities. Over the past 75 years the federal government has increasingly assumed a greater percentage of the cost for rehabilitation services while concurrently exerting more control over how those services were delivered. The current trend toward block grants and one stop-shopping clearly reflects an attempt to rebalance the state/federal relationship.

The second issue, vouchers, represents a profound break with the entire history of public rehabilitation. Vouchers promise to offer maximum consumer choice because people would be allowed to go to any qualified provider and purchase services. Proponents of vouchers assert that market forces will improve services and enhance outcomes. The envisioned outcomes are to "render the individuals employable and achieve an employment outcome" (Sec 104, i, Proposed Careers Act). If passed, this law will again solidify placement as the *raison d'être* for the vocational rehabilitation profession but, for the first time, services will be provided within a competitive, market-driven environment. Public rehabilitation counselors would be required to compete with other providers for vouchers.

The third factor, integrated workforce development areas, offers rehabilitation professionals the opportunity to reclaim the original mandate of the profession. It does so by addressing many of the same needs identified in 1918, and by weaving together all the government agencies that address the same concerns. The mandate: understanding, collaborating with, and integrating people with disabilities into the workforce, has remained much the same for 80 years, but the way each era shaped service delivery systems has varied. Rehabilitation counseling in its present form developed because the new industrialized labor market was complex and not readily negotiated by a person with a disability without extensive assistance. Despite this, the accepted knowledge base of the rehabilitation profession developed asymmetrically. Although knowledge about people with disabilities and the services they require has improved, little growth or evolution has occurred in the profession's understanding of labor market trends and the needs of employers. This has resulted in rehabilitation plans often being unresponsive to labor market data and employer needs (Gilbride & Burr, 1993). Further, rehabilitation professionals have been unable to document that they actually improve the financial status of even their successful clients (General Accounting Office, 1993). Beyond this, employers tend to view rehabilitation agencies as not cost effective (Gilbride & Stensrud, 1993).

The current situation necessitates some form of change within the rehabilitation profession, especially as it pertains to placement. The profession, however, has apparently neglected placement and there are no clear standards of performance or few empirically derived guides to effective practice. In a time when the profession's existence is challenged because it does not deliver adequate employment outcomes, little is know about how to improve this situation. What is known is that various models of placement have been developed and applied by practitioners. The utility of these models is largely untested. Current events may make many of them obsolete before they are allowed to demonstrate their effectiveness.

MODELS OF PLACEMENT

A comprehensive review of different models of placement was provided by Gilbride, Stensrud, and Johnson (1994). They divided placement models into two general categories: traditional models and new models. Traditional models are those that were used most often over the past decade and include counselor-provided placement, placement-specialist services, contracted services, and supported employment. New models are those that are experimental or derived from recent labor-market factors. These include marketing, team networking/mentoring, and demand-side placement.

Historically, traditional models of placement were derived from federal legislation. The two most common models have been vocational rehabilitation counselor-provided services and placement-professional-provided services. Both approaches offer the same services, which are similar to those described by Usdane in 1973. These services include job-seeking skills (clarification of job goals, preparation of resumés and portfolios, job-hunting strategies, interviewing skills, and job-search support), and employer development (contacting employers, matching employers with consumers, and providing postplacement follow-up). These activities account for most of the placement services provided to rehabilitation consumers.

Contracting for placement services has been used for several years in different forms. One form of contracted services is Projects with Industry (PWI), funded by legislation in 1968. In this approach, placement is contracted with organizations that are administered by employer councils. Such an approach moves placement responsibility closer to employers and involves them as collaborators in the rehabilitation process (Baumann, 1986; Kaplan & Hammond, 1982). PWIs exist as separate corporate entities that form a bridge between rehabilitation providers and employers. Because they are part provider and part employer, they understand the needs and concerns of both, thus making transition to work more effective. Contracting also can be used directly by rehabilitation agencies to secure outside entities that provide direct placement services. These services can be provided by any entity that markets itself as having placement capabilities, PWIs, nonprofit agencies, for-profit companies, or self-employed individuals. Because placement specialists have no professional credentialing process, there are no clear criteria that can be used to determine who is suitable to provide these services nor any standard compensation for the service.

Supported employment was authorized by the 1986 Amendments to the Rehabilitation Act (PL 99–506). Supported employment varies from other traditional models in that it applies a "place and train" approach rather than a "train and place" approach. This model is used most often for consumers with significant disabilities. Supported employees are assisted to secure employment with a cooperating business. On-site training and support are provided to the employee by a job coach who helps the employee learn how to do the job and how to function in different work roles. Job coaches may also work with employers to help them develop the capacity to effectively assimilate the supported employee into the workforce.

New models have emerged that supplement these traditional services. The new models differ from traditional ones in that the new ones derived from changes in the labor market rather than changes in federal legislation. New placement models include marketing, team networking/mentoring, and demand-side placement.

The marketing model of placement derived in large part from the efforts of the Job Placement Division of NRA. Members of JPD, in cooperation with some Regional Rehabilitation Continuing Education Programs and Drake University disseminated a marketing model of placement in the early and mid-1980s. This model was designed to go beyond the traditional sales calls made by job developers and create lasting relationships between placement specialists and employers. It offered the potential for rehabilitation personnel to target companies likely to employ people with disabilities and build long-term relationships that were in the best interests of consumers and employers. This was the first model to recognize that placement has two equally important clients: rehabilitation consumers and employers. Each has needs and expectations. Placement specialists who can effectively address the needs and expectations of both clients will provide quality placements. They also will open opportunities for future consumers to easily find jobs with those satisfied employers.

Team networking/mentoring is a model of placement that relies on current innovations in communication technology. In this approach, placement personnel create support networks comprised of employees with disabilities and employers who have successfully accommodated employees with disabilities. These people form a support network for consumers selecting employment (or training) and employers who are open to hiring people with disabilities but are uncertain how to do so effectively. Networked teams are linked via video or audio conferencing, the Internet, or some other distance medium. This approach uses untapped resources and allows the development of natural support networks, which should maintain themselves for years after the placement process is complete.

Demand-side placement recognizes that employers are the people most directly responsible for employing people with disabilities. Placement is seen as a consulting relationship with employers that increases their enthusiasm for hiring people with disabilities (Gilbride & Stensrud, 1992). As employers learn how to easily select and accommodate qualified applicants with disabilities, and as they learn to trust rehabilitation personnel as resources for their business, they should be more willing and better able to select people on the basis of job-related competence. Demand-side placement rests on the assumption that employment settings have a far greater need to be rehabilitated than do people with disabilities.

There is little empirical data concerning any of these models except supported employment. For this reason, the utility of each is uncertain. Gilbride et al., (1994) hypothesized that each model should be viewed as being appropriate in certain situations. They proposed that placement strategies should consider the situation in which it will be practiced. They summarized the situation-specific utility of each models as follows:

Counselor Provided Placement

This model may be most appropriate when

- Counselors have smaller case loads
- Clients require formal training or education, and some placement will be coordinated by the training program
- Rehabilitation counselors have placement training and have weekly time scheduled for employer development
- Clients live in rural areas in which other services are not available
- There are few employers available in the area
- Counselors have special case loads (i.e., learning disabilities, psychiatric disabilities)
- Placement may involve establishing self-employment, purchasing equipment, and subsequent technical assistance

Placement Specialist Provided

This model may be most appropriate when

- The specialist works from a large centralized office with a steady influx of placement-ready clients
- The area has a number of employers and varied industries
- The placement professional is specifically trained in placement and employer development
- Clients are geographically clustered

Contracted Placement

This model may be most appropriate when
- Rehabilitation counselors have large case loads
- There are well-trained rehabilitation professionals in the private sector with whom to contract

- VR agencies do not have adequate personnel to engage in consistent and ongoing employer development
- Referrals are made to services specializing in serving a specific group of consumers (such as clubhouses)

Supported Employment

This model may be most appropriate when

- Case loads consist of clients with severe disabilities
- Transition assistance is coordinated among rehabilitation and educational programs.
- Rehabilitation professionals have the capacity to train and supervise paraprofessionals, and provide employer development
- Ongoing funds and services are available to support clients postplacement

Marketing

This model may be most appropriate when

- Employers are generally not aware of rehabilitation services
- There is a major commitment of time, resources, and personnel by the agency to placement
- There are a number of varied businesses and industries in the area

Team Networking/Mentoring

This model may be most appropriate when

- There is at least a moderate number of people with disabilities in the area who are employed and willing to volunteer time
- Most employers in the area are inexperienced at hiring people with disabilities
- Computer technology is available to network members and

employers
- Rehabilitation professionals are trained in project management
- Few formal agencies or services are available in the area
- Clients require peer role models that help them develop appropriate vocational behaviors

Demand-Side Placement

This model may be most appropriate when

- A large number of employers are forced by events such as government regulation to consider employing people with disabilities
- There is a high demand for trained employees and an inadequate supply of applicants in the local market
- Employers are unfamiliar with hiring workers with disabilities, so they need access to technology and assistance in recruitment and accommodation
- Rehabilitation professionals are trained as business consultants and placement specialists
- There is a potential for a large and varied supply of placement-ready clients (Gilbride et al., 1994, pp. 229–230)

The practice of placement has advanced substantially since its origin in the early 20th century. Although placement was initially a simple train-and-place activity, innovative approaches are improving this approach in several ways. Place-and-train approaches are making better use of work-site-based education as a way to assist people with significant disabilities to develop work skills. Employer development has evolved to include approaches that offer innovative ways to involve employers in placement, build relationships between business and placement specialists, and show companies how they can benefit from the consulting expertise of rehabilitation personnel. These innovations offer promise in improving employment outcomes, consumer and employer satisfaction with rehabilitation services, and the impact of rehabilitation on society.

There is an unfortunate lack of adequate empirical research on different placement models which makes it difficult to determine how best to structure services. Despite the promise of recent innovations, too little is known about which model works best with specific consumers in specific labor markets. Gilbride et al., (1994) proposed an "aptitude-treatment interaction" (ATI) approach to assess placement models. This research strategy would compare different models in specific consumer–labor market combinations to determine the situation-specific effectiveness of each. From this research, rehabilitation counselors and placement professionals could have better information on which to base rehabilitation plans and employer development strategies.

Millington et al. (Millington, Asner, Linkowski, & Der-Stepian, 1996; Millington, Szymanski, & Johnston-Rodriguez, 1995) proposed a method for conceptualizing placement from the perspective of employers. This approach derived from the work of Vandergoot (1987, 1992) and extended his emphasis on rehabilitation professionals as "labor market intermediaries."

In the employer-focused model, "the employer" plays a management role within a business organization that is responsible for maximizing the productivity of the business' labor resources (Sartain & Baker, 1978). Employers manage change in the workforce or the marketplace through planning functions. They manage worker relationships through organizing functions, such as establishing a formal structure for the organization. They motivate workers to perform in predetermined ways through directing or leadership functions. They manage process and product standards through control functions. Most central to placement, employers manage the movement of applicants into the business organization, and the movement of workers within the business organization through staffing functions (Millington, Asner et al., 1996).

The staffing function includes recruitment, selection, and career development and support. Staffing activities are initiated when the employer perceives a long or short range labor need (Meyer & Donaho, 1979). This projection is based on analyses of market trends, available technologies, cost per hire, vacancy rates and turnover patterns within the organization. Once the need has been assessed and the staffing objective defined, the employer implements a selection process that recruits, screens, and hires applicants. Before external employment selection, managers look for other ways to use existing resources, consolidate work, automate activities, and make internal transfers.

The purpose of recruitment is to attract a pool of applicants who have self-selected the company based on meaningful criteria. Factors that affect recruitment are labor markets targeted for recruitment, demand for labor, budget constraints, immediacy of results, number of applicants desired, and company affirmative-action goals. Employers have two basic "intervention" strategies available in planning recruitment efforts: they can diversify the structure of the job, making it more flexible to accommodate target markets; or they can differentiate the avenues for deseminating information (advertising). Job-diversity strategies include flex time, telecommuting and home-based work, temporary employment, supplemental workforces, work sharing, and independent contracting (Arthur, 1991). Differentiating advertisement strategies include in-house job posting (Gutteridge, Leibowitz, & Shore, 1993), word-of-mouth, school recruitment, job fairs, open house, broad commercial media (want ads, radio, television) (Half, 1985), market-specific media (trade journals, professional publications), and private and governmental agencies.

The purpose of screening is to eliminate the "false positives" in the most economical way possible. Screening is not always formally defined in the selection process. It becomes necessary to formalize screening when the number of applicants in the recruitment pool presents an unacceptably high drain on the employer's resources. Because the objective is to expediently thin the applicant pool, screening criteria are negatively weighted and the decision-making process is kept simple. Screening strategies include structured phone interviews, application or resumé review, reference checks, and objective testing (Swan, 1989).

The purpose of hiring is to negotiate the best labor investment from the remaining applicants. Because the objective is to make thoughtful distinctions between desirable candidates, the criteria are generally positively weighted, and the process is more complex. The most prevalent method of hiring is the interview. Interviews are often centered around three concerns: ability to do the job, motivation, and manageability (Yate, 1987). Interviews may be structured or informal. In practice, interviews tend to be rather informal, and the decision process is relegated to subjective interpretation of the interviewer. Most hiring decisions are made by people conducting interviews only one or two times per year, thus making decision making less valid (Half, 1985).

When the applicants have been ranked according to desirability, the employer will approach the most desirable candidate and negotiate the close. This strategy is the employer's attempt to make the job attractive to the applicant, within the economic considerations of the business. Employers have offering strategies and may negotiate salary, perks, moving expenses, and other incentives (Wendover, 1989).

The final staffing function is career development and support. This function is controlled by a different set of decision-making and intervention strategies. By the time the employee enters the worksite, the organization has invested a considerable amount of resources and has established certain expectations for performance. Career development practices include training and development, job matching, and individual counseling (Gutteridge, Leibowitz, & Shore, 1993). Systems of rewards, in-house training and orientation programs are generally seen as effective interventions available to the employer that increase the productivity of their workers (Gutteridge et al., 1993).

This staffing knowledge base can improve our understanding of how rehabilitation professionals can effectively prepare consumers for employment. For example, the initial experiences of new workers suggest specific placement services that could improve job selection and retention. Cox (1993) found that new hires must integrate into the work culture via formal and informal socialization processes. Feldman (1981) identified three factors that enhance organizational socialization: developing work abilities, engaging in appropriate work role behaviors, and acquiring the values and beliefs of the workplace culture. Given this information, these would be the points at which placement efforts could design effective interventions. Rehabilitation placement plans, using one of several different placement models, could identify characteristics unique to an organization's culture and systematically prepare consumers to perform specific essential functions, demonstrate specific work-role behaviors, and do so in organizations whose values and beliefs are consistent with those of the consumer.

This information also demonstrates the importance of good consumer–employer matches. If, for example, the values of a consumer and an employer are inconsistent, we may be of better service by looking elsewhere for a placement rather than promoting a match that will lead to dissatisfaction by either client. Especially when some employers are less open to diversity, this matching of values and beliefs seems important for successful placements (Stensrud & Gilbride, 1994).

By combining the literature on rehabilitation placement and the literature on employer selection, new models and theories of placement should evolve. Research that tests these factors is critical if we are to improve our understanding of the placement process and deliver the employment outcomes expected by consumers and legislators.

EDUCATION FOR PLACEMENT COMPETENCIES

Neither of the two major accrediting bodies that affect rehabilitation recognize placement specialists as having independent professional status.

The Council on Rehabilitation Education (CORE), which accredits rehabilitation counselor education programs, and the Commission on Rehabilitation Counselor Certification (CCRC), which accredits individuals, both recognize rehabilitation counselors but not placement specialists. Both CORE and CRC include placement competencies in their evaluation criteria, which recognizes its importance for rehabilitation counselors. But the lack of any credentialing mechanisms has limited the growth of placement as a separate profession. Only a few graduate programs in the country offer education in placement as a specialization. This also limits the growth of the profession because few people with recognized graduate degrees in placement are available to work in rehabilitation.

Rehabilitation counselor education programs, although they include placement competencies in their curricula, often provide only one class on the subject during the coursework for a 2-year degree. This may not leave students with much understanding of how placement is done or how they can apply various placement strategies in their work as rehabilitation counselors. Rehabilitation educators without graduate degrees in rehabilitation (roughly 25% of all faculty) indicate they feel less competent to teach content related to placement (Ebener, Berven, & Wright, 1993). This also limits students' possible expertise in placement.

PLACEMENT IN THE FUTURE

The 1992 Reauthorization of the Rehabilitation Act resulted in an increased interest in placement. Current trends such as block grants, vouchering, and one-stop shopping also can be expected to expand interest in placement services. Each of these trends can be expected to increase the emphasis on employment as an outcome of rehabilitation. To the extent that this is the case, one can expect greater need for placement education and research among rehabilitation professions.

However governmental legislation proceeds, certain placement competencies will remain critical for rehabilitation professionals. Many of these, such as occupational and labor-market information, job analysis, job modification and restructuring, job-placement strategies, understanding employers, and client job-seeking and job-retention skills development (Szymanski, Linkowski, Leahy, Diamond, & Thoreson, 1993) already are known. Others will emerge as further research is conducted on the placement process.

CHAPTER 14

Systematic Practice: Case and Caseload Management

Jack L. Cassell, S. Wayne Mulkey, and Carrie Engen

T he practice of rehabilitation counseling rests on the confluence of two professional forces: counseling and management. *Systematic practice* by a professional in this arena is the result of these two forces working in synergy. No single professional force can be said to predominate, as synergy is only established through concepts and practice surrounding a "balance" principle. To espouse a "one foundation" profession is tantamount to preaching without a gospel or practicing without a guiding credo.

Although counseling and management come with equal forces directed toward building a competent professional practice, this chapter is confined to elaborations on the exposition of only the management force of the synergy. The counseling force of the synergy was thoroughly detailed in an earlier chapter. The systematic practice of rehabilitation counseling, then, is anchored in several elements and skills within a management paradigm. As noted by Cassell and Mulkey (1985) "it is evident that even *the most counseling-oriented rehabilitation practitioner cannot survive without implementation of at least minimal skills in management"* (p. xiv).

THE PARADIGM

The practice of rehabilitation caseload management (CLM) is based on a five-point model: boundary definitions (defines actions, micromanagement, macromanagement); skill clusters (planning, organizing, coordinating, directing, controlling); personal control (drives the system); action decisions (set objectives, proactive, outcome focus); and a systems approach (politico-mandated). When regularly practiced actions consistently emanate from these defining areas, the rehabilitation professional will be an effective caseload manager. This paradigm relies on several premises. Clearly, rehabilitation practitioners must:

- develop and become cognizant of the operational definitions that guide their job performance;
- develop competent responses in basic skill clusters that form the nucleus of a management approach dealing with a complex caseload of persons with disabilities;
- develop and rely on an internal referent for personal control when attempting to keep job parameters within manageable limits;
- become adept at issuing progressive, proactive action decisions that enhance success with stated objectives and projected outcomes; and
- develop a systems mentality for keeping complex arrays of information and data under management control.

BOUNDARY DEFINITIONS

Boundary Definitions are terms and concepts that provide a quality of comprehension, wholeness and objectivity to systematic practice. These terms provide a basic grounding on which to guide one's present understanding of practices and that enhance direction for ongoing development. Every individual in every profession creates and operates from sets and subsets of definitions. Personal and professional definitions of identity and purpose set psychological conditions that translate into boundaries and limitations that can facilitate or hinder outcomes. That is to say, because everyone at all times is forced to operate from a wide gamut of definitions, the kinds of definitions held by individuals has a direct influence on actions.

Consequently, a professional guided by accurate, unambiguous, descriptive definitions is much more likely to produce higher levels of performance. Conversely, ambiguous, negative-laden, incomplete definitions will produce a confused and stressed professional whose performance shall be diminished.

Manager

Rehabilitation counselors are managers even though many do not think of themselves as managers. Reeves (1994) notes there are managers without titles, and states, "You may not think of what you do as 'managing'. But if you are working through other people to achieve a purpose or goal, you are managing" (p.4). Indeed, at one time in history, the rehabilitation practitioner was titled a "rehabilitation administrator" rather than a counselor.

This definition or lack of it can be problematic. There is a premise in the field of management: if you do not *think* like a manager, you cannot *act* like a manager. Rehabilitation professionals who resist, repudiate, and expunge a management definition for themselves will experience system reprimands, practice disarray, and work force disharmony. Regardless, systematic practice will be unlikely.

Rehabilitation practitioners are counselors *and* managers (Cassell & Mulkey, 1985). This "two hat" philosophy is vital to developing a complete, systematic approach to practice. For example, various case management functions would emerge from the counseling role, whereas CLM functions essentially emanate from a managing role (Greenwood, 1992). The appropriate merging of "counseling" and "managing" skills results in outcomes that can be measured as actual performance.

Proactive Versus Reactive

In a broad sense, one's practice can be viewed as a dichotomy of actions stemming from a proactive or a reactive position. A person operating from a reactive definition would likely be low in initiative, nonanticipatory, and experience low personal control over the various aspects of managing a caseload. Such a person is likely to be stuck in a procrastinating mode.

The practitioner who operates from a proactive definition will likely be one who anticipates problems and deals with them before they become crises. A proactive definition produces a professional who is assertive, in charge, a risk-taker, and, wherever possible, a problem preventer (as opposed to merely a problem solver).

Case Management

Case management (CM) can be both a strategy and a philosophy. As a strategy, CM encompasses specific actions practiced by professionals in the public and private sectors. Professionals in both arenas of practice are mandated to focus on each individual case in order to reach an optimum level of adjustment for the consumer and satisfy other vested interests. As a philosophy, CM takes on differing qualities. Again, for both arenas, the basic regard for the consumer and support entities are paramount. For the public-sector professional, however, CM comes within the purview of caseload management practices. In fact, this professional is regarded as a caseload manager. In the private sector, CM is regarded as the orienting of professional practice, and this individual is generally referred to as a case manager. Although this section provides a focus on CM in the private sector, much of the noted information also pertains to the public-sector professional.

Case management emerged as a practice in the early 1900s (Case Management Society of America, 1995). Public health nurses and social workers who coordinated services through the public health sector are considered to be the early providers of case management services. The role of the case manager has evolved over time. Currently, case management services are provided by professionals trained in a variety of professions in a myriad of different practice settings.

In 1993, the Certified Case Manager (CCM) credential was introduced into the arena of case management, sponsored by the Certification of Insurance Rehabilitation Specialists Commission (CIRSC). At its 1996 Annual Meeting, the CIRSC approved a change of name for the Commission to Certification of Disability Management Specialists Commission (CDMSC). This, in turn, changed the name of the certification, formerly known as CIRS to Certified Disability Management Specialist (CDMS). The philosophy of case management as reported in the CCM Certification Guide is as follows:

Case management is not a profession in itself, but an area of practice within one's profession. Its underlying premise is that when an individual reached the optimum level of wellness and functional capability, everyone benefits: the individuals being served, their support systems, the health care delivery systems, and the various reimbursement sources. Case management serves as a means for achieving client wellness and autonomy through advocacy, communication, education, identification of services resources, and service facilitation. The case manager helps identify appropriate providers and facilities throughout the continuum of services, while ensuring that available resources are being used in a timely and cost-effective manner in order to obtain optimum value for both the client and the reimbursement source. Case management services are best offered in a climate that allows direct communication between the case manager, the client, and appropriate service personnel, in order to optimize the outcome for all concerned. Certification determines that the case manager possesses the education, skills, and experience required to render appropriate services based on sound principles of practice.

A basic definition of case management provided by the National Case Management Task Force is reported by Mullahy (1995):

> Case management is a collaborative process which assesses, plans, implements, coordinates, monitors and evaluates the options and services to meet an individual's health needs, using communication and available resources to promote quality, cost effective outcomes. (p. 9)

Case management is a highly effective strategy that assists in coordinating the needs of the consumer with the available resources in order to maximize the outcome for the consumer and effectively manage costs. The case manager should facilitate communication between all members of the treatment team, the consumer and support system, and the payer in order to minimize the fragmentation inherent in any delivery system, avoid duplication of services and waste in the system, and involve the consumer/support system in all decisions made on their behalf. The case manager is an advocate for the consumer as well as the payer (in some practice settings) in order to facilitate a win–win situation for the consumer, the treatment team, and the payer. The case manager is the link between the consumer and all other members of the delivery system involved in the care of that individual.

Goals of case management are reported by the Case Management Society of America (1995) in The Standards of Practice for Case Management as follows:

- Through early assessment, ensure that services are generated in a timely and cost-effective manner.

- Assist clients to achieve an optimal level of wellness and function by facilitating timely and appropriate health services.
- Assist clients to appropriately self-direct care, self-advocate and make decisions to the degree possible.
- Maintain cost effectiveness in the provision of health services.
- Appropriate expenditure of claims dollars and timely claim determinations.
- Enhance employee productivity, satisfaction and retention, when applicable. (p. 10)

The case management process, used to facilitate these goals, includes the following elements.

Case identification and selection is the first element. This process constitutes identifying individuals who will benefit from case management.

An in-depth *objective assessment* of the individual's needs is the next step for the case manager. Assessment areas may include: physical, psychosocial, functional, financial, spiritual, environmental, vocational, support systems, health expectations of the consumer, potential capabilities, resources, treatment options, prognosis, goals, and provider options.

Development of the plan of care, utilizing communication with the treatment team, the consumer and the payer, helps the case manager identify opportunities for effective intervention whereby consumer outcome can be positively influenced.

Implementation of the plan of care is a collaborative process as well. All elements of the case management team involved with the consumer need to be aware of the plan of care and what their roles are within the plan. The case manager is the facilitator, making sure that the rehabilitation plan is implemented in the most efficient way.

After the treatment plan is implemented, *monitoring and reevaluation of the plan of care* is ongoing. The case manager is continually evaluating the quality of care, the appropriate service and product delivery, and the impact of the treatment plan on the consumer and support system. The case manager must continuously evaluate whether the goals of the treatment plan (consumer) are being achieved and/or if the goals remain appropriate and realistic. The case manager must also assist with any revision to the treatment plan in conjunction with the treatment team and the consumer if the outcome or progress is not as anticipated, as well as provide support and any additional resources to the consumer and support system.

Within a case management perspective, goal-setting initiatives, objective setting, and process actions are generally micro-management specific.

Case management is characterized, for example, by supervising a client/patient appointment, arranging a service, and dealing with a customer's reservations/complaints/fears. Taking a particular case to satisfactory conclusions for all concerned is the end result sought by a case management process. Mullahy (1995) notes that the process of case management has at least eight stages:

1. case finding and targeting,
2. gathering and assessing information,
3. planning,
4. reporting,
5. obtaining approval,
6. coordination or putting the plan into action,
7. follow-up, and
8. evaluation.

Evaluation of the response of the consumer to the services and products delivered is the last essential element in the process of case management. Effectiveness of the plan of care, quality of service delivery, quality of providers, attainment of the goals of the consumer, appropriate resource allocation and quality-of-life improvements should be considered when evaluating a case. The outcome of the case should be measured against the case management goals, which are identified with the consumer, support system, and treatment team before the care plan is initiated.

Within the present context, skills directed toward case record management (Holmes & Karst, 1989) are also representative of a micro-management perspective. In this instance, "the case record has the important role of representing the client in the client's absence" (Holmes & Karst, 1989, p. 36). As the rehabilitation professional consistently maintains each case record and draws on it to ascertain consumers needs, the results reflect the effectiveness of the counseling methods that have been applied at a particular point in the rehabilitation process.

In summary, key concepts characterizing case management practice for the case manager in the private sector include:

- the focus on individuals, moving them through the system, coordinating service delivery to ensure that the goals of the individual are met;
- support and empowerment of the individual; and
- accountability for the outcome identified and consumer satisfaction involved in a single case.

Caseload Management

Definitions of caseload management are not replete. Some have ventured forward to define caseload management as being distinct from case management (Cassell & Mulkey, 1985; Gaines, 1979; Riggar & Patrick, 1984; Willey, 1978). For our purposes, caseload management can be defined as the systematic process of organizing, planning, coordinating, directing, and controlling for effective and efficient counselor and manager decision making to enhance a proactive practice. Indeed, CLM is a *process*. There are beginning stages, mid-stages, and ending stages. Beginning stages involve, for example, casefinding, fact finding, and eligibility determination. Mid-stages involve service provision, whereas case closure activities take place in the end stages. These aspects are true for nonprofit and private-for-profit rehabilitation practices; often, however, the actual tasks and duties differ. CLM involves application of at least the five listed management functions. Effective CLM is achieved through *counselor* and *manager* role interactions resulting in decision-making activity.

Henke, Connolly, and Cox (1975) described CLM without defining it. Their description of CLM reads:

> . . . how to work with more than one case at a time, how to select which case to work with, how to move from one case to another, how to establish a system to insure movement of all cases, and how to meet the objectives one has established, in terms of numbers served. (p. 218)

Contrary to some conceptualizations (e.g., Greenwood, 1992), case management is developed within the larger context of caseload management, not vice versa. This misunderstanding of case and caseload management extends to a larger scope and is perpetuated in some education/training arenas. Cassell and Mulkey (1992) surveyed the catalog-listed course offerings of Council on Rehabilitation Education (CORE) approved rehabilitation counselor education programs in the nation regarding the inclusion of CLM in their basic curricula. Strikingly, the finding revealed that less than 2% of the programs had a course devoted to CLM. Many reported CLM concepts were subsumed in case management instruction. Case management courses were available in 39% of the programs. If these findings represent instructional reality, graduates entering the field are likely doing so without the benefit of an orientation to systematic practice. To reiterate, CLM is the gestalt; case management is a process part within caseload management. The caseload manager, then, draws from successes in dealing with case management parts to achieve levels of outcomes.

The broader scope of CLM is evident when one considers that CLM involves a macro-management perspective dealing with multifarious, related elements. For example, related elements focus on case development (Szufnarowski, 1972), multicultural issues (Sheppard, Bunton, Menifee, & Rocha, 1995), and case management (Riggar & Patrick, 1984).

In summary, key concepts characterizing caseload management practice for the rehabilitation counselor include:

- the focus on the total caseload, the relationship and issues between and among the various cases,
- coordinating counselor practices with consumer and support service demands,
- coordinating counselor practices with agency/organization policies and procedures,
- taking multiple cases to logical conclusions in a timely manner, and
- accountability for outcome measures based on organizational standards and goals.

SKILL CLUSTERS

Skill clusters are patterns of actions that revolve around central themes or axes. A skill, of course, is a learned ability for doing something in a competent manner. Often the execution of one skill relies on another prerequisite skill. Thus, skills often occur in clusters, each skill relating to the other. Each cluster gathers together sets of specific actions that the caseload manager relies on for consistency of personal practices and for fulfilling organization standards. For managers of caseloads there are five major clusters: planning, organizing, coordinating, directing, and controlling.

Planning

Planning skills assist the caseload manager in anticipating future demands and help guard against the exogenous influences that interfere with daily efforts to produce desired outcomes. Webber (1975) declares the rationale for planning, "is not to show how precisely we can predict the future, but rather to uncover the things we must do today in order to have a future" (p. 268). Being in charge of the future (in a management sense) begins with good planning skills today.

Planning is intrasystemic. This means planning takes on its own system properties. Planning must be approached in a systematic way. Planning is neither ordinary insight nor foresight. The complete caseload manager is one who is adept at taking somewhat obscure or very incomplete information, then anticipating future developments of a case through "best bet" hypotheses or guesses. There are numerous planning methods, techniques, or skills. Several are listed below.

Skill One: Use a calendar

Consistently use a calendar or scheduling device. A rehabilitation practitioner is confronted with a multitude of elements and variables to keep within satisfactory operating limits (after all, this is what management is about). Therefore, a calendar of events is essential to observe and track the development of a case. Calendars or scheduling devices can follow the typical diary system using a week-at-a-glance notebook or the more sophisticated computer software available today. The Tickler System mentioned later is a planning method.

Skill Two: Use anticipatory decision making

Ackoff (1970) affirms that planning is anticipatory decision making. This skill assures the professional a future position of control and a higher level of ability to enact the proposed plans. Thus, anticipatory decision making is a crucial stimulus to readying the professional for making decisions and acting on them.

Skill Three: Make a habit of planning

Planning done daily and at the same time each day establishes consistency of actions. Thus, habitual planning takes on energizing characteristics that systematically stimulates a caseload manager into do-it-now responding. Like any habit, time and consistency are the key factors for building a response pattern that will withstand the onslaught of other "priority thieves." The skilled practitioner will soon be adept at utilizing the habits of successful people (Covey, 1989).

Skill Four: Follow strategic planning

Planning is strategy, not mere foresight. Strategy implies a weighing of best-bet alternatives and invoking actions to satisfy systematic intentions.

Planning has long been a basic strategy for managers. Recently the focus has become "strategic" planning (e.g. Cook & Fritts, 1994; Gibson & Mazur, 1995; Luther, 1995; Schoemaker, 1995; Tombazian, 1994), which means planning that is critical, vital, crucial, and essential. Webber (1975), prophetically, recognizes that dreams and visions are important to planning. Thus, a sense of where the caseload is and where one should be with it, is a part of strategic planning. An extension to this last perspective is Ackoff's (1970) contention that planning is anticipatory decision making. Although projected primarily on an organizational level, the strategic-planning process is applicable to the individual process as well. The steps projected for the individual level are (1) develop a personal vision; (2) write assumptions that shape a caseload; (3) from the assumptions list, state issues facing a caseload; (4) state objectives you want to achieve; (5) develop measures for objectives; and (6) choose strategies to satisfy objectives.

Finally, systemic planning requires the perspective that a common purpose exists among the activities to be accomplished in CLM. The activities are interlinked by a personal, professional, and an organizational philosophy of service to all concerns in a timely fashion. Planning is intrinsically linked with goal-setting activities. Remember, planning is not one goal, but is instead a direction. It is a common direction in which the caseload manager, the consumer, and the program are moving. Planning is not the setting of one plan, but the conscious selection of successive plans, one building inherently on the other.

Organizing

The cluster of skills involved in organizing all have a central focus of establishing the next priority to engage the caseload manager. The intersystemic nature of the five skill clusters (i.e., planning, organizing, coordinating, directing, and controlling) is evident when one considers the very basic question that must be posed for the organizing function of management. That question is, "What are the activities that must be accomplished?" This question is, of course, answered through the enumerations from the planning stage (e.g., through a constructed list of activities to be accomplished).

Organizing, then, is priority setting. How chaotic it would be for a caseload manager to complete an activity and not have a next priority work activity. How self-deceiving and stress producing it is for caseload managers to be working on an activity a very short time, switch to another set of actions, switch again a few minutes later, all the while falsely assessing themselves to be working on the next priority each time.

Skill One: Set ABC priorities

Lakein (1973) suggests an effective manager will take demands confronting the individual and divide them into ABC levels of immediacy. "A" actions require primary focus and need to be responded to systematically. "C" actions are low in priority and should be left to solve themselves or done in a block timing effort (i.e., save and deal with all at one time). "B" priorities should be put into either an "A" or "C" category. Activities are either worth a manager's time or not. "B" actions will translate into procrastination if not dealt with in a timely manner.

Skill Two: Learn to ICE caseload management problems

There are at least three elements that help the rehabilitation practitioner become skilled at establishing priorities. The acronym ICE forms these elements: *Insulate:* The practitioner must be in charge of controllable time and be selectively unavailable to be in a position to do all the things required to manage a caseload. *Concentrate:* In light of the 80–20 Principle, the practitioner must concentrate efforts on the 20% of activities that will produce the greatest outcomes. Also, practitioners must consolidate their activities with a skill such as block timing. *Eliminate:* Avoid nonessential activities, selectively neglect low-priority activities, and sometimes practice saying "NO."

Skill Three: Use the tickler system

Some form of a tickler system is important for organizing. A tickler system is a device or method for jogging one's memory. This can be a file system or calendar system that serves as a stimulus to bring an activity to one's attention in a *timely* manner. There are several variations on the tickler-system approach. One especially effective one is given later in this chapter.

Coordinating

Since C. H. Patterson (1957) first posed the question, rehabilitation professionals have long wondered whether they are counselors or coordinators. Patterson, of course, was solely interested in skill clusters focused on counseling. Therefore, those educators and trainers who followed this lead (even to the present day) disparage management functions when, in fact, these are crucial to the counselor–manager equation. Without either, the equation is worthless and the rehabilitation professional is lost in a myriad of confusing priorities.

The skills necessary for coordinating assist the practitioner in recognizing community resources and becoming the link between consumer needs and the wide range of possible services available to meet those needs. Coordinating skills involve being competent with public relations in order to interpret organizational philosophies, policies, programs, and practices of managers to the various rehabilitation constituents (Seitel, 1984).

Patterson's lack of a gestalt perspective is hardly excusable. Present-day educators and human resource developers likewise must share the burden of providing the complete rehabilitation practitioner with comprehensive skills that enhance performance and personal functioning.

Skill One: Continuity

Skills within clusters take on many forms. Continuity as a skill is the learned ability of competently bringing together the assessed needs of consumers and developed resources available to meet the needs. Continuity connotes smoothness, flow, and progression of the case from the last developed stage to the next logical stage or state. Caseload managers who do not have a systematic approach to bringing together numerous other professionals and services to satisfy rehabilitation program requirements will find themselves unable to fulfill the *timeliness* principle of effective caseload management.

Skill Two: Concatenation

Although continuity skills satisfy urgency or timeliness elements, concatenation skills function to satisfy linking elements. That is, the professional must be knowledgeable and alert to the many rehabilitation entities that will cost effectively meet the established objectives for the various program strategies on the caseload. This potent skill cluster has historically served as the inclusive descriptor of the functioning of the rehabilitation professional. As a link between and among the myriad responsibilities required of a present-day rehabilitation practitioner, credence for such a premise is established.

Skill Three: Power communication.

Coordination and linking activities bring the professional into contact with numerous persons in a wide variety of positions within other organizations. Many of these individuals are accustomed to interacting on high levels within their organizations. Therefore, powerful communication interactions are replete. The rehabilitation professional must be equipped with the basic patterns and skills that contribute to power communications.

Finally, a clear threat to systematic caseload management exists when incorporating coordinating skill clusters into practice. The threat arises from the application of the strength of these skills in excess. That is to say, coordinating is a process of paving rehabilitation roads for consumers to travel on, (i.e., doing for others). At times, the "counselor hat" with all its devotion to the helping behaviors, attempts to be all things to all people. Thereby, professionals coordinate themselves into system suicide as they rob the consumer of self-initiation development through doing too much for each consumer in an overcrowded caseload.

Directing

Once again the system and synergy aspects of these skill clusters become evident when one considers that planning plus organizing gives the practitioner the bases for making and *enforcing* decisions. Directing skill clusters provides the action from which the previous skill clusters operate. The "best bet" estimates from planning are acted on through the directing skills. Directing is probably the weakest of the skill clusters in a population of rehabilitation caseload managers. Logically, this is evident because directing skills endowed with pointing, steering, leading, instructing, regulating, and administering behaviors are perceived as an antagonist to counseling orientations imbued with helping, supporting, and empathic behaviors. The subtle power of directing a consumer to become his or her own powerful self through internally generated goal setting and objective achievement is overlooked by professionals heavily weighted by a pure counselor orientation.

Skill One. Assertiveness.

Experience advises that one of the most pervasive concerns of professionals working with individuals on their caseloads is the inability to say "NO" appropriately. A common phrase in the assertiveness field rings true, "Too much 'yes' leads to stress." If the coordinating skill clusters are not functioning at a high level, the caseload manager will attempt to be "all things to all people." This, of course, is the unbalanced equation in which the counselor role is practiced at the expense of the managing role.

Skill Two: Do It Now!

Much of the time, true management of a caseload is simply overcoming action inertia. Professionals often get caught in a maelstrom that stymies motivation and direction. Analogous to overcoming inertia in the physical sciences, psychological inertia must be surmounted. Rehearse the command to oneself to "Do It Now!" (Lakein, 1973) until it becomes automatic. Then, act on the command with aggressive action. This self-initiating stimulus will lead to action chaining until the task is accomplished.

Skill Three: Five levels of initiative.

Oncken and Wass (1974) instruct the manager regarding the effective guiding of initiative on the part of individuals on a caseload. The rehabilitation caseload manager must learn how to transfer initiative to consumers. Oncken and Wass identify five levels of consumer initiative:

1. Waiting to be told what to do.
2. Asking, "What is the next thing to be done?"
3. Recommending a course of action—then taking some form of action.
4. Actually taking action on one's own, but reporting immediately to the caseload manager the initiatives taken.
5. Acting on one's own and only reporting on a routine basis.

The focus of directing actions on the part of the caseload manager is to guide the consumer to achieve level 5. Caseload managers with 20% to

40% of individuals on a caseload in levels 1 and 2 are involved in excessive doing-*for*-consumers rather than doing-*with*-consumers in a counselor–manager–consumer interaction cycle. Once level 5 is achieved the consumer is very close to the closure stage in the rehabilitation process.

Directing involves other patterns of action as well. These include effective communicating, appropriate leading, and motivating consumers of services. Directing is a style that can be learned. However, directing often requires a paradigm shift from pure counseling orientations to instructing and channeling constructive actions on the part of the consumer or patient. This permits the consumer or patient to experience the rewarding opportunity of establishing internal control over her or his processes, thereby enhancing stable, lasting rehabilitation results.

Controlling

Controlling is the last of the skill clusters. Controlling skills work to keep the previous skills within operational boundaries. Controlling operates to weave among the previous skill clusters and pull them together into a system of codependent patterns of choice making, action initiating, results assessing, and insuring consistent repetition of the cycle.

A Tickler System

An excellent example of how the skill clusters described above translate into practice come with the use of tickler systems (Elliott & Santner, n.d.). Again, a tickler system can be an organized way to jog memory, to serve as a reminder to bring matters to one's attention in a timely manner. One common tickler which has been implemented in many rehabilitation offices is the Planning Tickler System. This system is implemented in the following manner:

Step 1 Prioritize cases. I: cases needing immediate attention; II: cases in which the caseload manager has been receiving many outside calls; III: cases needing to be closed; IV: cases needing more than one hour of attention at one time; V: cases on the fringes that are not seen frequently; VI: cases long established and that may need follow-up only every 60 or 90 days.

Step 2 Set up a weekly cycle for the entire caseload. Take the total number of cases and divide by a number that will give approximately 15. This figure gives the number of weeks for a caseload to become completely cycled. For example, for a caseload of 120 this yields a system of three cases tickled up per day for eight weeks. Thus, in an 8-week cycle every case will have been tickled up and processed to some degree. The 8-week cycle and three per day can be adjusted for larger or smaller caseload sizes. Steps one and two are preparatory. These should be done only once, that is, at the initial setup stage.

Step 3 Initiate the tickler system. Obtain a week-at-a-glance type of calendar. Fill in all scheduled activities presently known to the caseload manager. Now, spread the cases from the priority order in Step 1 throughout the calendar as follows: (a) Spread cases in #I and #II into the first 2 weeks (these are high-priority cases needing immediate attention); (b) Schedule #III next (schedule early in the month); (c) Schedule # IV (put an asterisk by these cases; this avoids scheduling too many of these in a single week); (d) Date the cases in # IV and # V (make time for a call or write a letter to make contact with these long-term cases).

Step 4 Initiate a cycle and keep the cycles going. On the first day of the week, have an assistant pull cases for necessary action. Work these cases into the week along with the other appointments first entered in Step 3. When a case is tickled up, be sure all cases have a specific activity toward achieving goals set for the case. When finished with the case, redate it and put it on the calendar according to the need to accomplish the next objective. Finally, write a narrative for activities that will be accomplished by the next tickler date.

There are recognizable benefits to the caseload manager for implementing such a planned tickler system. Elliott and Santner (n.d.) argue that a tickler system (a) establishes a regular occurring cycle for the entire caseload, (b) prevents "loss" of cases on large caseloads, (c) copes with tendencies toward overscheduling, (d) thwarts the "urgency equals emergency syndrome" (every case will be tickled up and given its due attention over time), (e) makes plans for systematic closing of cases that are not moving (helps manage caseload size), and (f) affords high concentration, which should translate to quality case work.

This specific tickler can be used in its entirety, or caseload managers can use it as a model to develop their own systems. The concept is that there must be a system if the caseload manager is to manage large, complex, caseloads in a quality manner.

PERSONAL CONTROL

Personal control is a key ingredient in the systems paradigm. If skill clusters are the mechanical works of an entity termed professional practice, then personal control is the fuel needed to drive the entity. Personal control is the energy or force required to take charge of elements poised to go in divergent directions, contrary to intended and anticipated end results. Personal control may be illustrated as those intrapersonal processes that allow the practitioner to take charge of situations and events that would override the practitioners assessed best-bet actions, that is, actions that would produce the desired outcome to benefit the consumer on that professional's caseload. Control as an organizational/structural variable does not fall within the purview of the present discussion.

Focus on personal control is given by internal versus external control orientations (Rotter, 1966, 1975). This extensively researched area provides a broad-based set of concepts from which the caseload manager can operate. In general, the perception that one's own behavior produces the majority of outcomes experienced defines an internal control expectancy. Whereas, the belief that outcomes and happenings are not the result of one's own actions leads to expectancies that one has little effect on those outcomes. The caseload manager who cannot develop the perspective that his or her actions had a significant effect on outcomes will not be in a position to exert managerial actions through the previously described skill cluster.

The person with an internal orientation is more able to take charge, take risks, manage time appropriately, respond assertively, and apply self-motivation and rewards for outcomes. The person with an external orientation is likely to experience greater confusion over which priorities to act on, procrastinates on making choices, is not a risk taker, can be manipulated by assertive or aggressive others, and is unable to establish systematic caseload management. Further, with control localized within the caseload manager, this individual is more likely to be in a position to model the kind of control orientation that will be teachable to consumers who can draw on this orientation to stabilize themselves at the conclusion of strategic programs of rehabilitation.

Action Decisions

There are basic common threads (Marshall & Oliver, 1995) to the decision-making problems encountered by rehabilitation caseload managers.

To achieve a desired objective or rehabilitation outcome, the decision maker must select from any number of alternative choices of actions. The Apex Decision (Cassell & Mulkey, 1985) is the initial choice (decision) between doing nothing and doing something. Procrastination (i.e., doing nothing) is the greatest threat to any action decision.

Action decisions require rehabilitation caseload mangers to (1) set objectives, (2) be proactive, and (3) maintain an outcome focus. This process can be visualized through a travel analogy. When one determines the destination of a city to visit (objective), anticipatory action (proactive response) dictates the necessary planning, while keeping on the road in a timely manner seeks completion of the trip (outcome focus). Action decisions provide a means for evaluating competing demands (desired sideroads, or stops) and potential alternatives (change directions or city) to assure effective results.

There is an ever-increasing emphasis placed on assisting caseload managers in making decisions on the basis of accurate and adequate information (Cassell & Mulkey, 1985; Mittra, 1986). Compromise is an important concept relative to understanding the selection of decision variables. Caseload managers must represent a philosophy or viewpoint that integrates or separates decision variables that influence the outcome focus. Thus, the decision approach used by any caseload manager determines the adequacy of case movement.

To illustrate, it is important to set obtainable objectives initially. These objectives must be Specific, Measurable, Achievable, Relevant, and Time specific. The acronym SMART can also translate into structural events for all participants who will experience the decision. Objectives and intentions must never be determined as equal. It is critical that achievable objectives be established at the initial stage of planning. Remember, before event outcomes can reach fruition, action decisions must be selected. There will always be levels of uncertainty, but the effective caseload manager will act on the best possible information for yielding desired and appropriate results.

SYSTEMS APPROACH

A systems approach within this paradigm signifies that without an adopted or self-constructed system of operations, effective practices will never evolve. All successful caseload managers employ a system or series of interconnected subsystems on which to base action and practice. A systems approach runs the gamut from something as simple as a diary system of appointments and timely scheduled actions all the way to elaborate computer-based management information systems. Regardless, having a systems frame of mind is the only approach that will sustain a caseload manager in the face of multiple demands in the multifaced profession of rehabilitation.

In an environment crowded with a diversity of variables, many of which cannot be controlled but must be managed, the rehabilitation professional cannot survive without a modus operandi emanating from a systems perspective. "By the seat of the pants" caseload management is asynchronous with a politico-mandated rehabilitation environment. Demands on the rehabilitation caseload manager are multifarious and competing. For example, the rehabilitation organization has goals and objectives to be served. Then, consumer populations have advocate forces readily questioning the efficacy of professional decision making. Also, adjunctive sociolegal groups and organizations that consumers apply to and/or hire contend for the caseload manager's action decisions. All this suggests that priority setting and action initiating can only come from some systematic weighing and sometimes juggling of competing demands. If there were only one principle of an effective caseload manager, it would be that *the rehabilitation professional must operate from a self-constructed system of operations.* The rehabilitation professional must construct, adopt, or retool a system for doing caseload management. Of course, this system must interface with the parameters of organizational policy. There is no other alternative to survival in an environment in which *quantity* of demands significantly outstrips *quality* responses. For caseload management and case management practices, consistency and effectiveness are synonymous with system ideology.

CHAPTER 15

Role of Technology: Engineering and Computers

William Crimando

S
ince the passage of the Rehabilitation Act Amendments of 1992 (P.L. 102–569), assistive technology devices and assistive technology services have been included as part of rehabilitation technology. Public Law 100–407, the Technology-Related Assistance for Individuals with Disabilities Act of 1988, defines assistive technology devices as "any item, piece of equipment, or product system, whether acquired commercially or off the shelf, modified or customized, that increases, maintains, or improves functional capabilities of individuals with disabilities" (Cook & Hussey, 1995, p. 5). Assistive technology services, defined in the same law, are "any service that directly assists an individual with a disability in the selection, acquisition, or use of an assistive technology device" (Cook & Hussey, 1995, p. 6).

Technology serves persons with disabilities in several ways: First, assistive or rehabilitation technology enhances the ability to perform basic life functions, such as ambulating, eating, dressing, and self-care. Second, it provides a means of achieving greater levels of independence and employment. Finally, technology promotes a better quality of life for persons with disabilities, with specialized software, and in the mundane but time-saving functions such as word processing, database maintenance, and spreadsheet manipulation that able-bodied persons also perform.

This chapter discusses assistive technology and its use by rehabilitation consumers. The roles of the rehabilitation engineer and rehabilitation technologist are examined, because they have the primary function of providing assistive technology services. Specific examples of assistive technology are provided. The use of the computer is highlighted and is expanded to discuss more fully the potential impact the computer has on the lives of persons with disabilities. The use of computers by rehabilitation practitioners, other than with their consumers, will not be discussed.

REHABILITATION ENGINEERING AND ASSISTIVE TECHNOLOGY

Rehabilitation engineering is the "systematic application of technologies, engineering methodologies, or scientific principles to meet the needs of and address the barriers confronted by individuals with handicaps in areas which include education, rehabilitation, employment, transportation, independent living, and recreation" (P.L. 102–569, 1986, pp. 4–5). Puckett (1996) identified the types of services or products that might be secured through rehabilitation engineering and included these: prosthetics and orthotics, sensory aids, adaptive driving controls or vehicles, mobility devices, custom seating and postural positioning, communication devices, and adapted worksites and tools. Thus, those engaged under the broad title of rehabilitation engineering can be called on to meet a variety of consumer needs. Rehabilitation engineering is a broad title, as it is unclear who can call themselves rehabilitation engineers (Puckett, 1996). Scheck (1990) suggests that the name be reserved for those who hold a degree in engineering, using other terms for those who do not, such as rehabilitation technologist, adaptive equipment specialist, or assistive devices specialist. Puckett (1996) avers that the training and professional competence the individual has in assistive technology are more important than the title. Thus, the services are often rendered informally, by those without the professional credential. Indeed, many assistive devices, some crude and some sophisticated, are developed by those with a knowledge of tools or industrial design, and consumers themselves.

The 1992 Amendments (P.L. 102–569) included the terms rehabilitation engineering, assistive technology devices, and assistive technology services under the broad rubric of "rehabilitation technology" (Rehabilitation Services Administration, 1993). The function of those providing rehabilitation technology is described in P.L. 100–407, and includes:

- the evaluation of the needs of consumers, including functional evaluation in their customary environments;
- providing for the acquisition of assistive technology devices by consumers;
- selecting, designing, fitting, customizing, adapting, applying, maintaining, repairing, or replacing assistive technology devices;
- coordinating or using other interventions, therapies, or services with assistive technology devices, such as those associated with existing education and rehabilitation plans;
- training and technical assistance for consumers or their families; and
- training and technical assistance for professionals (including those providing education or rehabilitation services), employers, or others who provide services to employ, or are otherwise substantially involved in the major life functions of persons with disabilities.

According to Cook and Hussey (1995), assistive technology practitioners (their names for persons providing such services) include engineers, occupational therapists, physical therapists, recreation therapists, special educators, speech pathologists, and vocational rehabilitation counselors. "Each professional has a contribution to make to the industry based on his or her unique background" (p. 34).

Delivery of Assistive Technology Services

The development and implementation of assistive devices are highly individualized. Though some devices are produced in quantity, they must be customized for each individual user. Cook and Hussey (1995) describe these steps in the "customized" service delivery process:

1. Referral and Intake: The consumer, or someone acting for the consumer, identifies a need for technology and makes a referral to an assistive technology professional (ATP). (Puckett, 1996, lists considerations in determining such need.) The ATP gathers basic data to decide whether a match exists between the type of service he or she provides and the consumer's needs.

2. Initial Evaluation: A more detailed description of the consumer's technology needs is developed. The consumer's language, cognitive, physical, or sensory skills may be thoroughly evaluated. Finally, potential devices are selected, and the consumer tries them out. The ATP identifies modifications that need to be made.

3. Recommendation and Report: Evaluation results are summarized in a written report. This report includes recommendations for technologies, based on the consensus of those involved in the referral and evaluation steps. The report is used to justify funding for the purchase of devices and further services.

4. Implementation: The equipment is ordered and modified, or fabricated if necessary. It is set up and delivered to the consumer, who receives training on its use.

5. Follow-up: Besides providing routine maintenance and repair of devices, the ATP determines whether the goals of the referral have been met, and whether the consumer is satisfied with the system.

6. Follow-along: A system is set in place by which regular contact can be made with the consumer to identify the need for further assistive technology intervention, which would restart at step 1.

Examples of Assistive Technology Devices

The literature is full of examples of assistive technology devices. Those interested may browse *Assistive Technology*, a journal published by the Rehabilitation Engineering Society of North America (RESNA), the *IEEE Transactions on Rehabilitation Engineering*, and the *Journal of Rehabilitation Research and Development*. The following is a description of a few devices:

Prostetics and Orthotics

Prosthetic devices provide a replacement for a body part or function, whereas orthotics augment an existing function. Speech prostheses, or augmentative communication devices, for example, are designed for those whose disability results in diminished communication ability. Typical approaches involve the introduction of technology that provides: alternative access (e.g., through a switch, keyboard, or other means); a vocabulary set that consists of letters, words, phrases, and icons; and output such as synthetic speech (cf. Cook & Hussey, 1995). In the past, mechanical leg braces have been prescribed to assist standing and walking but are often abandoned because of the high physical effort required for the small functional gain (Rehabilitation Engineering, 1995). In recent years, researchers have shown the feasibility of electrically stimulating the nervous system below the level of the spinal lesion to produce muscle contractions useful for locomotion. Neuroprosthetic systems have been developed comprising: (a) implanted or skin-surface electrodes, (b) sensors mounted on the body, (c) manual controls mounted on walking-aid handgrips, and microcomputer-based control systems. More recently advanced neuroprostheses called "Hybrid Systems" allow practical standing and walking, and involve the development of sensors, adaptive control methods, and (d) new lightweight bracing incorporating motion control mechanisms (Rehabilitation Engineering, 1995).

Wheelchairs and Mobility Devices. Puckett (1996) notes that new designs and materials have changed the appearance and functionality of wheelchairs and mobility devices. "The choice for mobility aids range from versatile motorized scooters for individuals who can ambulate . . . to full-size, power-base wheelchairs [that] can accept a number of specialized seating units" (pp. 170–171). These chairs can be operated by joystick, chin control, head control, foot control, and breath control, as appropriate for the user. Standard seating systems, often not acceptable to the person with decubiti problems, certain spinal-cord injuries, scoliosis, or other problems, can be replaced by seats made of plywood, foam, vinyl, custom-formed plastics, and mold-injection foam products (Puckett, 1996).

Adaptive Worksites and Tool Modifications

Starting with the passage of the Rehabilitation Act of 1973 (P.L. 93–112), and more recently the Americans with Disabilities Act (ADA: P.L. 101–336), the concept "reasonable accommodation" has become more salient to the business and rehabilitation communities. A reasonable accommodation is a modification of a job, worksite, employment practice, and so on, that (a) allows an otherwise qualified handicapped person to hold a job, and (b) does not impose a financial hardship on an employer or potential employer. Although both parts of this definition are arbitrary, the technology exists. Puckett (1996) defines the goal of worksite modification as "maximiz[ing] the individual's functional capability and independence, in the safest and most cost-efficient manner possible" (p. 172). This may include making architectural modifications to remove barriers to the job site, or modifying the job site itself. Modifications may include "low-tech" and low-cost manipulation aids (e.g., mouthsticks, head pointers, reachers, and modified tool handles), or "high-tech," potentially high-cost items such as electronic environmental control units and robotics. Cook and Hussey (1995) describe, for example, the Desktop Vocational Assistant Robot (DeVAR). This system uses an over-head-mounted robot arm programmed to perform a wide range of daily living, self-care, and vocational tasks, both routine or planned, or non-routine, unanticipated tasks. The DeVAR includes speech recognition for user control, multiaxis joystick control, a color monitor to display command prompts and robot status, and voice synthesis for providing feedback to the user.

COMPUTERS

Few recent innovations have received as much attention as have the introduction of the computer in our everyday lives. Although the impact of computers is arguable, the "hype" alone has changed the way we talk, think, and work. Computers and software have appeared in rehabilitation literature since about 1980, and discussions include their use in services to consumers (Crimando & Godley, 1984, 1985; Crimando & Sawyer, 1983a; McKee & Chiavaroli, 1984), computer-assisted instruction (Crimando & Baker, 1984), and computerization of professional practice (Crimando & Bordieri, 1991; Crimando & Sawyer, 1983b).

Computers and computer software, as discussed in this section, should more properly be referred to as examples of rehabilitative or educational technology (Cook & Hussey, 1995). Rehabilitative, or educational technology, is technology used as a tool for remediation or rehabilitation rather than being a part of one's daily life or functional activities.

Cognitive Rehabilitation

After a severe head injury, a person may experience cognitive deficits such as impaired memory and judgment, incompleteness of thought and action, and impaired problem solving and concentration. Cognitive rehabilitation consists of activities by which the person with severe brain injury tries to acquire these lost functions.

Whiteside (1995) discussed the use of computers in cognitive rehabilitation. She gave these advantages, among others:

- Tasks can be presented in an attention-maintaining gamelike format.
- Computers allow consumers to work independently at their own pace.
- Users tolerate making mistakes better when facing a computer than when they face a therapist.
- Computers allow simultaneous supervision of several consumers.

- Computers provide immediate, consistent feedback.
- Task difficulty can be adjusted dynamically, according to the user's performance.

Whiteside (1995) identified 16 software programs that are commonly used for cognitive rehabilitation. Examples include Computer Programs for Neuropsychological Testing and Cognitive Rehabilitation, which features monitoring of the user's fatigue level to determine automatically when rest periods are needed, and COGREHAB, Volumes 1–4 (Whiteside, 1995).

Telecommuting

Telecommuting is the use of remote terminals, personal computers, telephone, fax, and electronic mail—usually in the worker's home—to send, receive, and perform work assignments (cf. Crimando & Godley, 1985). Telecommuting has also been referred to as telework (The 'far out' success of teleworking, 1995) and distributed work (Grantham & Nichols, 1994–1995). It is estimated that approximately 4.3 million persons perform at least part of their work assignments under these arrangements (Grantham & Nichols, 1994–1995), and telecommuters are in skilled, professional, and managerial jobs—some of which are upper-level. Telecommuting has been proposed as a means to increase the representation of persons with severe disabilities in the work force (Crimando & Godley, 1985).

Grantham and Nichols (1994–1995) insist that distributed workers are engaged almost exclusively in "knowledge work." They cite Drucker's definition: "any work that requires the use of mental power rather than muscle power" (Grantham & Nichols, 1994–1995, p. 32). They suggest that although such work is usually attributed to software engineers, writers, financial analysts, and consultants, parts of nearly everyone's job could be done in a distributed way. Thus, its viability for improving the employment opportunities of persons with disabilities is apparent. Crimando and Godley (1985) describe two examples: "a severely disabled person who is completely homebound may be able to secure and hold employment, and a person who has to undergo kidney dialysis three times a week could work a full week through telecommuting" (p. 278).

Internet Resources

Commonly referred to as "the Information Superhighway" the Internet is the name for a group of worldwide information resources (Hahn & Stout, 1994). The resources consist of text, sound, or graphic files, databases, software, multimedia files, and so on, residing on numerous computer networks—called servers—around the world. In one sense, the various users of the Internet become its resources also, because they put the files there to begin with, and continue to be accessible through electronic mail (e-mail) or other means. These resources can be accessed with special software, called client software, by anyone with a computer and a connection to the network.

One of the most common uses of the Internet is information retrieval, that is, finding all the information available on specific topics. Three sources for information are bulletin board systems (BBSs), gopher servers, and World-Wide Web (WWW) servers. BBSs are repositories for messages and files, often around a single topic or a number of related topics (Hahn & Stout, 1994). They are each maintained by a single person or organization, and exist on a single server. Gopher servers and software provide a series of menus from which one can access virtually any type of textual information. Gopher servers are also searchable by keyword, through a program called Veronica. Through Veronica, one enters a keyword, and then Gopher servers are searched for documents that mention the keyword in their titles. Although the server itself is maintained by one organization, the documents produced by the search are housed on many servers. For example, a keyword search on the word "disability" might produce Disability Information (from University of Minnesota), Trace Center: Disability and Computer Access Information, and the Cornucopia of Disability Information. The World-Wide Web also allows keyword searches, but its output will be files, or "pages" that contain network links to other text, graphic, sound, and multimedia files, and programs. Special WWW software, called *browsers* and *viewers*, allows access to these links, and enables the user to see or hear the information/file provided.

A complete explanation of all of the different types of servers, software, and files available on the Internet, if it were possible, would dominate this chapter. Those interested are invited to read any of the many books written about the Internet. The discussion below describes a few of the types of resource of which persons with disabilities might avail themselves.

Disability-Related Support Groups

Benshoff (1993) writes that "peer self-help groups have grown to occupy a prominent place in the retinue of available community services. . . . They are typified by their absence of formal, professional leadership, [and] acceptance of all comers who indicate an interest in change" (p. 57). The Internet offers its share of self-help groups. Access to these groups is provided through electronic mail, electronic bulletin boards, and the WWW. Some are "USENET" groups or discussion groups, consisting of people with similar interests who carry on long-term discussions by computer around a particular topic (Hahn & Stout, 1994). Specialized programs called *newsreaders* are used for this purpose. USENET groups form and disband daily, and at the writing of this chapter there were over 10,000 different groups. Support groups, primarily existing under the "alt.support" heading, include groups for persons with arthritis, cancer, attention deficit, depression, learning disabilities, multiple sclerosis, and Tourette's syndrome.

   "BITNET" groups are similar to USENET groups, except that these groups carry on their discussions by e-mail. This is accomplished through a centralized program called a *listserver*, which, among other things, keeps e-mail addresses for all "subscribers" of these groups, and automatically distributes mail to them. BITNET groups, like USENET groups, form and disband daily. Examples include the groups bit.listserv.down-syn (Down's Syndrome), and bit.listserv.deaf-l. Finally, a number of self-help and advocacy groups maintain WWW pages. These include the National Alliance of Mental Illness (NAMI, 1995), Deaf World (About Deaf, 1995), the Association for Retarded Citizens (Welcome to the ARC's, 1995), and Alcoholics Anonymous (Welcome to Online AA,1995).

Project Enable and St. John's University

Project Enable, housed at the West Virginia Rehabilitation Research and Training Center, is a BBS providing information and software relating to disability, rehabilitation, employment, and education (WVRRTC's Project Enable, 1995). It also maintains WWW pages. The BBS is the locus of more than 150 special interest discussion groups and more than 5,000 files and searchable databases. Using either the Web site or the BBS, one can access software for adaptive computing (software and hardware modifications for use by persons with disabilities), commercial demonstrations of software products for persons with disabilities, government documents, and compressed copies of a number of disability newsletters.

The Gopher Server at St. John's University is similar to Project Enable. St. John's is the "home" of "Equal Access to Software and Information" (EASI), a discussion group for persons seeking or wishing to provide information on adaptive computing. They have an electronic journal *Information Technology and Disabilities,* which frequently has articles on job accommodations, exemplary training or university programs, adaptive technology, and other resources of interest.

Miscellaneous Online Resources

Numerous additional resources exist on the Internet in which people with disabilities may be interested. These include:

- Access to libraries—A number of libraries maintain their catalogs and some of their holdings online. These can be accessed from one's home through BBSs or the World Wide Web.
- Disabilities Mall—Maintained by Evan Kemp Associates, the Disabilities Mall (1995) provides information on new assistive technology available from commercial sources.
- Job Search—There are a number of online job-search services. For example JobHunt (1995) lists job search and retrieval systems, and places to submit résumés in its listings.

Adaptive Computing

Off-the-shelf computer hardware and software requires the user to have certain psychomotor and sensory skills, such as finger dexterity, vision and, sometimes, hearing. Thus, the functions discussed above—cognitive rehabilitation, telecommuting, and Internet use—may not be accessible to persons with impaired finger use, vision, or hearing. The special devices and modifications made to hardware and software for such persons are referred to as adaptive computing. Although the computer consists of a number of devices working together, the only devices requiring adaptation are those used for input and output.

Alternate Input Devices

Standard input devices on most computers are the keyboard and mouse. Large print and Braille overlays allow persons who are blind or visually impaired to use the standard keyboard. Although keyboards can be used with head sticks, chin sticks, sip-and-puff switches, and so on, a common problem is that some computer and software functions can only be accessed through key combinations. Stick input would not allow two or sometimes three keys to be pressed simultaneously. However, software adaptations such as Access Pack for Windows (Microsoft, Inc.) and Easy Keys, built into the operating system for the Macintosh, convert simultaneous key combinations into sequences. Those who cannot use a keyboard at all may benefit from voice recognition hardware and software, or from a virtual keyboard (Cook & Hussey, 1995). A virtual keyboard uses a video image of the keyboard on the video screen together with a cursor, which is used to inform the computer which key is to be "pressed." The cursor can be placed using a number of options, such as a camera trained on the user's eye, and software to identify the coordinates of keys the user stares at.

Output Devices

Standard computer output devices include the visual display device, or monitor, and printers. The computer also emits auditory beeps at times to alert the user. Persons with visual impairments can benefit from large (i.e., 21–26 inch screens) monitors, monitors with enhanced contrast or color, or from hardware/software combinations that read the screen. The latter option is obtained through a voice synthesizer and screen reader software, such as Flipper or VOS, both designed for the DOS-based machines, or from outSPOKEN for Macintosh and Windows. outSPOKEN (Berkeley Systems, 1995) transforms the graphical user interface of the Macintosh or Windows environment into an audible interface for users with visual impairments and learning disabilities. It takes advantage of the Macintosh's built-in speech capabilities to read the text and graphics of standard Macintosh applications. Most printers are capable of larger typefaces, and some produce raised-dot Braille output. Finally, users with hearing impairments may benefit from programs that substitute light indicators for audible beeps, such as Access Pack for Windows (Microsoft, Inc.).

The potential for technology to enhance the lives and possibilities of persons with disabilities is tremendous. From low-tech adapted tools and adaptive switches, to the now-ordinary personal computer and Internet, to high-tech prosthetic, orthotic, and robotic systems, technology exists or can be designed to help persons with disabilities perform functions that previously were not imagined possible. The strongest limitations may be those imposed by funding and lack of knowledge. Some of these technologies are very expensive, and in the age of decreased funding and managed care may be accessible to only a privileged few. Rehabilitation practitioners and advocates should do what they can to influence legislatures to provide adequate levels of funding. At the same time, consumers, practitioners, and advocates alike should make sure that they keep their knowledge up with the technology, make appropriate use of the services available, and help assistive technology specialists design the best, most useful, and most cost-effective technology they can.

CHAPTER 16

Quality Assurance: Administration and Supervision

James T. Herbert

T he success of rehabilitation agencies and facilities in meeting the needs of persons with disabilities is largely dependent on having a well-qualified professional staff. In assuring that effective, efficient, and timely services are provided, it is the challenge of rehabilitation administrators and supervisors to manage personnel who share in the mission of improving the quality of life for persons with disabilities. Given the current political climate, which demands that rehabilitation service delivery and supporting programs be scrutinized, and the recent national report by the General Accounting Office (GAO, 1993), which criticized the effectiveness of the federal vocational rehabilitation program, it is especially critical that rehabilitation administrators, managers, and supervisors find ways to ensure quality service delivery. Important issues such as examining how improvements in rehabilitation service delivery programs can be made, having staff who are able to meet the needs of a culturally diverse clientele, adopting a life-long commitment to learning beyond that obtained on the job so that professional competence expands, and developing new leaders who have a clear vision and can inspire others represent formidable challenges for rehabilitation administrators. These issues as well as influences resulting from changes and innovations, regulatory mandates, and professional leadership initiatives will have a profound effect on the future of rehabilitation administration, management, and supervision (Brabham & Emener, 1988).

This chapter reviews the available literature concerning characteristics that typify effective supervision, training needs of rehabilitation administrators and supervisors, and several important issues that confront rehabilitation administration and supervision practice. Given the scope of professional practice of rehabilitation counselors elucidated in the previous chapters, this chapter will focus on the subsequent stages of professional development that many rehabilitation counselors eventually experience during their careers.

Before examining qualities that differentiate effective from less than effective administrative and clinical supervision, it is necessary to first define each domain. In succinct terms, administrative supervision is generally intended to increase the efficiency of agency services (Haimann & Hilgert, 1977), whereas clinical supervision is directed to developing personal and professional growth of staff personnel (Emener, 1978). Although these domains can be distinctly different (Ross, 1979), in general, basic supervision tasks consist of planning, organizing, leading, evaluating, and staffing (Riggar, Crimando, & Bordieri, 1991).

QUALITIES OF EFFECTIVE ADMINISTRATORS AND SUPERVISORS

A number of characteristics that are applicable to both administrative and clinical supervision frameworks have been cited in the literature. These characteristics include someone who demonstrates creativity (Emener & Jernigan, 1985), encourages independent thought in others (Bozarth & Emener, 1981), respects individual differences and provides ongoing support (Webb, 1983), enhances greater sensitivity among supervisees (Critchley, 1987), exemplifies sincerity, sets a good example for others, acknowledges good performance among staff (Woodruff, 1989), and generates a positive image about self and work (Graham, 1981). As is evident in these citations as well as reviews of clinical supervision (e.g., Herbert, 1995), most of the available literature concerning supervision is either anecdotal or some compilation of subjective experience. Although efforts to examine clinical supervision within preprofessional training programs have emerged (e.g., Herbert, Hemlick, & Ward, 1991; Herbert & Ward, 1989, 1990; Herbert, Ward, & Hemlick, 1995), there is very little information regarding actual administrative and clinical supervision practices and how they impact on counselor skill development. What is available has addressed staff preferences for specific supervisory behaviors.

Empirical Studies of Supervision Effectiveness

Studies that have examined what qualities supervisees seek in their supervisors reveal that rehabilitation counselors want supervisors to demonstrate a genuine concern for others, personal honesty, flexibility, efficiency, decisiveness, and leadership (English, Oberle, & Byrne, 1979). Clearly defining tasks and assignments to supervisees, soliciting their opinions, displaying enthusiasm, giving negative feedback in private, and encouraging employees are further helpful supervisor behaviors (Clark et al., 1985). Knowledge of policies, procedures, regulations, agency goals and purposes, good problem-solving skills, high ethical standards, fair treatment of all staff, and an ability to teach and train others are characteristics specifically desired by vocational rehabilitation personnel who work in state–federal agencies (Tucker, McNeill, Abrams, & Brown, 1988).

Although research investigating the quality of supervision that rehabilitation personnel receive is limited and somewhat dated, a comprehensive study by English et al. (1979) provides some indication of the quality of supervision received in state–federal programs provided by "first-line" vocational rehabilitation supervisors. This study revealed that the majority of vocational rehabilitation counselors rate the quality of supervisor case consultation in job placement and development, personal adjustment, and vocational counseling as being either "poor" or "fair." In working environments such as those found in private sector, for-profit agencies, satisfaction with supervisors is higher than that reported in public, nonprofit rehabilitation facilities and agencies (Farruggia, 1986). Studies examining supervisory practices, supervisor needs, and supervisory influence on job satisfaction of front-line staff in vocational evaluation, work adjustment, and the private-for-profit sector have been absent. This void as well as more recent data concerning the state–federal program and other nonprofit rehabilitation facilities represents an important area for further research.

Effective Supervision and Relationship to Job Satisfaction

Although a distinction between administrative and clinical supervision has been offered, Ross (1979) contends that the principles that guide effective clinical supervision are the same ones guiding effective organizational supervision. Both supervision forms are therefore highly compatible as "the same principles that make people effective as individuals also make them effective at work" (Ross, 1979, p. 18). These principles include: (a) creating an atmosphere of warmth, consideration, and responsiveness while providing direction and structure to subordinates; (b) assisting staff to accept responsibility for their actions and associated outcomes; (c) helping staff to identify clear, concrete, and difficult work goals; and (d) assisting employees to identify and obtain rewards that are of value to them. Stated more succinctly, "subordinates [should] know how to perform, have incentives to perform, work sufficiently, and achieve adequate success" (Riggar et al., 1991, p. 136).

Given the aforementioned desired characteristics by rehabilitation personnel, it is clear that supervisory personnel, whether they provide administrative or clinical functions, can have a profound effect on the professional development of those they supervise. This relationship, according to several earlier investigations (e.g., Aiken, Smits, & Lollar, 1972; Smits, 1972) is often more important than motivator concerns (determiners of job satisfaction such as the nature of work itself, advancement, recognition, achievement) and other hygiene aspects (factors that by themselves cannot cause satisfaction but are necessary for avoiding dissatisfaction, such as interpersonal relationships, working conditions, salary) (cf. Herzberg, 1966). In fact, Bordieri and Riggar (1989) concluded from their research on job satisfaction of rehabilitation facility personnel that motivating factors may be enhanced by the quality of supervision that service workers receive. There is support for the belief that staff turnover is influenced as a result of the nature of supervision received (e.g., Crimando, Hansen, & Riggar, 1986; Crimando, Riggar, & Hansen, 1986; Riggar, Hansen, & Crimando, 1987). Additional evidence also suggests that although satisfaction with supervision does not determine staff job satisfaction, it appears that supervisory interactions influence employee satisfaction and productivity (Clark et al., 1985). This influence suggests the importance that supervisory personnel need to be better trained in carrying out their job duties (Garske, 1995).

TRAINING NEEDS OF ADMINISTRATORS AND SUPERVISORS

A major concern for administrators and supervisors is how to obtain consistent, high levels of performance from their staff. In an earlier survey of training needs of vocational rehabilitation agency administrators, Hutchinson, Luck, and Hardy (1978) found that managing personnel problems constituted the most critical training need. A subsequent study of top, middle, and first-line supervisors who worked in nonprofit rehabilitation facilities and state–federal rehabilitation agencies was conducted by Matkin, Sawyer, Lorenz, and Rubin (1982). Among rehabilitation facility administrators, the following training need hierarchy was reported: program planning and evaluation, fiscal management, public relations, general personnel management, production management, professional management, marketing, labor relations, research, and purchasing. A similar rank of training priorities was reported by state agency administrators as well, with the exception that research was in the middle and rank ordering and production management were in the lower third group of training need priorities.

In the most comprehensive study assessing training needs, Menz and Bordieri (1986) surveyed over 1,600 rehabilitation facility administrators that included executive directors, assistant directors, and program managers. Menz and Bordieri found that training needs were similar for 13 of 20 content categories across the three administrative levels. Consistent training needs were seen in the following areas: organizational planning, business operations—production efficiency and contract development, community image/fund raising, personnel administration and management, management techniques, access, control, and utilization of information systems, effective use of "core" work force, administrative responsibilities, risk prevention and control, fiscal procedures, physical design and facility layout, and organizational continuity, consistency, and stability. These results as well as those noted by Matkin et al. (1982) indicate that supervisory management issues such as personnel evaluation and selection, labor relations, staff retention and promotion, marketing, organizational planning, business operations, fund raising, risk prevention, fiscal procedures, and organizational stability represent areas in which continual, ongoing training is needed.

EDUCATIONAL OPTIONS TO ENHANCE REHABILITATION ADMINISTRATION AND SUPERVISION COMPETENCE

Providing training to develop and enhance administrative and supervisory competence must be conducted in a format that is accessible, useful, and cost-efficient. Two options exist for persons seeking training in rehabilitation administration and supervision. One option is to pursue a preservice, graduate degree program in rehabilitation administration. Such programs have been available for nearly 40 years yet, in comparison to rehabilitation counseling programs, there has been minimal growth. A study by Riggar, Crimando, Bordieri, and Phillips (1988) identified 10 rehabilitation administration programs. Currently, there are eight programs with member institutions affiliated with the National Council on Rehabilitation Education (NCRE, 1995–1996). Although there is no accreditation of rehabilitation administration programs, Matkin et al. (1982) proposed a curriculum for those persons seeking professional degree training in rehabilitation administration. Using national data from rehabilitation administrators employed in private nonprofit and state–federal agencies, Matkin et al. suggested the following required coursework: program planning and evaluation, fiscal management, general personnel management, and public relations. Other recommended coursework included: professional management, production management, research, marketing, and labor relations. Matkin (1982) also proposed that training in administrative and supervisory functions become part of the preprofessional educational experience of all rehabilitation counselors. This training would help beginning counselors to become better "informed consumers" so that a more complete understanding of management and supervision practices results (Emener, 1986b). Exposure to rehabilitation supervision and training issues would further prepare students beyond the initial years as rehabilitation counselors (Bordieri, Riggar, Crimando, & Matkin, 1988).

Although a number of authors (e.g., Beardsley, Riggar, & Hafer, 1984; English et al., 1979; Matkin et al., 1982; McDonald & Lorenz, 1977; Scalia & Wolfe, 1984) contend that preservice training is the most effective way to address training needs, it seems clear that obtaining a professional degree prior to assuming management duties remains the exception rather than the rule (e.g., Lorenz, Nelipovich, & Wainwright, 1984; Riggar & Matkin, 1984). Consequently, there is a clear choice for the second option to develop rehabilitation management and supervision competence. This option is what Stephens and Kneipp (1981) referred to as the "learn-by-doing method." This preference is not surprising given that much of what an administrator learns is acquired through personal experience (McDonald & Lorenz, 1977; Sawyer & Schumacher, 1980; Wainwright & Sanders, 1988). Further, many personnel do not wish to participate in protracted, generalized training and instead prefer short-term, learning by doing methods (Menz & Bordieri, 1987).

In conjunction with acquiring direct experience while learning how to become an effective administrator, manager, or supervisor, a number of inservice staff training options exist. These options, designed to accommodate working professionals so that careers disruptions can be minimized, include self study, job rotation, mentoring, individualized projects, and workshops (Smith & Bordieri, 1988). The most popular formats according to Smith and Bordieri are workshops, seminars, and self-instructional materials. For administrative personnel who work in state–federal agencies and nonprofit rehabilitation facilities, the Rehabilitation Continuing Education Program (RCEP) may be in the best position to provide continuing education (Riggar & Hansen, 1986). When considering the complexity of skills required by administrative and supervisory personnel, Menz and Bordieri (1987) believe that some training efforts are "doomed to fail" because certain knowledge requires time and experience to develop, refine, and synthesize the information before it can be applied. As a result, these investigators found that inservice training will more likely succeed if training is structured to address facility staff development needs, offered in places that keep costs to a minimum, and conducted in concise, content-specific presentations.

Technological advances available through distance education programs affiliated with universities may provide a mechanism for working professionals to receive more formalized, rigorous training without leaving their homes and jobs (Eldredge, Gerard, & Smart, 1994). Further, Regional Rehabilitation Continuing Education Programs play a prominent role in not only offering distance education programs but in providing a number of technological advances including assistive computer technology, computer-assisted instruction, electronic bulletin boards, interactive multimedia systems, local area networks, and management information systems (Cassell, Colvin, & Hannum, 1991).

Whether administration and supervision personnel acquire expertise through professional graduate training, direct experience, inservice training, or some combination of these approaches, it is incumbent that all supervisory personnel recognize that they serve as models for those they supervise. With respect to training, supervisory personnel must realize that training is a lifelong process (Patterson & Pankowski, 1988). Supervisors who do not model this type of commitment to improve professional competence should not be surprised when their subordinates display similar disinterest in professional development activities (Stephens & Emener, 1988). Although some critics (e.g., Conour, 1982) contend that as one climbs the administrative ladder, the likelihood of participating in any training decreases, data from Menz and Bordieri (1987) indicate that the overwhelming majority of executive directors intend to pursue ongoing training. Reliance on inservice training through continuing education opportunities, however, means that supervisors and administrators are aware of the need and responsibility to seek training. This assumption, as Riggar et al. (1988) indicated, does not best serve the rehabilitation administration profession.

Perhaps, as Patterson and Pankowski (1988) recommend, training administrators, managers, and supervisors requires a shared and coordinated effort among rehabilitation administrators, continuing education personnel, preservice educators, and staff-development specialists. As these authors noted, "Better utilization of existing resources would improve the quality of training available, ensure the availability of such training to all practitioners, and ultimately enhance the delivery of rehabilitation services to clients" (p. 120).

IMPORTANT ISSUES CONCERNING ADMINISTRATION AND SUPERVISION PRACTICE

The issues raised in this section relate to maintaining a well-trained workforce as well as those concerned with advancing the profession of rehabilitation administration and supervision. The transition for the professional who previously functioned as an effective service provider to one who now supervises/manages other service providers presents a unique set of challenges. Successfully meeting these challenges is largely dependent on the quality of inservice and preservice training received, the nature of supervision that the newly promoted supervisor/administrator experienced throughout one's professional career, the existing work culture that characterizes the way employees and supervisors interact with one another, and the capacity and ability to serve as an effective leader.

Making the Transition from Service Provider to Supervisor

Several studies (e.g., Matkin, 1982; Riggar & Matkin, 1984) have found that advancement from practitioner to supervisor occurs within several years, whereas others (e.g., Crimando et al., 1986) have found that longer periods are required. Promotion to supervisory, managerial, or administrative positions often occurs as a result of demonstrating years of providing effective service delivery. The assumption that if one is an effective service provider then one will also be an effective supervisor is fallacious, however (Riggar et al., 1988). There is little empirical evidence that indicates skills required for successful service delivery are the same for those needed to be an effective manager and supervisor (Stephens & Emener, 1988). This myth fails to acknowledge that supervision represents a unique set of knowledge, skills, and abilities (McCarthy, DeBell, Kanuha, & McLeod, 1988).

Although longitudinal research of effective counselors who were later promoted to supervisory and eventual administrative positions has not been conducted, a review of the role and function studies of rehabilitation administrators (e.g., Coffey & Hansen, 1978) in comparison to those of rehabilitation counselors (e.g., Rubin et al., 1984), suggests that unique knowledge, skills, and competencies are required to effectively perform these work roles. This does not require, however, that practitioners who are promoted to higher administrative, management, or supervisory positions forego their initial identity as rehabilitation counselors to forge a new one (Szymanski, 1988). As noted earlier, the review of literature regarding what interpersonal qualities rehabilitation counselors seek in effective administrators and supervisors are also ones that, in all likelihood, effective practitioners demonstrate with clients they serve.

In order to make a successful transition to higher administrative levels, Latta (1981) believed that a necessary attitudinal shift was needed if one was going to be equally successful in managing other rehabilitation professionals. Accordingly, effective administrators should subscribe to a number of managerial presumptions, such as:

> The primary goal of the manager is to maintain a productive organization, not a "happy family"; To exist as a manager is to influence; "Person power" is generally more effective than "position power"; Good performance-review and feedback is central to the management process; and, problem finding skills are more important than problem-solving skills. (pp. 53–56)

These presumptions may be particularly relevant for the recently promoted first-line supervisor who may experience an "identity conflict" (Wells, 1978). As a new supervisor or manager, this professional now encounters a whole range of new work situations, such as supervising previous coworkers (Farrant, 1989), training new employees (Lansing, 1989), retaining good employees (Thomas & Thomas, 1989), motivating workers who have plateaued (Karp, 1989; Kurtz, 1989), establishing mentoring relationships (Patterson & Fabian, 1992; Viranyi, Crimando, Riggar, & Schmidt, 1992), resolving ethical dilemmas (Patterson, 1989), and managing a culturally diverse work force (Abramms-Mezoff & Johns, 1989; Lowrey, 1983). Such interpersonal situations for new managers and administrators can be quite difficult to negotiate and, as a result, may lead to occupational stress (e.g., Riggar, Godley, & Hafer, 1984; Sawyer & Schumacher, 1980). Further, success in negotiating a potentially stressful transition from service provider to subsequent supervisory and administrative positions will be greatly influenced by the existence of strong organizational support. This support serves as a buffer to mediate job stress among all rehabilitation personnel (Kelley & Satcher, 1992).

Staff Performance Appraisal

Staff evaluation is a critical component to maintaining quality assurance of rehabilitation service delivery programs (Christian, 1981). This evaluation process constitutes a primary supervisory function that is embedded in recruitment, selection, placement, evaluation, promotion, transfer, training, and development of rehabilitation staff (Sample, 1984). Staff performance appraisal, however, is one that is often perceived as a negatively charged experience despite the potential benefits it offers (Lorenz, 1979; Weinburger, 1977). Part of the reason for this negative perception is that many rehabilitation personnel are uncertain of the exact purpose of the assessment (Dale & McDonald, 1982). Although there has been an increasing effort for accountability in rehabilitation services, evaluating individual performance against such standards often produces anxiety, conflict, and resistance among employees (Lorenz, 1979) and represents one of the most difficult tasks a supervisor must perform (Bordieri, Crimando, Riggar, & Schmidt, 1992). Whether the performance–appraisal system in place is perceived as positive or punitive often depends on: (a) the administrator developing a mind-set that emphasizes the benefits of appraisal, (b) a recognition that the process must be carried out to benefit both individual needs and organizational requirements, and (c) a resulting document that is technically defensible (Phillips, Puckett, Smith, & Tenny, 1985).

A number of pragmatic suggestions that can facilitate performance evaluations have been cited throughout the rehabilitation and supervisory management literature. These suggestions include: (a) that the supervisor and each staff member participate in the employee job-performance-evaluation process and be able to do so on a more frequent, ongoing basis (e.g., Dale & McDonald, 1982; Graham, 1981; Phillips et al., 1985; Taylor et al., 1989); (b) inservice training on how to conduct performance appraisal be given to both supervisory and employee staff (Dale & McDonald, 1982; Graham, 1981); (c) employees be given specific written standards against which to rate their performance on each factor (Graharn, 1981; Taylor et al., 1989); (d) performance goals be established that are specific, measurable, realistic, and agreed on by both individual supervisor and staff person (Knippen & Green, 1989); (e) written evaluations are characterized by objective data based on actual observation of work performance (Graham, 1981) and not subjective trait information (Lawrie, 1989; Sample, 1984); (f) evaluation criteria specify what, when, who, and how evaluations are conducted (Bordieri et al., 1992); (g) in addition to the supervisor and employee having input as to evaluating performance, other sources such as colleagues and rehabilitation consumers should also be considered (Dale & McDonald, 1982; Emener & Placido, 1982); (h) different evaluations should be used for staff development training needs versus personnel decisions (Dale & McDonald, 1982); (i) individualized criteria should be used when considering performance measures (Rice, 1981); and (j) an employee development plan outlining specific objectives for improvement, required resources, contingencies, target dates, and monitoring procedures should be completed jointly by supervisor and employee (Graham, 1981). Given the proposed characteristics of conducting an effective appraisal system and the unique working environments of rehabilitation practice, it may partially explain why there is no widely accepted appraisal system used in rehabilitation facilities (Phillips, Bordieri, Buys, & Sabin, 1987).

Although there has been a great deal of discussion as to the difficulty in developing objective work-performance criteria (e.g., Bordieri et al., 1992), it is interesting that little, if any, mention has been offered to use the extensive data accumulated in the role-and-function studies of rehabilitation counselors (e.g., Rubin et al., 1984), vocational evaluators, (Gannaway & Sink, 1979), work-adjustment specialists (e.g., Eillien, Menz, & Coffey, 1979) and rehabilitation administrators and supervisors (e.g., Coffey & Hansen, 1978) as a base for developing performance standards. Surely, the extensive work devoted to what rehabilitation personnel do during work and what information is required to perform these job duties (e.g., Leahy, Shapson, & Wright, 1987) offer a way to develop a more objective, standardized appraisal system.

Professional Credentialing

Professional credentialing has the potential to assure that competent personnel are providing quality services although at the same time it may promote elitism and stifle innovation (Thomas, 1993). As the debate for professional credentialing and specialization has continued in the field of rehabilitation counseling (e.g., Goodwin, 1992; Irons, 1989), a similar discussion exists within the field of rehabilitation administration. This debate essentially concerns whether minimal standards should be established for rehabilitation administrators, managers, and supervisors, what those standards should involve, and what criteria should be used in establishing such standards. Proponents (e.g., Lorenz et al., 1984) contend that certification of administrators and supervisors helps to recognize that such professions do, indeed, exist. In addition, certification provides some evidence of minimal competence necessary to perform supervisory and administrative tasks and that one adheres to a set of ethical standards. Whether certification is, in fact, a valid measure of professional competence is debatable. Within the rehabilitation counseling field, this issue has been questioned with respect to competence (e.g., Scofield, Berven, & Harrison, 1981; Thomas, 1987) as well as whether this credential results in more employment opportunities, quicker promotions, higher salaries, and greater job security (Irons, 1989), and professional pride (Goodwin, 1992). To the extent that these same criticisms are applicable to professional credentialing of rehabilitation supervisors, administrators or managers have not been evaluated empirically or articulated fully in the recent supervision literature. Despite calls for encouraging professionalism through certification and training (e.g., Phillips & Wainwright, 1986; Wainwright & Sanders, 1988), there is no strong mandate by members of the National Rehabilitation Administration Association (NRAA) to develop and implement such standards (Lorenz et al., 1984). At present, upgrading professional standards in administration and supervision remains a laudable goal (e.g., Wainwright, Newman, & Phillips, 1995).

One initiative toward examining the need for certification standards would be to undertake similar research that has demonstrated the efficacy of master's level rehabilitation counselor training and rehabilitation outcome (e.g., Szymanski, Herbert, Parker, & Danek, 1992). An examination of what combination of training and experience is related to human resource development outcomes such as employee job satisfaction (e.g., Garske, 1995), staff turnover (e.g., Crimando et al., 1986), service delivery costs and benefits (e.g., Simon, 1982), quality of work life (e.g., Emener & Stephens, 1982), and staff productivity (e.g., Simon, 1987) could be undertaken. Further, supervisor personality characteristics, behaviors, leadership styles, and working alliance with rehabilitation counselors represent interpersonal aspects that influence counselor effectiveness and may ultimately affect service delivery outcomes. Understanding these interpersonal dynamics between administrators and managers and supervisors and counselors may help advance the rehabilitation administration and supervision research literature. As Riggar et al. (1988) commented, it is within these administration, management, and supervision boundaries that "all rehabilitation administration is developed, research is conducted, and roles and functions performed" (p. 96).

SUMMARY

Supervisors and administrators serve as gatekeepers in assuring that quality programs are available to persons who require rehabilitation services. Effective administrative personnel serve to empower staff and inspire them to constantly test their limits. Although the transition from rehabilitation counselor to later supervisory and administrative positions can be challenging, with appropriate training and experience rehabilitation leaders are in a unique position to make a positive impact on the scope of professional practice. Certainly, rehabilitation counseling has evolved because of the effective leadership provided by administrators who had a vision for the future, could articulate it to others, and made the necessary commitment for this vision to be realized.

CHAPTER 17

Issues and Perspectives: Profession and Practice

T. F. Riggar and Dennis R. Maki

T
he evolution of rehabilitation counseling has been governed by a variety of factors. Not the least of these factors have been the federal laws that virtually created the system and the profession. As we have seen in Chapter 3—*History and Systems*—legislative action guides the focus of rehabilitation counseling particularly concerning consumer groups and their involvement. At the same time, as evidenced by private-sector rehabilitation, the profession seeks its own place in the structure of business and society. Another variable that influences our profession is the constant, ongoing, myriad changes in our society. Given that rehabilitation counselors assist approximately 49 million Americans with disabilities (Mariani, 1995) as detailed in Chapter 9—*Public and Private Rehabilitation Counseling Practices*—it is clear that the largest single minority group in the United States today is Americans with disabilities. Chapter 8—*Cultural Pluralism*— makes it clear that the same stereotypes, prejudices, and so on that abound when considering ethnic or specific cultural groups still persist and are prominent in today's society, especially concerning the status and functional ability of people with disabilities.

We do not have far to go to appreciate the paradigms of rehabilitation counseling practice, in fact, Chapter 2—*Theory and Philosophies*— eloquently details the basis of our profession today. But what of yesterday and the future? To help us examine perspectives in rehabilitation counseling and the issues of the past as they relate to the present and the future we are indebted to Brubaker (1981) who over a decade and a half ago conducted an interview with Dr. Daniel Sinick. Dr. Sinick, was a President of the American Rehabilitation Counseling Association and the Council of Rehabilitation Counselor Educators (now NCRE), who had recently retired from George Washington University where he became Director of the RCE program in 1967 after more than a decade at San Francisco State University. Dr. Sinick's interview, among other things, told us that "Rehabilitation Counseling is moving sufficiently fast to deal with non-vocational aspects of counseling" (p. 179). But that "rehabilitation counselors ought to gain expertise in the vocational potential of people of *all* ages. . . . It's obvious that other disciplines, such as social work and psychology, broadly lack that kind of vocation orientation" (p. 180). Although he noted a decade and a half ago that "part-time, temporary or volunteer work. . . . Ours is still a work-oriented society" (p. 180). This is currently confirmed in Chapter 13—*Placement.* Dr. Sinick foresaw the "dual orientation toward the vocation and the independent living areas" (p. 180) as noted in several chapters herein. He predicted rehabilitation counseling's expansion in private-sector rehabilitation, increased involvement with special education, and even commented concerning the combination of ARCA and NRCA—"I think the merger is a must" (p. 184). In 1993 the Alliance for Rehabilitation Counseling created a formal organizational structure by the ARCA and NRCA to "marshal the strengths of both professional organizations into powerful, meaningful, unified professional voice for rehabilitation counseling" (Kirk & La Forge, 1995, p. 49). In all of these areas and more, perspectives and issues have continued, expanded, and become part of the vital ongoing profession of rehabilitation counseling. As we will see, our past evolves to our present and becomes our future.

In a more contemporary view, in 1985, Dr. Edna Mora Szymanski, then the 28th president of ARCA, in a Presidential Address, declared that:

> The profession of rehabilitation counseling is grounded in basic beliefs in human rights, the value of work, and a partnership with persons with disabilities. Its focus is on individuals and their potential. (p. 2)

In her address she quoted Salvatore DiMichael, the first ARCA president, who predicted that rehabilitation counselors were "not only professional enthusiasts but even secular missionaries" (DiMichael, 1969, p. 9

cited in Szymanski, 1985, p. 2). Dr. Szymanski detailed the positive thinking and cooperative action that would lead the profession as it journeyed into the future:

- If the profession is to be true to its foundation and its potential, it must engage in a full partnership with citizens with disabilities.
- All professional rehabilitation counselors must be firmly grounded in a belief in and respect for human rights and individual dignity.
- Professional rehabilitation counselors need to remain firmly committed to and able to visualize human and societal potential.
- The profession must actively recruit the best and brightest students to meet the challenges of the future.
- The profession must continue to improve its ability to serve persons with disabilities through ongoing research which assists in identifying those competencies most necessary for specific settings and populations.
- Individual rehabilitation counselors will need to take seriously their professional responsibility to continuously upgrade their skills.
- Individual rehabilitation counselors will also need to recognize professional association membership and participation as a professional responsibility.
- Rehabilitation counselors will need to exhibit pride in their profession. (pp. 4–5)

Subsequently Dr. Kenneth R. Thomas was requested by ARCA President Dr. Szymanski to work with other past ARCA presidents to reflect on the future of rehabilitation counseling. Ken Thomas, Salvatore DiMichael, Donald Linkowski, Stanford Rubin, and Richard Thoreson combined to examine the profession, education, research, and practice of rehabilitation counseling. These are the same content areas we will examine herein; providing status updates and new perspectives on these issues.

PROFESSION

As Thomas (1991a) explains "a complication in computing the number of rehabilitation counselors relates to how one specifically defines the term"

(p. 180). With over 120,000 people employed as counselors, and over 25,000 of those who list their positions as "rehabilitation counselor" the number "compares favorably with other rehabilitation professions such as occupational therapy (33,000) and recreation therapy (26,000)" (p. 180) but does not approach 100,000+ psychologists or 380,000+ social workers as an occupation. The debate of the ARCA past-presidents dealt primarily with who and what is a "rehabilitation counselor" and how the term "qualified" is determined. These discussions concerning who, what, and how as relates to rehabilitation counseling often depend on orientation. Thomas (1991a) commented that when he started in rehabilitation over 25 years ago that employment was generally limited to state vocational rehabilitation agencies, nonprofit rehabilitation facilities, state institutions, or half-way houses. Clearly employment trends have changed, and as will be seen further on they have changed considerably in the 75+ years since the inception of rehabilitation counseling. Not just private-sector rehabilitation and specialty counseling areas, that is, addictions counseling, but the whole advance of an individual rehabilitation counselors' career into management or administration will be accounted.

One may see that as the decades pass many of the same issues, perspectives, and questions remain. Because of the constant, ongoing shifting bureaucratic and societal basis of rehabilitation counseling these issues often are answered not by specific, detailed proposals but by guidelines, options, or questions. Thomas (1991a) detailed that as rehabilitation counseling faced the 1990s and beyond it had a variety of options:

- It could remain a broad-based, but fragmented profession whose loyalties are split between counseling and rehabilitation, with the scale tilting increasingly toward rehabilitation.
- It could view itself as a specialization within generic counseling and join with other counselors in the development of counseling as a profession equivalent to psychology or social work.
- It could view itself as a specialization within rehabilitation along with vocational evaluation, job placement, and rehabilitation administration and work toward the development of a profession that would assumedly be called rehabilitation (Reagles, 1981).
- The two national rehabilitation counseling professional associations (ARCA and NRCA) along with NCRE could merge to form an independent association of rehabilitation counselors (Rasch, 1979).

- Or it could view itself as an applied area of psychology and encourage master's level practitioners to join the APA (American Psychological Association) as associate members and doctoral-level practitioners and academics to join APA as members and to obtain psychology licenses. (p. 182)

Even now in the latter part of the decade, rehabilitation counseling as a profession has not found closure on many of these issues. Leahy and Szymanski (1995) recently said that "the question of whether rehabilitation counseling should be conceptualized as a profession or as a specialty area of counseling practice remains unresolved" (p. 166). Part of this continuing debate revolves around whether rehabilitation counselors become "qualified" by becoming CRCs or some other certification process (NBCC, MAC, etc.), whether they join ACA/ARCA, NRA/NRCA, or APA Division 17 (Counseling Psychology) or Division 22 (Rehabilitation Psychology), or whether they were originally a CRC and then became trained and employed as a Vocational Evaluator (CVE), or Certified Case Manager (CCM), or as is becoming increasingly apparent, promoted to supervisor and then as administrator enrolling in the NRA as an NRAA member. All of these options and avenues of employment depend on training, education, employment settings, and populations. What can be said with certainty is that "although the central role of the rehabilitation counselor has remained quite consistent over the years, the functions and required knowledge and skill competencies of the rehabilitation counselor have expanded" (p. 163).

Whatever perspective, whatever the issue, it is incumbent on rehabilitation counseling to become proactive. Change-management principles tell us that we must not just react to events, but through our professional organizations, large consumer groups, and rehabilitation facilities and agencies begin to chart our own course for the future. We "may need to garner necessary financial and human resources, develop temporary management structures, empower project champions, and most certainly, provide end-users a legitimate role in planning for change" (Crimando, Riggar, & Bordieri, 1988, p. 22). Because rehabilitation has always been about change, whether it is the change in life-styles and livelihood of persons with disabilities, or the changes faced by rehabilitation service delivery systems we must manage our change proactively:

We must first and foremost refine our skills in planning. At the very basic level we must be able to articulate who we will serve, how, when, and why. . . . Finally, we must develop our abilities to plan scenarios that reflect those impacts, and develop alternatives to deal with them. (Lorenz, Larsen, & Schumacher, 1981, p. 364)

EDUCATION

In Chapter 16—*Quality Assurance*—Dr. James T. Herbert declared that "the success as to whether rehabilitation agencies and facilities meet the needs of persons with disabilities is largely dependent upon having a well-qualified professional staff." The continuing debate in rehabilitation as to what constitutes a qualified rehabilitation professional continues unabated. Part of the problem with determining qualifications, that is, training, education, experience, degree level, and so on, depends on specific employment settings, consumer populations, expanded job opportunities and requirements, and short- and long-term follow-up studies of rehabilitation counseling graduates, including role and function studies. With rehabilitation education programs of various types and levels approaching 100 in number, and with 31 identified doctoral programs in the U.S. (Bieschke, Bishop, & Herbert, 1995), the breadth and depth of such programs is only rarely examined and even then university, state, regional, federal, and consumer feedback alters their characteristics. Recent events, for example, have caused many rehabilitation education programs to expand their offerings in the addictions counseling arena to accommodate those students and employment settings now requiring addictions counseling certification (Page & Bailey, 1995; Shaw, MacGillis, & Dvorchik, 1994). Additionally rehabilitation education programs are becoming more and more aware that their graduates are seeking and finding employment in private-for-profit rehabilitation. While contending that "there is strong evidence that the profession is distinct and different than other counseling areas; roles and functions of both public and private sector rehabilitation counselors delineate this distinction" (Havranek & Brodwin, 1994, p. 370), they call on rehabilitation education programs to modify their curricula and respond to the changes and challenges that have, are, and will occur in the future as private-for-profit job opportunities for rehabilitation counselors expand dramatically.

No examination of education can be complete without at least briefly touching on perhaps the most asked question in rehabilitation—Who is qualified? In a recent thoroughly comprehensive study, Szymanski, Herbert, Parker, and Danek (1992) revealed:

Recent research in the Arkansas (Cook & Bolton, 1992), Maryland (Szymanski & Danek, 1992), New York (Szymanski & Parker, 1989), and Wisconsin (Syzmanski, 1991) state vocational rehabilitation agencies demonstrated that rehabilitation counselors with relevant preservice education (i.e., master's degrees in rehabilitation counseling or a closely related discipline) had better competitive rehabilitation outcomes for clients with severe disabilities than did counselors with unrelated bachelor's and master's degrees. The results of these studies also suggested that work experience did not adequately substitute for education. (pp. 108–109)

An additional issue concerning education, one that has increasingly come to the fore in the past decade, concerns multiculturalism. As indicated in Chapter 8—*Cultural Pluralism*—considerable effort and education will be required in the future to assure that rehabilitation counselors do not "favor negative client factors over positive ones" (Strohmer, Pellerin, & Davidson, 1995, p. 82). One method to diminish, alleviate, and abolish inequities is to "address the educational and service needs of the growing number of minorities, who will not only be entering the field in record numbers, but also constituting an increasing number of client referrals" (Thomas, 1991a, p. 187). As the problem now stands inequity and injustice still occurs:

Data revealed that a disproportionate number of African Americans received inadequate services in all major categories of DVR. A large percentage . . . were not accepted for service. Among applicants accepted . . . a larger percentage of African American cases were closed without being rehabilitated, and . . . closed as "successfully rehabilitated" were more likely than European Americans to be in the lower income levels. (Feist-Price, 1995, p. 119)

Although education is surely the key, the professions themselves must take an active stand in solving many of the problems detailed in Chapter 8. One immediate action could be the appropriate modification of the existing Code of Professional Ethics for Rehabilitation Counselors. As espoused by McGinn, Flowers, and Rubin (1994), this organizational position would assist to promote more equitable, just, and effective services to individuals from various racial, ethnic, and cultural minority groups.

Long-Distance Learning

No discussion of rehabilitation counselor education in the future or the future of rehabilitation counselor education would be complete without mention of Long-Distance Learning. As detailed by Dr. William Crimando in Chapter 15—*Role of Technology: Engineering and Computers*—technology now exists to enable the availability of almost all information that exists. McFarlane and Turner (1995) tell us that several elements will affect our work, personal, and social lives:

- information will continue to expand at a geometric rate;
- economic, political, and organizational demands will increase in each of our professional settings;
- "consumers and customers" are expecting increased productivity, improved quality; and
- continued responsiveness; and
- continuous, lifelong learning is fundamental to our professional and personal viability. (p. 327)

These elements and the increasing availability of long-distance learning provides a harmonious blending of needs and resources. McLaren (1995) lists some of the more dominant rationales for long-distance learning:

- Alleviate geographical isolation.
- Resolve scheduling conflicts.
- Distribute scarce or unique instructional resources.
- Provide equal educational opportunity for students who are unable to attend traditional classes due to disability. (p. 262)

All of these considerations make it obvious that long-distance learning, especially Interactive Television (ITV) are not just especially pertinent for rehabilitation counselor education but in fact for rehabilitation consumers and customers. These technological methodologies have reached such a state of reality and applicability that they are already in use in a variety of settings. Many educational institutions have and are conducting ongoing classes using a variety of long-distance learning technology. These schools include, but are certainly not limited to: Queensborough Community College of the City University of New York, External Education Program for the Homebound; *Rehab*Leadership Project, University of

Northern Colorado; Department of Rehabilitation Counseling at Sargent College of Allied Health Professions, Boston University; Distance Learning Through Telecommunication Interwork Institute, San Diego State University; Utah State University; the Rehabilitation Institute, Southern Illinois University; and a variety of programs in the states of Maine, Arizona, Kentucky, Iowa, and Indiana.

RESEARCH

Science is both qualitative and quantitative. As detailed by Newman and Benz (in press) "scientific inquiry is both an inductive and deductive process, with feedback loops that effect the inductive and deductive procedures and which are self-correcting." They relate that the two methodologies are neither mutually exclusive nor are they interchangeable but rather should be seen as interactive places on a methodological continuum. Rehabilitation research is an excellent example of this methodological continuum. Although there is one professional journal that deals exclusively with rehabilitation education issues, *Rehabilitation Education*, there are a wide variety of journals that examine the entire field of rehabilitation counseling. Journals such as *Rehabilitation Counseling Bulletin, Journal of Applied Rehabilitation Counseling, Journal of Counseling and Development, Journal of Rehabilitation,* etc. each focus on diverse areas of rehabilitation and rehabilitation counseling and are often willing to present articles of general interest to professionals as well as emerging or topical special issues that devote whole publications to areas of specific interest. The wide variety of journals of interest to rehabilitation professionals matches the equally varied interests, job requirements, and content needs of practicing professionals. Aside from psychology, rehabilitation is perhaps the most diverse of the human services, with its practitioners found in a myriad of employment settings. These needs and requirements, as well as content and site mandates, explain the role and function of wide-ranging research in rehabilitation. One need only examine the Reference Section of this book to view the considerable number of individual and disparate journals that have published rehabilitation and rehabilitation-counseling-related articles.

A result of this research, in addition to aiding professional functionability in the field, is the provision of data to maintain current, valid criteria and standards for accreditation, certification, and licensing. Leahy and Szymanski (1995) relate that "in an era of increased public scrutiny . . . a strong research program is vital for professional credibility. Rehabilitation counseling is perhaps in the forefront of the counseling professions in the research area" (p. 165).

As most rehabilitation research is produced through universities a constant issue is the applicability of the result of esoteric research. Although the call always exists for practitioners to publish it is usually only university and university-related personnel who have the education, experience, resources, and perhaps most importantly, time to conduct elaborate, long-term research. Even in the rarefied environments of academia controversy exists concerning rehabilitation research. Thomas (1991b) feels that "too much emphasis has been placed on programmatic research and too many resources allocated to large rehabilitation research institutes and research and training centers at the expense of basic research and the individual researcher" (p. 189). Anyone, particularly a practitioner, who has ever attempted to gain governmental support to examine an important problem (research proposal) knows how daunting and demanding the process can be. In many cases obtaining the resources is more difficult than actually conducting the research. Perhaps in the future those bureaucrats (rarely researchers) (Matkin & Riggar, 1991) who disseminate grants will heed the words of Thomas (1991b) who discovered that:

> Great ideas spring from the minds of creative, independent men and woman, and they are seldom in areas that governments and society would necessarily wish to be explored . . . great thinkers and discoverers also tend to be individuals who are well-read and informed in a variety of fields. They are not trained; rather, they are educated. (p. 189)

PRACTICE

Although the core, the foundation, the basis of rehabilitation counseling has not changed over the years, the demands on rehabilitation counselors as professionals has expanded considerably. At issue herein are perspectives about the future course of rehabilitation and rehabilitation counseling. These perspectives primarily involve employment settings. As the skills and abilities of rehabilitation counselors have become known, an increasing number of human services, indeed even corporate employers, seek their knowledge. The practice has, is, and will always be directed to the traditional markets of state vocational rehabilitation agencies, non-profit rehabilitation facilities, and state/federal hospitals, institutions, agencies, and organizations, but will also continue to expand into other areas that continue to involve more and more qualified rehabilitation counselors; namely, psychology/counseling, private for-profit rehabilitation, and administration/management/supervision.

Psychology/Counseling

Rehabilitation counseling has grown beyond the traditional vocational counselor emphasis and today, within the natural progression of a profession, after all the other requirements of the profession are met, has evolved into a goodly number of specializations and certifications (Hosie, 1995; Matarazzo, 1987). More and more, however, we find that qualified rehabilitation counselors are moving into school-based transition programs, university services for students with disabilities, disability-management programs within employer settings, and various types of clinics (Leahy & Szymanski, 1995; Thomas, 1991b), as well as marriage and family counseling, clinical mental health, group private practice, pastoral and substance abuse counseling (Mariani, 1995). All of these content areas are but a normal progression and transition of the work of traditional rehabilitation counselors. Those with an interest and willingness to gain more training and education, based on their rehabilitation counseling foundation, easily transition into many of these employment areas. One area of import, particularly as it continues to absorb so many qualified rehabilitation counselors, is the private-for-profit arena.

Private Rehabilitation

Chapter 9—*Public and Private Rehabilitation Counseling Practices*—provides us with an excellent overview of the status and potential future of private rehabilitation counseling today. Dr. Ralph E. Matkin details the causes and nature of the rapid increase in private, for-profit rehabilitation employment settings by examining (1) mandatory provisions of state workers' compensation statutes, (2) insurance-based disability systems and practices, (3) the changing nature of the clients served by public rehabilitation agencies (i.e., severely disabled, developmental disabilities), and (4) increasing client caseloads with an increasing average duration per case when funding allocations to agencies were not keeping pace with the increasing costs required to serve clients with the most severe disabilities. Coupled with the knowledge that in the health care arena, "rehabilitation is growing faster than any other discipline" (McMahon, Shaw, & Mahaffey, 1988; cited in Kilbury, Benshoff, & Riggar, 1990) and that "clearly the most growth has taken place in the private-for-profit sector, especially in the private rehabilitation companies" (Thomas, 1991a, p. 192) makes it clear that "rehabilitation is in a state of transition shifting from the traditional State/Federal system to a diversified growth-oriented competitive business system model" (p. 196). A unique indicator of the rise of private-sector rehabilitation is the proliferation of articles that specifically comment on the private sector's effect on training programs (Matkin & Riggar, 1988b) and how rehabilitation education should respond (Kilbury et al., 1990).

In 1986 Dr. William G. Emener provided for us a snapshot perspective of rehabilitation in America through a comparison of the history of the public and private sectors. That information, adapted and updated herein, reveals the transition and stages of both portions of rehabilitation (see Table 17.1).

The current Era of Empowerment (mentioned in Chapter 2—*Theory*

Table 17.1. A Snapshot Perspective of Rehabilitation in America:
Public and Private Sectors

Public sector	Eras	Private Sector
Trial and development	1914–1935	
Establishment and permanence	1930s	
Rehabilitation medicine	1940s	
Growth and expansion	1950s	
Civil rights advancements	1960s	Infancy stage
Cutback and retrenchment (high tech)	1970s	Expansion, threat, and intimidation
Litigation "Holding on" (redirection)	1980s	Continued growth and maturation
Empowerment ADA/civil rights reinforcement	1990s	Health care (management) and consulting
Computers and engineering	2000s	Diversification

Adapted and updated from Emener, W. G. (1986a). Future perspectives on rehabilitation in America. *Journal of Private Sector Rehabilitation, 1*(2), 59–70.

and Philosophies) can be determined as a strengthening of self-efficacy—
one's belief in his or her effectiveness to perform a task (Barrett,
Crimando, & Riggar, 1993; Conger, 1989; Conger & Kanungo, 1988;
Olney & Salomone, 1992). The empowering nature of the ADA, strength-
ening the self-efficacy of professionals and consumers alike, is well
detailed in Chapter 4—*Policy and Law*, and Chapter 5—*Ethical and
Legal*. Although there is thorough examination of the ADA herein, the
Civil Rights Act of 1991, as we will see further on, does and will have just
as great an impact on the field of rehabilitation as did the initial Civil
Rights Act of 1964.

Considerable mention has ensued concerning private-sector, for-profit
rehabilitation, especially employment content settings for qualified rehabilitation counselors. Table 17.2 provides an adapted and updated review
of current job opportunities in this expanding employment arena. As
noted in Table 17.1 the private sector portion of rehabilitation will continue to expand. Although at this juncture many rehabilitation counselors
are based increasingly in health care fields and as consultants, especially
with the advent of the ADA, the future for private sector rehabilitation
appears to be continued expansion and diversification into other functional and content areas. New laws bringing with them potentially new
rehabilitation populations and changes in the structure of business and
society will open new employment settings and expanded job opportunities for qualified rehabilitation personnel. During these upcoming times,
the 21st century, it is expected that the public portion of rehabilitation
will be changed by the advent of computers and engineering, including
long-distance learning (Bitter, 1991). Chapter 15—*Role of Technology:
Engineering and Computers*—provides an excellent review of the potential of technology to impact favorably on the lives of Americans with
disabilities. So great is this potential that House (1995) predicted that "In
one sense, innovations in electronic technology may accomplish more
than our legal system to provide equal opportunities to people with disabilities" (pp. 269–270).

Administration

Although CORE-accredited and other rehabilitation counseling programs
seek to produce trained and educated rehabilitation counselors who will
qualify for CRC and other certification and licensing they often neglect to

Table 17.2 Rehabilitation Content Settings

Insurance—entitlement
- Disability management/
  Medical review coverage/
  billing mechanisms
- Vocational testimony
  - SSI-SSDI
    - Tort-Personal injury,
      Divorce
  - Labor market surveys/
    Job placement
  - Law firms/Labor unions/
    Insurance

Employee assistance
programs (EAP)
- Counseling
  - drug/alcohol
  - personal
  - disability
  - marital
  - career
  - financial/bankruptcy

Consulting
- Training/human resource
  development (HRD)

- Management assistance
- Computer applications
- Board of Directors
- Marketing, image
- Private clinical practice

Facilities—hospitals
- Comprehensive outpatient
  rehabilitation facilities (CORF)
- Profit-making hospitals not
  covered by diagnostic regimental
  grade for services (DRGS)
- Head injury programs

Personnel
- Hiring, orientation
- Affirmative Action/EEOC
- Disability concerns
- Career development
- Employee turnover reduction
- Legal rights
- Drug testing

Health
- Stress reduction
- Health awareness
- OSHA

Adapted and updated from Riggar, T. F., Crimando, W., Bordieri, J., & Phillips, J. S. (1988). Rehabilitation administration preservice education: Preparing the professional rehabilitation administrator, manager, and supervisor. *Journal of Rehabilitation Administration, 12*(4), 93-102; and Kilbury, R. F., Benshoff, J. J., & Riggar, T. F. (1990). The expansion of private sector rehabilitation: Will rehabilitation education respond? *Rehabilitation Education, 4*(3), 163-170.

consider one vital body of research. Whereas some consider it inappropriate to include administration/supervision course work in RCE programs (Herrick, 1983) the need for such knowledge and skills among RCE graduates has been clearly seen. In 1982 Sullivan reported that promotion of RCE graduates to management positions comes very early in their professional careers; Matkin (1982) cited an informal study conducted among RCE graduates from a midwestern university program that indicated promotion to supervisory levels occurred within 18 months following graduation; Emener (1983) estimated that one-third of RCE graduates assume administrative roles and functions within 5 years of graduation; and Riggar and Matkin (1984) in examining graduates over a 5-year period at four rehabilitation programs at three different rehabilitation schools ($N = 66$, effective response rate = 72.5%) discovered that 74.2% of graduate-level rehabilitation graduates advanced, on the average, within 14.25 months to administrative or supervisory positions. They found that many of these quickly promoted individuals continued a caseload with 54.6% performing management activities for 20 or more hours per week.

> Yet, as rehabilitation counselors, especially those with master's degrees, advance up the career ladder, they encounter management responsibilities that their training did not prepare them to perform. As a result, rehabilitation counselors are often confronted with administrative responsibilities beyond their level of expertise which may cause high anxiety and stress and be a contributing factor to professional burnout. (Matkin, 1982, p. 21)

Two significant factors seem to be causal with rehabilitation counselors who matriculate to administrative/supervisory positions. The first part has to do with the qualified nature of their performance and impact of graduate-level education, and the second relates to rehabilitation employee organizational withdrawal behavior (turnover). Often RCE graduates become employed in positions where few other master's-degree level personnel are working. Because of the education, experience, and knowledge required for their advanced degree they are perceived to be equipped to inform, teach, and lead other less qualified employees. Frequently an RCE's first position postgraduation involves supervising bachelor level, and high school, or even GED employees who have been employed at the agency, facility, or organization for many years. Often spending 50+% of their time performing administration and supervision, for which they received no formal training or education, may lead to the problems quoted above by Matkin (1982). Not being able to be full-time human service providers with direct contact with consumers, and less time processing paperwork, their level of personal accomplishment is diminished (Gomez & Michaelis, 1995).

Stress and burnout contribute to RCE graduates ascending to administrative and supervisory positions by causing the withdrawal of potentially competitive workers. Biggs, Flett, Voges, and Alpass (1995) found that organizational conflict, age, and length of service were significant predictors of job satisfaction; whereas level of education was significantly related to distress. It is clear that burnout and little job satisfaction are directly related to turnover (Riggar, 1985; Riggar, Godley, & Hafer, 1984). A decade ago it was discovered that turnover in state/federal rehabilitation agency offices in two Rehabilitation Services Administration (RSA) regions included nearly 1 out of every 10 counselors (Crimando, Hansen, & Riggar, 1986). Many of these studies culminated in an examination of exactly why rehabilitation employees were leaving their employment. Riggar, Hansen, and Crimando (1987) followed up on 78 individuals who withdrew from rehabilitation employment within six selected states over a 12-month period. Results indicated that the number one reason (18.3%) why people were leaving their rehabilitation job was "Little Advancement Potential," the next highest ranked reason (15.2%) was 'Little Job Satisfaction," and third reason for leaving (12.2%) was 'Stress/Burnout." In a current ongoing study within the 6 states of Region V concerning turnover it has been found that for supervisory/management personnel the turnover rate is 18.3% (range 9%–32%), and for direct service personnel the turnover rate is 28.6% (range 15%–57%) (K. Barrett, personal communication, December 1, 1995). In those settings in which promotion does not seem likely due to turnover, advancement may well be best attained by seeking another job (15.2%—Little Advancement Potential).

Whatever the reasons it is clear that RCE graduates who are well-qualified rehabilitation counselors soon advance into positions of administration and supervision for which they may be ill equipped because of their sole concentration on CORE-related knowledge. Although there are considerable transferable skills from counseling to supervision, the basics of human service or rehabilitation administration (planning, organizing, leading, evaluating, and staffing) (Riggar & Lorenz, 1986) are in fact a separate specialty in rehabilitation that contains its own track, requirements, roles, and functions, and has in fact its own NRA division and professional journal. Perhaps in the future NCRE mandates will no longer do RCE graduates an injustice by failing to minimally introduce an area of competence into which so many will matriculate relatively quickly.

LAW

In 1993, for the first time, the Centers for Disease Control reported rates of overall disability among all Americans 16 or older based on 1990 U.S. census data. The results indicated that 43.2 per 1,000 people had a disability that prevented them from leaving home alone, and 47.7 per 1,000 had a disability that prevented them from caring for themselves at home (Associated Press, 1993) The 49+ million Americans with disabilities constitute the largest single minority group in the United States. For this group of Americans, composed of varied constitutient groups, a vast array of laws have been passed by the federal government.

Two of these acts, the Americans with Disabilities Act of 1990 and the Civil Rights Act of 1991, profoundly influence the practice of rehabilitation and the lives of these 49+ million Americans. The ADA referred to as the "Emancipation Proclamation for those with disabilities" (Elsasser, 1989, p.1) was based in part on the "Civil Rights Act for the Disabled" Rehabilitation Act of 1973 and the Civil Rights Act of 1964. A year later the 1991 Civil Rights Act was passed in part to "expand the scope of relevant civil rights statutes in order to provide adequate protection to victims of discrimination"(Riggar, Maki, & Flowers, 1991, p.36). These two acts, and the Rehabilitation Act Amendments of 1992, constitute the current federal rehabilitation mandate and govern our rehabilitation counseling practice today.

Recent research (Boone & Wolfe, 1995), however, has shown that 43% of 70 community employers and employees had never heard of the ADA. In 1994 a survey conducted for the National Organization on Disability found that people aged 16–64 who had disabilities had an employment rate of 33% in 1986 and 31% in 1994 (Casper, 1995; Homes, 1994; Manning, 1994). More recently (Henry, 1995) reported on an ARC (national advocacy group) study which found that 1992–1993 state data showed that 66% of children with mental retardation were still segregated in separate classes, schools, or residential facilities. It was noted that the Department of Education found the figures misleading as the Department indicated that 26.7% of students with mental retardation spent some time in regular classrooms, but not whole days. Despite the clear legislative intent of the Rehabilitation Act of 1973, the ADA, the Education for All Handicapped Children's Act of 1975, the Developmental Disabilities Assistance and Bill of Rights Act of 1976, and the Individuals With Disabilities Education Act Amendments of 1990, as applied to the above circumstances, it is clear that inequity and injustice still occurs.

Of particular concern to many rehabilitation professionals are the unexpected responses, reactions, and consequences to many of these laws. For example, some contend that the ADA has spawned numerous "absurd and lunatic" lawsuits so outrageous that ADA could be said to stand for Attorneys' Dreams Answered (Bovard, 1995). From 1992 when the ADA went into effect to 1993 the EEOC (Equal Employment Opportunities Commission) had received over 14,000 charges of discrimination. Of these 18.6% were filed by individuals with back impairments and nearly half the complaints were brought by people who had been fired (Frum & Brennan, 1993). Even among rehabilitation professionals there are words of caution concerning that which surrounds the ADA. In example, Arokiasamy and Millington (1994) mentioned that:

> The rights-based approach, because it is dependent on legislation and its enforcement by courts, is invariably adversarial, resulting in win–lose situations instead of the win–win propositions that traditionally lead to successful satisfaction of both parties. . . . In such a confrontational environment, what is guaranteed is employment for lawyers and a new breed of professionals spawned by the law, called ADA consultants. What is not guaranteed is willing and genuine involvement of employers in providing access and employment of persons with disabilities. (p.93)

The EEOC, whose job it is to enforce rights-based legislation, estimated that it had 97,000 unresolved cases in 1994, 24,000 more than in 1993, and more than double the number in 1990 (Kilborn, 1994). However backlogged the EEOC still appears to maintain a formidable presence. Noble (1994) reported in a study of 300 companies with at least 250 employees in New York, New Jersey, and Connecticut that companies were indeed hiring from "targeted" groups. When queried as to how and why it was discovered that women were hired 56.9% of the time because of affirmative action concerns, 23.5% because of regulations and only 6.9% because of productivity. For minorities it was found that 56.8% were hired because of affirmative action concerns, 21.6% because of regulations, and 7.2% for productivity. For "disabled workers" it was reported that 22.1% were hired because of affirmative action concerns, 68.5% because of regulations, and only 1.7% for productivity. Surely Noble is correct when she reports that employers are in the dark about diversity.

Although these results are seemingly contrary to the intent and letter of the laws it must be remembered that not many years ago, before these laws, the picture was much bleaker. Today "75% of Americans with disabilities say access to public facilities has improved, 63% see improved attitudes toward people with disabilities, and 60% say access to public transportation is better" (Manning, 1994, p.5D). These laws and the current status are excellent beginning points on which today's rehabilitation counselors can proceed to improve. Much as the ADA and the Rehabilitation Act Amendments of 1992 improved and expanded on the Rehabilitation Act of 1973, and the Civil Rights Act of 1991 improved and expanded on the Civil Rights Act of 1964, rehabilitation counselors today have unique opportunities not available just a few decades ago. For the first time rehabilitation has the real opportunity of assuring the fair-opportunity rule as a part of American public policy on disability:

> The *fair opportunity rule* under the principle of justice states that no persons should be denied the benefits generally available to members of a society, such as the right to participate fully in the social, cultural, and political aspects of community life, because of handicapping characteristics involuntarily acquired. (Beauchamp & Childress, 1983, cited in Rubin & Millard, 1991, p. 14)

Appendixes

History of Rehabilitation and Rehabilitation-Related Laws, and Legislation

1880   **Employers' Liability Act (England).** Modified the old common law defenses between masters and servants.

1886   **Civil Rights Act.** Granted all persons the right to make and enforce contracts, including employment contracts.

1906   **Federal Employers' Liability Act (FELA).** For protection and for reform of the old common law rules of employers' liability; railroad related.

1908   **Federal Employers' Compensation Act (FECA).** Workers' compensation law for federal employees.

1910   New York State instituted first compulsory workers' compensation law.

1913   Federal income tax established.

1916   **National Defense Act.** Preparing soldiers for returning to civilian life after enlistment.

1917   **Smith-Hughes Act.** Established the federal/state program in vocational education; emphasis on vocational rehabilitation of veterans; provided a basis for a system of vocational rehabilitation; matching funds—federal/state.

1918   **Soldier's Rehabilitation Act.** Provided programs for vocational rehabilitation of disabled veterans. Known as the **Smith–Sears Veterans Rehabilitation Act,** and later provided a basis for vocational rehabilitation for civilians.

1920 **Vocational Rehabilitation Act (Smith–Fess Act).** Provided for the civilian vocational rehabilitation program. Federal/state 50/50 matching funds. Funds for vocational guidance, vocational education, occupational adjustment, placement services, prostethics/restoration services, and vocational training for individuals with physical disabilities; minimum age 16.

1921 **Veteran's Bureau Act.** Established the Bureau, which later became the Veterans Administration.

1927 **Longshore and Harbor Workers Compensation Act.** Developed from the interaction of maritime and state laws.

1935 **Social Security Act.** First permanent basis for the federal vocational rehabilitation program; provided for continuous authorization of funds.

1936 **Randolph–Sheppard Act.** Authorized states to license qualified blind persons to operate vending stands.

1938 **Wagner–O'Day Act.** Compulsory for the federal government to buy certain products from workshops that employed blind persons.

1938 **Fair Labor and Standards Act.** Established a minimum wage and provisions for overtime labor as well as prohibits child labor.

1938 **Railroad Unemployment Insurance Act.** Benefits; expanded and detailed regulatory powers of the Railroad Retirement Board, linked with the Social Security Act.

1943 **Vocational Rehabilitation Act Amendments (Barden–LaFollette Act).** Provided a specific definition of vocational rehabilitation. Expanded services to mental disabilities and mental illness.

1943 **Disabled Veterans' Rehabilitation Act.** The VA was authorized to carry out all necessary services to assist disabled servicemen to adjust to the world of work following their honorable discharge.

1944 **Servicemen's Readjustment Act.** "G.I.Bill" provided training and education assistance for those whose education had been interrupted by military service.

1952 **Veterans' Readjustment Assistance Act.** "G.I.Bill" provided education and training for Korean War veterans.

1954 **Social Security Disability Insurance.** Enacted a federal income support program for the blind, poor, aged, and disabled; referred to as supplemental security income.

1954 **Vocational Rehabilitation Amendments.** Expanded the role of state agencies and provide them with more funding (federal 60% matching funds) and program options.

1956   **Social Security Act Amendments.** Authorized Social Security disability allowances for individuals with disabilities.

1962   **Public Welfare Amendments.** Emphasis on making people tax payers instead of tax consumers via vocational training and social services. Formal interaction between Departments of Public Assistance and Vocational Rehabilitation.

1963   **Equal Pay Act.** Prohibits employers from discriminating between employees with respect to wage on the basis of gender.

1964   **Economic Opportunities Act.** Philosophy of combating dependency among poor by promoting self-help and reeducation programs.

1964   **Civil Rights Act.** Prohibits discrimination against any individual with respect to hiring, discharge, compensation, terms, conditions, or privileges of employment because of such individual's race, color, religion, gender, or national origin. As amended includes the Pregnancy Discrimination Act. The Act created the Equal Opportunity Enforcement Commission (EEOC)

1965   **Social Security Amendments.** Enabled state DVR to be reimbursed for providing VR services to persons eligible for SSDI.

1965   **Vocational Rehabilitation Act Amendments.** Expanded services to persons with socially disabling conditions such as alcoholism; introduced extended evaluation. Federal funding 75%. National Commission on Architectural Barriers authorized.

1967   **Executive Order 11246 as amended by Executive Order 11378.** Prohibits job discrimination on the basis of race, color, religion, gender, or national origin and requires *affirmative action* to insure equality of opportunity in all aspects of employment. Applies to employers holding federal contracts or subcontracts of $100,000 or more.

1967   **The Age Discrimination in Employment Act.** Insures that persons over the age of 40 are not discriminated against on the basis of age.

1967   **Vocational Rehabilitation Act Amendments.** Established the National Center for Deaf–Blind Youths and Adults. Grants to VR agencies for pilot projects for provision of VR services to migratory agricultural workers and to members of their families.

1968   **Vocational Rehabilitation Amendments.** Added follow-up services to maintain employment and services to family members. Expanded use of vocational evaluation and work adjustment services. Federal 80% of match.

1970   **Occupational Safety and Health Act.** Establishes federal standards for a safe and healthful working environment.

1972 **Education Amendments.** Forbids discrimination on the basis of gender in all federally assisted education programs.

1972 **Equal Employment Opportunity Act.** Insures that state and local governments, governmental agencies, and political subdivisions and departments offer equal employment opportunities to all persons.

1973 **Rehabilitation Act.**
Section 501—Affirmative Action in federal hiring.
Section 502—Accessibility
Section 503—Prohibits job discrimination on the basis of disability and requires affirmative action to employ and advance in employment individuals with disabilities who, with reasonable accommodation, can perform the essential functions of the job.
Section 504, subpart B—Insures that decisions concerning employment are made in such a manner that discrimination on the basis of handicap does not occur and may not limit, segregate, or classify applicants or employees in any way that adversely affects their opportunities or status because of handicap.

1973 **Health Maintenance Organization Act.** Encourages the development of health maintenance organizations (HMOs) in their initial stages.

1974 **Employment Retirement Income Security Act.** Regulates private pension funds and employer benefits programs. Forbids the firing of employees in order to keep premiums on group health insurance plans from increasing.

1974 **Vietnam Era Veterans' Readjustment Assistance Act.** Prohibits job discrimination and requires affirmative action to employ and advance in employment qualified Vietnam era veterans and qualified special disabled veterans.

1974 **Rehabilitation Act Amendments.** Extended appropriations of the Rehab Act of 1973. Strengthened the program for the blind authorized by the Randolph-Sheppard Act of 1936.

1975 **Age Discrimination Act.** For programs or activities receiving federal financial assistance, prohibits discrimination on the basis of age.

1975 **Education for All Handicapped Childrens' Act.** Mandated that all handicapped children have available to them a free appropriate public education that emphasizes special education and related services designed to meet their unique needs and to assure the rights of handicapped children and their parents or guardians are protected.

1976 **Developmental Disabilities Assistance and Bill of Rights Act.** Assures that developmentally disabled persons receive appropriate services.

1976 **Vocational Education Amendments.** Placement of an individual in vocational training is a group decision.

1978 **Targeted Jobs Tax Credit.** Encourages the hiring of specific disadvantaged groups with high levels of unemployment; referrals from VR agencies.

1978 **Equal Employment Opportunity Commission, U.S.Office of Personnel Management, Departments of Labor and Justice Uniform Guidelines on Employment Selection Procedures.** Fairness applied to employment testing and other selection procedures used as a basis for any employment decision such as hiring, promotion, demotion, memberships (as in labor organizations), referral, retention, licensing and certification, or training or transfer (if these led to any of the previous decisions).

1978 **Civil Rights Commission Amendments.** Expanded the jurisdiction of the Civil Rights Commission to include protection against discrimination on the basis of handicap.

1978 **Rehabilitation, Comprehensive Services, and Developmental Disabilities Act.** Provided comprehensive independent living services. Bill of Rights Act was added to Title V; National Council on the Handicapped established; Interagency Committee on Handicapped Research was developed.

1979 **Department of Education Organization Act.** Established a Department of Education; mandated the Office of Special Education and Rehabilitative Services (OSERS).

1979 **Standards for a Merit System of Personnel Administration.** Recruitment efforts are to be planned and carried out in such a manner that assures open competition and open consideration of qualified applicants.

1979 **Fringe Benefit Regulation Prohibition.** Allowed tax deductions for businesses that removed barriers to handicapped persons.

1980 **Education Amendments.** Created a new special education teachers' training program.

1980 **Personal Assistance for Handicapped Employees' Act.** Permits executive agencies and the Library of Congress to employ personal assistance for handicapped federal employees both at their regular duty stations and while on travel status.

1980 **Civil Rights of Institutionalized Persons.** Gives the U.S. Department of Justice authority to initiate civil suits against states to protect the rights of persons who are mentally ill, retarded, or chronically ill or handicapped or other institutionalized persons.

1981 **Housing and Community Development Act.** The act required HUD to provide study on housing needs and conditions of the handicapped.

1982 **Voting Rights Act Amendments.** Provides that any voter who requires assistance to vote by reason of blindness, disability, or inability to read or write may be given assistance by a person of the voter's own choice.

1982 **Telecommunications for Disabled Act.** Provide reasonable access to telephone service for persons with impaired hearing and to enable telephone companies to accommodate persons with other physical disabilities.

1982 **Job Training and Partnership Act (JTPA).** Replaces CETA; program to prepare youth and unskilled adults to move into the labor force and to afford job training to economically disadvantaged individuals and those in special need of training.

1984 **Rehabilitation Amendments.** Extended Act of 1973 and 1978. A handicapped individual was further defined as one who had reached the age of 16. Client Assistance Programs (CAP) established. National Council on the Handicapped was removed from DOE to become an independent agency. Rule that 51% of consumer control of independent living facilities required.

1984 **Voting Accessibility for the Elderly and Handicapped Act.** Requires that registration and polling places for federal elections be accessible to persons with disabilities.

1986 **Air Carrier Access Act.** Section 504 also pertains to the action of air carriers operating at federally funded airports. Prohibits discrimination against persons with disabilities by all air carriers and provided for enforcement under the Department of Transportation.

1986 **Immigration Reform and Control Act.** Prohibits discrimination based on national origin or citizenship status; does not extend to aliens who are not authorized to work in the United States.

1986 **Rehabilitation Act Amendments.** Provides for individuals with handicaps to maximize their employability, independence, and integration into the pubic and the community.

1987 **Civil Rights Restoration Act.** Restores the scope of coverage and clarifies the application of various laws. Determined that small providers are not required to make significant structural alterations to their existing facilities for the purpose of assuring program accessibility, if alternative means are available. Individuals with handicaps in the employment context does not include those who have a currently contagious disease or infection . . . who would constitute a direct threat to the health or safety of other individuals . . . or who are unable to perform the duties of the job.

1988 **Technology-Related Assistance for Individuals with Disabilities Act.** Provided financial assistance to states to help develop and implement a consumer-responsive program of technology-related assistance.

1988 **Fair Housing Act Amendments.** First federal law to extend the antidiscrimination mandate for persons with disabilities into the private sector: to include housing which had not been the recipient of federal subsidies or funds.

1990 **Americans with Disabilities Act.** Civil rights protection to individuals with disabilities like those provided to individuals on the basis of race, gender, national origin, and religion. Guarantees equal opportunity.

Title I—Employment. Required to provide "reasonable accommodation." Only "undue hardship" or "direct threat to oneself or others" as employer defense.

Title II—Public Accommodations. Auxiliary aids and services provided; physical barriers removed; alterations must be accessible.

Title III—Transportation. Buses purchased on or after August 26, 1990 must be accessible; comparable paratransit or other special transportation must be offered; all new bus stations must be accessible. New rail cars must be accessible if purchased on or before August 26, 1990; existing rail systems must have one accessible car by July 26, 1995; all rail systems must be accessible when new constructed or remodeled.

Title IV—Telecommunications. Telephone companies must offer telephone relay services to individuals who use telecommunication devices designed for the hearing impaired.

Title V—Miscellaneous provisions. State and local government facilities, services and communications must be accessible. Coverage has been extended to Congress. Individuals are granted the right to bring private actions.

1990 **Revenue Reconciliation Act.** Provided a 50% tax credit for the first $10,000 of eligible costs for complying with the ADA. A tax deduction of up to $15,000 for removal of physical barriers.

1991 **Civil Rights Act.** The Act overturns a series of U.S. Supreme Court decisions that were adverse to the interests of victims of employment discrimination and provides for increased damages and jury trials in cases of intentional gender, religious, and disability bias.

Requires the EEOC to establish a Technical Assistance Training Institute to provide educational and outreach activities for individuals who historically have been the victims of job bias. Establishes a Glass Ceiling Commission to study barriers to the advancement of women and minorities in the workforce.

1991 **Individuals with Disabilities Education Act (IDEA) (retitled the Education for All Handicapped Children Act-1975).** State must implement procedures for identifying, locating, and evaluating all its children with disabilities; education with children without disabilities to the greatest extent possible.

1992 **Rehabilitation Amendments.** Changed eligibility requirements so that the rehab agency has to demonstrate that an individual cannot benefit from services; increased consumer control over the IWRP. Enhanced access, accountability, and procedural regularity.

REHABILITATION ACRONYMS

SELECTED ORGANIZATIONS

ACA   American Counseling Association

Subdivisions of the ACA

AAC   Association for Assessment in Counseling
AADA   Association for Adult Development and Aging
ACCA   American College Counseling Association
ACEG   Association for Counselors and Educators in Government
ACES   Association for Counselor Education and Supervision
AHEAD   Association for Humanistic Education and Development
AMCD   Association for Multicultural Counseling and Development
AMHCA   American Mental Health Counselors Association
ARCA   American Rehabilitation Counseling Association
ASCA   American School Counselor Association
ASERVIC   Association for Spiritual, Ethical and Religious Values in Counseling
ASGW   Association for Specialists in Group Work
IAAOC   International Association of Addiction and Offender Counselors

IAMFC International Association of Marriage and Family
Counselors
NCDA National Career Development Association
NECA National Employment Counseling Association

NRA National Rehabilitation Association

Subdivisions of the NRA

NAIL National Association for Independent Living
NAMCRC National Association of Multicultural Rehabilitation
Concerns
NARI National Association of Rehabilitation Instructors
NARS National Association of Rehabilitation Secretaries
NASPPR National Association of Service Providers in Private
Rehabilitation
NRAA National Rehabilitation Administration Association
NRAJPD National Rehabilitation Association of Job Placement
Development
NRCA National Rehabilitation Counseling Association
VEWAA Vocational Evaluation and Work Adjustment Association

Other Organizations

AA Alcoholics Anonymous
AAMFT American Association of Marriage and Family Therapists
ACRM American Congress of Rehabilitation Medicine
ADARA American Deafness and Rehabilitation Association
APA American Psychological Association
  Division 17 Rehabilitation Psychology
  Division 22 Counseling Psychology
ARA American Rehabilitation Association
ARC Alliance for Rehabilitation Counseling
ARC Association for Retarded Citizens
ASHA American Speech–Hearing Association
CARP Canadian Association of Rehabilitation Personnel
CMSA Case Management Society of America
CSAVR Council of State Administrators of Vocational Rehabilitation
IAPRS International Association of Psychosocial Rehabilitation
Services

FRER Foundation for Rehabilitation Education and Research
NAMI National Alliance of Mental Illness
NANWRW National Association of Non-White Rehabilitation
Workers
NARPPS National Association of Rehabiitation Professionals in the
Private Sector
NCRE National Council on Rehabilitation Education
NCIL National Council of Independent Living
NOD National Organization on Disability
PVA Paralyzed Veterans of America
RESNA Rehabilitation Engineering Society of North America
WHO World Health Organization

SELECTED JOURNALS

APM&R *Archives of Physical Medicine and Rehabilitation* (ACRM)
AR *American Rehabilitation* (RSA)
IJRR *International Journal of Rehabilitation Research*
ITD *Information Technology and Disabilities*
JARC *Journal of Applied Rehabilitation Counseling* (NRCA)
JCD *Journal of Counseling and Development* (ACA)
JJP *Journal of Job Placement* (NRAJPD)
JR *Journal of Rehabilitation* (NRA)
JRA *Journal of Rehabilitation Administration* (NRAA)
JRRD *Journal of Rehabilitation Research and Development* (DVA)
JVR *Journal of Vocational Rehabilitation*
RCB *Rehabilitation Counseling Bulletin* (ARCA)
RE *Rehabilitaiton Education* (NCRE)
Rehab BRIEF *Bringing Research Into Effective Focus* (NIDRR)
RP *Rehabilitation Psychologist* (APA, Division 17)
VEWA BULLETIN *Vocational Evaluation and Work Adjustment
Bulletin* (VEWAA)
VR&CPR *Vocational Rehabilitation and Counseling Professional
Review*

CERTIFICATION BODIES/CREDENTIALS

AASCB American Association of State Counselor Licensure Boards

CRCC   Commission for Rehabilitation Counselor Certification
   CRC   Certified Rehabilitation Counselor
   CRC-MAC   Certified Rehabilitation Counselor—Master's in
                 Addictions Counseling
   CCRC   Certified Canadian Rehabilitation Counselor
CIRSC   Certification of Insurance Rehabilitation Specialists
        Commission; now known as Certification of
        Disability Management Specialists Commission (**CDMSC**)
   CIRS   Certified Insurance Rehabilitation Specialists; now known as
        Certified Disability Management Specialist (**CDMS**)
CCMC   Commission for Case Manager Certification
   CCM   Certified Case Manager
CCWAVES   Commission on Certification of Work Adjustment and
        Vocational Evaluation Specialists
   CVE   Certified Vocational Evaluator
NBCC   National Board for Counselor Certification
   CCMHC   Certified Clinical Mental Health Counselor
   NCC   National Certified Counselor
   NCCC   National Certified Career Counselor

CAC   Certified Addictions Counselor
COPA   Council on Postsecondary Accreditation
COTA   Certified Occupational Therapy Assistant
CRRN   Certified Rehabilitation Registered Nurse
FACP   Fellow of the American College of Physicians
FACS   Fellow of the American College of Surgeons
LPC   Licensed Professional Counselor
LPCC   Licensed Professional Clinical Counselor
LPMHC   Licensed Professional Mental Health Counselor
MAC   Master Addictions Counselor
OTR   Registered Occupational Therapist
PT   Physical Therapist
PTA   Physical Therapist Assistant
RPRC   Registered Professional Counselor—California

ACCREDITATION BODIES

CACREP   Commission on the Accreditation of Counseling and
        Related Educational Programs

CARF   Commission for Accreditation of Rehabilitation Facilities
CORE   Council on Rehabilitation Education
JCAHO   Joint Commission on the Accreditation of Healthcare
Organizations

GOVERNMENTAL/LEGISLATIVE

ABA   Architectural Barriers Act
ADA   Americans with Disabilities Act
ADAAG   Americans with Disabilities Act Accessibility Guidelines
ATBCB   Architectural and Transportation Barriers Compliance Board
CAP   Client Assistance Projects
CDC   Center for Disease Control
CIL   Center for Independent Living
CRA   Civil Rights Act
DBTAC   Disability Business and Technical Assistance Centers
DOE   Department of Education
DOJ   Department of Justice
DOL   Department of Labor
DOT   Department of Transportation
DOT   *Dictionary of Occupational Titles*
DVA   Department of Veterans Affairs
DVR   Division/Department of Vocational Rehabilitation
EEOC   Equal Employment Opportunity Commission
FCC   Federal Communications Commission
GAO   General Accounting Office
GOE   Guide to Occuptional Exploration
HEW   Department of Health, Education and Welfare
HHS   Department of Health and Human Services
HUD   Department of Housing and Urban Development
IDEA   Individuals with Disabilities Education Act
IEP   Individual Evaluation/Education Plan
IL   Independent Living
ILR   Independent Living Rehabilitation
ILRU   Independent Living Research Utilization
IWRP   Individual Written Rehabilitation Plan
JAN   Job Accommodations Network
NARIC   National Rehabilitation Information Center
NCD   National Council on Disability

NCHRTM   National Clearninghouse on Rehabilitation Training
      Materials
NCMRR   National Center for Medical Rehabilitation Research
NIDRR   National Institute on Disability and Rehabilitation Research
NIH   National Institutes of Health
NIMH   National Institute of Mental Health
NOD   National Organization on Disability
OPM   Office of Personnel Management
OSERS   Office of Special Education and Rehabilitation Services
OSEP   Office of Special Education Programs
OSHA   Occupational Health and Safety Administration
PCEPD   President's Commission on the Environment of Persons
      with Disabilities
PWI   Projects with Industry
QRP   Qualified Rehabilitation Professional
RCEP   Regional Continuing Education Program
R&D   Research and Development
RSA   Rehabilitation Services Administration
RTC   Research and Training Center
SSA   Social Security Administration
SSDI   Social Security Disability Insurance
SSI   Supplemental Security Income
UAF   University Affiliated Facility
VA   Veterans Administration
VBA   Veteran's Benefits Administration
VHA   Veteran's Health Administration
VR&C   Vocational Rehabilitation and Counseling
WID   World Institute on Disability

MISCELLANEOUS

ATI   Attitude-Treatment Interaction
ATP   Assistive Technology Professional
CAI   Computer Assisted Instruction
CEU   Continuing Education Unit
CLM   Caseload Management
DD   Developmental Disability
DSM-IV   Diagnostic and Statistical Manual

EAP   Employee Assistance Program
EASI   Equal Access to Software and Information
ICD   International Center for Disability
ITV   Interactive Television
LDL   Long Distance Learning
LTD   Long Term Disability
OJT   On-the-Job Training
OJE   On-the-Job Evaluation
PDR   *Physician's Desk Reference*
RCE   Rehabilitation Counselor Education
RCT   Rehabilitation Counselor Training
RFP   Request for Proposals
RTW   Return to Work
TDD   Telecommunication Devices for the Deaf
TTY   Teletypewriters
VDARE   Vocational Diagnosis and Assessment of Residual
Employability

Scope of Practice for Rehabilitation Counseling

I. ASSUMPTION

1. The Scope of Practice Statement identifies knowledge and skills required for the provision of effective rehabilitation counseling services to persons with physical, mental, developmental, cognitive, and emotional disabilities as embodied in the standards of the profession's credentialing organizations.

2. The several rehabilitation disciplines and related processes (e.g., vocational evaluation, job development and job placement, work adjustment, case management) are tied to the central field of rehabilitation counseling. The field of rehabilitation counseling is a specialty within the rehabilitation profession with counseling at its core, and is differentiated from other related counseling fields.

3. The professional scope of rehabilitation counseling practice is also differentiated from an individual scope of practice, which may overlap, but is more specialized than the professional scope. An individual scope of practice is based on one's own knowledge of the abilities and skills that have been gained through a program of education and professional experience. A person is ethically bound to limit his/her practice to that individual scope of practice.

II. UNDERLYING VALUES

1.   Facilitation of independence, integration, and inclusion of people with disabilities in employment and the community.

2.   Belief in the dignity and worth of all people.

3.   Commitment to a sense of equal justice based on a model of accommodation to provide and equalize the opportunities to participate in all rights and privileges available to all people; and a commitment to supporting persons with disabilities in advocacy activities to enable them to achieve this status and empower themselves.

4.   Emphasis on the holistic nature of human function, which is procedurally facilitated by the utilization of such techniques as:

- interdisciplinary teamwork;
- counseling to assist in maintaining a holistic perspective;
- a commitment to considering individuals within the context of their family systems and communities.

5.   Recognition of the importance of focusing on the assets of the person.

6.   Commitment to models of service delivery that emphasize integrated, comprehensive services which are mutually planned by the consumer and the rehabilitation counselor.

III. SCOPE OF PRACTICE STATEMENT

Rehabilitation counseling is a systematic process that assists persons with physical, mental, developmental, cognitive, and emotional disabilities to achieve their personal, career, and independent-living goals in the most integrated setting possible through the application of the counseling process. The counseling process involves communication, goal setting, and beneficial growth or change through self-advocacy, psychological, vocational, social, and behavioral interventions. The specific techniques and modalities used within this rehabilitation counseling process may include, but are not limited to:

assessment and appraisal;

diagnosis and treatment planning;

career (vocational) counseling;

individual and group counseling treatment interventions focused on facilitating adjustments to the medical and psychosocial impact of disability;

case management, referral, and service coordination;

program evaluation and research;

interventions to remove environmental, employment, and attitudinal barriers;

consultation services among multiple parties and regulatory systems;

job analysis, job development, and placement services, including assistance with employment and job accommodations; and

the provision of consultation about, and access to, rehabilitation technology.

IV. SELECTED DEFINITIONS

The following definitions are provided to increase the understanding of certain key terms and concepts used in the Scope of Practice Statement for Rehabilitation Counseling.

Appraisal: Selecting, administering, scoring, and interpreting instruments designed to assess an individual's attitudes, abilities, achievements, interests, personal characteristics, disabilities, and mental, emotional, or behavioral disorders as well as the use of methods and techniques for understanding human behavior in relation to coping with, adapting to, or changing life situations.

Diagnosis and Treatment Planning: Assessing, analyzing, and providing diagnostic descriptions of mental, emotional, or behavioral conditions or disabilities; exploring possible solutions; and developing and implementing a treatment plan for mental, emotional, and psychosocial adjustment or development. Diagnosis and treatment planning shall not be construed to permit the performance of any act that rehabilitation counselors are not educated and trained to perform.

Counseling Treatment Intervention: The application of cognitive, affective, behavioral, and systemic counseling strategies, which include developmental, wellness, pathologic, and multicultural principles of human behavior. Such interventions are specifically implemented in the context of a professional counseling relationship and may include, but are not limited to: appraisal; individual, group, marriage, and family counseling and psychotherapy; the diagnostic description and treatment of persons with mental, emotional, and behavioral disorders or disabilities; guidance and consulting to facilitate normal growth and development, including educational and career development; the utilization of functional assessments and career counseling for persons requesting assistance in adjusting to a disability or handicapping condition; referrals; consulting; and research.

Referral: Evaluating and identifying the needs of a counselee to determine the advisability of referrals to other specialists, advising the counselee of such judgments, and communicating as requested or deemed appropriate to such referral sources.

Case Management: A systematic process merging counseling and managerial concepts and skills through the application of techniques derived from intuitive and researched methods, thereby advancing efficient and effective decision making for functional control of self, client, setting, and other relevant factors for anchoring a proactive practice. In case management, the counselor's role is focused on interviewing, counseling, planning rehabilitation programs, coordinating services, interacting with significant others, placing clients and following up with them, monitoring a client's progress, and solving problems.

Program Evaluation: The effort to determine what changes occur as a result of a planned program by comparing actual changes (results) with desired changes (stated goals), and by identifying the degree to which the activity (planned program) is responsible for those changes.

Research: A systematic effort to collect, analyze, and interpret quantitative or qualitative data that describe how social characteristics, behavior, emotions, cognition, disabilities, mental disorders, and interpersonal transactions among individuals and organizations interact.

Consultation: The application of scientific principles and procedures in counseling and human development to provide assistance in understanding and solving current or potential problems that the consultee may have in relation to a third party, be it an individual, group, or organization.

Code of Professional Ethics for Certified Rehabilitation Counselors and CRCC Guidelines and Procedures for Processing Complaints

CODE OF PROFESSIONAL ETHICS

The Commission on Rehabilitation Counselor Certification has adopted a Code of Professional Ethics for its Certified Rehabilitation Counselors. The following organizations have adopted the same Code for their memberships: the American Rehabilitation Counseling Association, the National Rehabilitation Counseling Association, and the National Council on Rehabilitation Education. Portions of the Code are derived from the American Psychological Association's Ethical Principles of Psychologists.

Preamble

Rehabilitation counselors are committed to facilitating the personal, social, and economic independence of individuals with disabilities. In fulfilling this commitment, rehabilitation counselors work with various people, programs, institutions, and service delivery systems. Rehabilitation counselors recognize that their actions (or inaction) can either aid or hinder clients in achieving their rehabilitation objectives, and they accept this responsibility as part of their professional obligations. Rehabilitation counselors may be called upon to provide various kinds of assistance including: counseling; vocational explorations; psychological and vocational assessments; evaluations of social, medical, vocational, and psychiatric information; job placement and job development activities; and other types of rehabilitation services. They are required to do so in a manner that is consistent with their education and experience. Moreover, rehabilitation counselors must demonstrate their adherence to ethical standards and ensure that these standards are vigorously enforced. The Code of Professional Ethics (henceforth referred to as the Code) is designed to facilitate the achievement of these goals.

The primary obligation of rehabilitation counselors is to their clients (defined in the Code as individuals with disabilities who are receiving services from rehabilitation counselors). The objective of the Code is to promote public welfare by specifying and enforcing ethical standards of behavior expected of rehabilitation counselors. Accordingly, the Code contains two kinds of standards: Canons and Rules of Professional Conduct.

The Canons are general standards of an aspirational and inspirational nature that reflect the fundamental spirit of caring and respect which professionals share. They are maxims designed to serve as models of exemplary professional conduct. The Canons also express general concepts and principles from which the more specific Rules are derived. Unlike the Canons, the Rules are exacting standards intended to provide guidance in specific circumstances.

Rehabilitation counselors who violate the Code are subject to disciplinary action. A violation of a Rule is interpreted as a violation of the applicable Canon and the general principles it embodies. Since the use of the Certified Rehabilitation Counselor (CRC) designation is a privilege granted by the Commission on Rehabilitation Counselor Certification (CRCC), the Commission reserves unto itself the power to suspend or revoke this privilege or to impose other penalties for a Rule violation. Disciplinary penalties are imposed as warranted by the severity of the offense and its attendant circumstances. All disciplinary actions are undertaken in accordance with published procedures and penalties that are designed to ensure proper enforcement of the Code within a framework of due process and equal protection under the law.

When there is reason to question the ethical propriety of specific behavior, individuals are encouraged to refrain from such behavior until the matter has been clarified. CRCs who need assistance in interpreting the Code should write to the Commission to request an advisory opinion. Counselors who are not certified should request such opinions from their own professional organizations.

CANON 1: MORAL AND LEGAL STANDARDS

Rehabilitation counselors shall behave in a legal, ethical, and moral manner in the conduct of their profession, maintaining the integrity of the Code and avoiding any behavior that would cause harm to others.

Rules of Professional Conduct

R1.1   Rehabilitation counselors will obey the laws and statutes of the legal jurisdiction in which they practice, and are subject to disciplinary action for any violation to the extent that such violation suggests the likelihood of professional misconduct.

R1.2   Rehabilitation counselors will be thoroughly familiar with and observe the legal limitations of the services they offer to clients. They will discuss these limitations as well as all benefits available to clients with the persons they serve in order to facilitate open, honest communications and avoid unrealistic expectations.

R1.3   Rehabilitation counselors will be alert to the legal parameters relevant to their practices as well as to any disparities that may exist between legally mandated ethical or professional standards and the Code. Where disparities exist, rehabilitation counselors will follow the legal mandates and formally communicate such disparities to the appropriate committee on professional ethics. In the absence of any legal guidelines, the Code is ethically binding.

R1.4   Rehabilitation counselors will not engage in any act or omission of a dishonest, deceitful or fraudulent nature in the conduct of their professional activities. They will not allow the pursuit of financial gain or other personal benefits to interfere with the exercise of sound professional judgment and skills, nor will they abuse the relationship with a client to promote their personal or financial gain or the financial gain of an employer.

R1.5   Rehabilitation counselors will understand and abide by the Canons and Rules of Professional Conduct prescribed in the Code.

R1.6   Rehabilitation counselors will not advocate, sanction, participate in, cause to be accomplished, carry out through another or condone any act which they themselves are prohibited from performing by the Code.

R1.7   Moral and ethical standards of behavior are a personal matter for rehabilitation counselors to the same degree as they are for any other citizen, except as such standards may compromise the fulfillment of the individual's professional responsibilities or reduce public trust in rehabilitation counselors.

R1.8   Rehabilitation counselors will respect the rights and reputation of any institution, organization or firm with which they are associated when making oral or written statements. In those instances where they are critical of current policies, they will attempt to effect changes through constructive action within the organization.

R1.9   Rehabilitation counselors will refuse to participate in employment practices that are inconsistent with moral or legal standards regarding the treatment of employees or the public. Rehabilitation counselors will not condone practices that result in illegal or otherwise unjustifiable discrimination on any basis in hiring, promotion or training.

CANON 2: COUNSELOR–CLIENT RELATIONSHIP

Rehabilitation counselors shall respect the integrity and protect the welfare of the people and groups with whom they work. The primary obligation of rehabilitation counselors is to their clients (defined as individuals with disabilities who are receiving services from rehabilitation counselors). At all times, rehabilitation counselors shall endeavor to place their clients' interests above their own.

Rules of Professional Conduct

R2.1   Rehabilitation counselors will make clear to clients the purposes, goals, and limitations that may affect the counseling relationship.

R2.2   Rehabilitation counselors will not misrepresent their role or competence to clients. If requested, they will provide information about their credentials, and will refer clients to other specialists as the needs of the clients dictate.

R2.3   Rehabilitation counselors will be continually cognizant of their own needs and values as well as of their potential influence over clients, students, and subordinates. They will avoid exploiting the trust or dependency of such persons. Rehabilitation counselors will make every effort to avoid dual relationships that could impair their professional judgment or increase the risk of exploitation. Examples of dual relationships include, but are not limited to research with and treatment of employees, students, supervisors, close friends or relatives. Sexual intimacy with clients is unethical.

R2.4   Rehabilitation counselors who provide services at the request of a third party will clarify the nature of their relationships to all involved. They will inform all parties of their ethical responsibilities and take other action as appropriate. Rehabilitation counselors who are employed by third parties as case consultants or expert witnesses, where there is no intent to provide rehabilitation counseling services directly to clients (beyond file review, initial review and/or assessment) will clearly define, through written or oral means, the limits of their relationship (particularly in the areas of informed consent and legally privileged communications) to all involved. When serving as case consultants or expert witnesses, rehabilitation counselors have an obligation to provide unbiased, objective opinions.

R2.5   Rehabilitation counselors will honor the rights of clients to consent to participate in rehabilitation services. They will inform the clients or their legal guardians of factors that may affect the clients' decision to take part in rehabilitation services, and they will obtain written consents once the clients or their guardians are fully informed of these factors. Rehabilitation counselors who work with minors or other persons who are unable to give informed, voluntary consent will take special care to protect the interests of their clients.

R2.6   Rehabilitation counselors will avoid initiating or continuing consulting or counseling relationships if it appears there can be no benefit to the client; in these cases, the rehabilitation counselor will suggest appropriate alternatives to the client.

R2.7   Rehabilitation counselors will recognize that families are usually an important factor in the client's rehabilitation and will strive to enlist their understanding and involvement as a positive resource in achieving rehabilitation goals. The client's permission will be secured prior to any family involvement.

R2.8   Rehabilitation counselors and their clients will work together to devise integrated, individualized rehabilitation plans that promise reasonable success and are consistent with each client's circumstances and abilities. Rehabilitation counselors will continually monitor such plans to ensure their ongoing viability and effectiveness, remembering that clients have the right to make their own choices.

R2.9   Rehabilitation counselors will work with their clients in evaluating potential employment opportunities, considering only those jobs and circumstances that are consistent with the client's overall abilities, vocational limitations, physical restrictions, general temperament, interests and aptitudes, social skills, education, general qualifications, and other relevant characteristics and needs. Rehabilitation counselors will neither place or participate in the placing of clients in positions that could damage the interests and welfare of either the client or the employer.

CANON 3: CLIENT ADVOCACY

Rehabilitation counselors shall serve as advocates for individuals with disabilities.

Rules of Professional Conduct

R3.1   Rehabilitation counselors will be obligated at all times to promote better access for individuals with disabilities to facilities, programs, transportation, and communication media so that clients will not be excluded from opportunities to participate fully in rehabilitation, education and social activities.

R3.2   Rehabilitation counselors will ensure that programs, facilities and employment settings are appropriately accessible before referring clients to them.

R3.3   Rehabilitation counselors will strive to understand the accessibility problems of individuals with cognitive, hearing, mobility, visual and/or other disabilities, and to demonstrate this understanding in the practice of their profession.

R3.4   Rehabilitation counselors will strive to eliminate attitudinal barriers, including stereotyping and discrimination, toward individuals with disabilities and to increase their own awareness and sensitivity to such individuals.

R3.5   Rehabilitation counselors will remain aware of the actions taken by cooperating agencies on behalf of their clients and will act as the advocates of such clients to ensure effective service delivery.

CANON 4: PROFESSIONAL RELATIONSHIPS

Rehabilitation counselors shall act with integrity in their relationships with colleagues, organizations, agencies, institutions, referral sources, and other professions in order to provide clients with optimum benefits.

Rules of Professional Conduct

R4.1   Rehabilitation counselors will ensure that there is a mutual understanding of the rehabilitation plan by all agencies involved in the rehabilitation of clients and that all rehabilitation plans are developed with such mutual understanding.

R4.2   Rehabilitation counselors will abide by and help to implement "team" decisions when formulating rehabilitation plans and procedures, even if not in personal agreement with such decisions, unless they constitute a breach of ethical conduct.

R4.3   Rehabilitation counselors will not commit receiving counselors to any prescribed course of action in relation to clients they may transfer to other colleagues or agencies.

R4.4   Rehabilitation counselors will promptly supply all information needed for a cooperating agency or counselor to begin serving a transferred client.

R4.5   Rehabilitation counselors will not offer ongoing professional counseling or case management services to clients who are receiving such services from another counselor without first notifying that individual. File reviews and second-opinion services are not included in the concept of professional counseling and case management services.

R4.6   Rehabilitation counselors will secure appropriate reports and evaluations from other specialists when such reports are essential for rehabilitation planning and/or service delivery.

R4.7   Rehabilitation counselors will not discuss the competency of other counselors or agencies (including the judgments made, methods used or quality of rehabilitation plans) in a disparaging way with their clients.

R4.8   Rehabilitation counselors will not use their professional relationships with supervisors, colleagues, students or employees to exploit them sexually or otherwise. Neither will they engage in or condone sexual harassment (defined as deliberate or repeated comments, gestures, or physical contacts of a sexual nature that are unwanted by the recipients).

R4.9   Rehabilitation counselors who know of an ethics violation by another counselor will attempt to resolve the issue informally with that person provided the misconduct is minor in nature and/or appears to be due to a lack of sensitivity, knowledge or experience. If the violation is more serious or not amenable to an informal resolution, the counselor will bring it to the attention of the appropriate committee on professional ethics.

R4.10   Rehabilitation counselors possessing information of an alleged violation of this Code will reveal such information to the Commission or another authority empowered to investigate or act upon the alleged violation, if requested to do so. This does not apply to information that is protected by law.

R4.11   Rehabilitation counselors who employ or supervise students or other professionals will provide appropriate working conditions, timely evaluations, constructive consultations, and suitable experience opportunities to facilitate the professional development of these individuals.

CANON 5: PUBLIC STATEMENTS/FEES

Rehabilitation counselors shall adhere to professional standards in establishing fees and promoting their services.

Rules of Professional Conduct

R5.1   Rehabilitation counselors will consider carefully the value of their services and the financial resources of their clients in order to establish reasonable fees for their professional services.

R5.2   Rehabilitation counselors will not accept a fee or any other form of remuneration for their work from clients who are entitled to their services through an institution, agency or other benefit structure, unless the client has been fully informed of the availability of such services from those sources.

R5.3   Rehabilitation counselors will neither give nor receive commissions, rebates or any other form of remuneration when referring clients for professional services.

R5.4   Rehabilitation counselors who describe the counseling and other services offered to the public will present such information fairly and accurately, avoiding misrepresentation through sensationalism, exaggeration or superficiality. Rehabilitation counselors will be guided by their primary obligation to aid the public forming valid opinions and making informed choices and judgments.

CANON 6: CONFIDENTIALITY

Rehabilitation counselors shall respect the confidentiality of information obtained from clients in the course of their work.

Rules of Professional Conduct

R6.1   Rehabilitation counselors will inform clients of the limits of confidentiality at the onset of the counseling relationship.

R6.2   Rehabilitation counselors will take reasonable direct action, inform responsible authorities or warn those persons at risk if the condition or actions of a client indicate there is clear and imminent danger to the client or others; counselors will take such actions only after advising the client of what must be done. Consultations with other professionals may be used where appropriate. Such assumptions of responsibility for a client must be taken only after careful deliberation, and clients must be permitted to resume responsibility as quickly as possible.

R6.3   Rehabilitation counselors will not forward any confidential information to another person, agency or potential employers without the written permission of the client or the client's legal guardian.

R6.4   Rehabilitation counselors will ensure that the agencies which cooperate in serving their clients have specific policies and practices in place to protect client confidentiality.

R6.5   Rehabilitation counselors will safeguard the maintenance, storage, and disposal of client records so unauthorized persons cannot gain access to them. Any non-professional who must be given access to a client's records will be thoroughly instructed about the confidentiality standards to be observed by the rehabilitation counselor.

R6.6   Rehabilitation counselors will present only germane data in preparing oral and written reports, and will make every effort to avoid undue invasions of privacy.

R6.7   Rehabilitation counselors will obtain written permission from clients or their legal guardians prior to taping or otherwise recording counseling sessions. Even if a guardian's consent is obtained, counselors will not record sessions against the expressed wishes of their client.

R6.8 Rehabilitation counselors will persist in claiming the privileged status of confidential information obtained from their clients where communications between counselors and clients have been accorded privileged status under the law.

R6.9 Rehabilitation counselors will provide only relevant information about clients seeking jobs to prospective employers. Before releasing any information that might be considered confidential, the counselor will secure the permission of the client or legal guardian.

CANON 7: ASSESSMENT

Rehabilitation counselors shall promote the welfare of clients in the selection, use and interpretation of assessment measures.

Rules of Professional Conduct

R7.1 Rehabilitation counselors will recognize that different tests require different levels of competence to administer, score and interpret; they will also recognize the limits of their competence and will perform only those functions for which they are trained.

R7.2 Rehabilitation counselors will carefully consider the specific validity, reliability, and appropriateness of tests when selecting them for use in a given situation or for particular clients. They will proceed with caution in attempting to evaluate and interpret the performance of individuals with disabilities, members of minority groups or persons who are not represented in standardized norms. Rehabilitation counselors will take into consideration the effects of socio-economic, ethnic, disability, and cultural factors on test scores.

R7.3 Rehabilitation counselors will administer tests under the standardized conditions. When non-standard conditions are required to accommodate clients with disabilities, or when irregularities occur during the testing session, those circumstances will be noted and taken into account when interpreting the test results.

R7.4 Rehabilitation counselors will ensure that instrument limitations are not exceeded, and that periodic assessments are made to prevent client stereotyping.

R7.5 Rehabilitation counselors will inform clients of the purpose of any testing and the explicit use of the results before administration. Recognizing the right of clients to their test results, counselors will explain such results in language the clients can understand.

R7.6 Rehabilitation counselors will ensure that specific interpretations accompany any release of individual data. The client's welfare and explicit prior permission from the client will determine who is to receive test results. Assessment data will be interpreted on the basis of the particular goals of the evaluation.

R7.7 Rehabilitation counselors will attempt to ensure that the interpretations produced by computerized assessment programs or procedures have been validated through appropriate research. Public offerings of automated test interpretation services will be considered as professional-to-professional consultations. In these instances, the formal responsibility of the consultant is to the consultee, but the ultimate and overriding responsibility is to the client.

R7.8   Rehabilitation counselors will recognize that assessment results may become outdated and will make every effort to avoid the use of obsolete measures.

CANON 8: RESEARCH ACTIVITIES

Rehabilitation counselors shall assist in efforts to expand the knowledge needed to serve individuals with disabilities more effectively.

Rules of Professional Conduct

R8.1   Rehabilitation counselors will ensure that research data meet rigid standards of validity, accuracy, and protection of confidentiality.

R8.2   Rehabilitation counselors will be aware of and responsive to all pertinent guidelines on research with human subjects. When planning such research, counselors will ensure that the project, design, and execution are in full compliance with such guidelines.

R8.3   Rehabilitation counselors who present case studies in classes, professional meetings or publications will confine the content to information that can be sufficiently disguised to ensure full protection of client identity.

R8.4   Rehabilitation counselors will credit those who contribute to publications in proportion to the size of their contribution.

R8.5   Rehabilitation counselors recognize that openness and honesty are essential to relationships between counselors and research participants. When a study's methodology requires concealment or deception, the counselor will ensure that participants understand the reasons for such action.

CANON 9: COMPETENCE

Rehabilitation counselors shall establish and maintain their professional competence at a level which ensures their clients will receive the benefit of the highest quality of service the profession is capable of offering.

Rules of Professional Conduct

R9.1   Rehabilitation counselors will function within the limits of their defined role, training and technical competency, accepting only those positions for which they are professionally qualified.

R9.2   Rehabilitation counselors will continuously strive, through reading, attending professional meetings, and taking courses of instruction, to remain aware of developments, concepts and practices that are essential in providing the highest quality of services to their clients.

R9.3   Rehabilitation counselors, recognizing that personal problems may interfere with their professional effectiveness, will refrain from undertaking any activity in which such problems could lead to inadequate performance. If they are already engaged in such a situation when they become aware of a problem, they will seek competent professional assistance to determine if they should limit, suspend or terminate their professional activities.

R9.4   Rehabilitation counselors who are educators will perform their duties based on careful preparation so that their instruction is accurate, up-to-date, and scholarly.

R9.5   Rehabilitation counselors who are educators will ensure that statements made in catalogs and course outlines are accurate, particularly in terms of subject matter, basis for grading, and nature of classroom experiences.

R9.6   Rehabilitation counselors who are educators will maintain high standards of knowledge and skill by presenting information in their field fully and accurately, and by giving appropriate recognition to alternative viewpoints.

CANON 10: CRC CREDENTIAL

Rehabilitation counselors holding the designation of Certified Rehabilitation Counselor (CRC) shall honor its integrity and respect the limitations placed on its use.

Rules of Professional Conduct

R10.1   Certified Rehabilitation Counselors will use the designation only in accordance with the relevant Guidelines promulgated by the Commission on Rehabilitation Counselor Certification (CRCC).

R10.2   Certified Rehabilitation Counselors will not claim a depth or scope of knowledge, skills or professional capabilities that are greater than warranted simply because they have achieved the CRC designation.

R10.3   Certified Rehabilitation Counselors will not make unfair comparisons between persons who hold the designation and those who do not.

R10.4   Certified Rehabilitation Counselors will not write, speak or act in such a way as to lead another to reasonably believe the counselor is an official CRCC representative unless authorized to do so in writing by the Commission.

R10.5   Certified Rehabilitation Counselors will not claim possession of unique skills or devices not available to others in the profession unless the existence and efficacy of such skills or devices has been scientifically demonstrated.

R10.6   Certified Rehabilitation Counselors will not initiate or support the candidacy of an individual for certification if that individual is known to engage in professional practices that violate this Code.

Acknowledgements

Referenced documents, statements, and sources for the development of this revised Code are as follows: National Rehabilitation Counseling Association Code of Ethics, National Academy of Certified Clinical Mental Health Counselors, and the Ethical Standards of the American Association for Counseling and Development. Portions of the Code are also derived from the "Ethical Principles of Psychologists" of the American Psychological Association.

CRCC GUIDELINES AND PROCEDURES
FOR PROCESSING COMPLAINTS
Adopted April 1995

Section A: General

1.   The Commission on Rehabilitation Counselor Certification, hereafter referred to as the "Commission" or "CRCC," is dedicated to the international promotion of professional rehabilitation counselor certification through credentialing to advance the quality of service provided to persons with disabilities.

2.   The Commission, in furthering its objectives, administers the Code of Professional Ethics for Rehabilitation Counselors that has been developed and approved by the Commission.

3.   The purpose of this document is to facilitate the work of the CRCC Ethics Committee ("Committee") by specifying the procedures for processing cases of alleged violation of the CRCC Code of Professional Ethics for Rehabilitation Counselors, enumeratinging options for sanctioning certificants, and stating appeals procedures. The intent of the Commission is to monitor the professional conduct of its certificants to promote sound ethical practices. CRCC does not, however, warrant the performance of any individual.

4.   Throughout this document and for the purposes of this document, "accused" does not imply either guilt or innocence.

5.   In the event that the CRCC receives a complaint concerning an individual who does not possess a CRC designation, a representative of CRCC will inform the complainant and may refer the complainant to an appropriate authority.

6.   Any failure to disclose pertinent information or any misleading disclosure by a CRC with respect to an ethics charge, criminal case, disciplinary proceeding, or similar matter, concerning him/her, may constitute a violation.

Section B: Ethics Committee Members

1.   The Ethics Committee is a standing Committee of the Commission. The Committee consists of at least four (4), but not more than five (5) members, appointed by the Chair of the Commission and confirmed by a majority vote of the Commission, including the individual appointed as Chair of the Committee. Any vacancy occurring on the Committee will be filled by the Chair of the Commission.

2.   A quorum of three members of the Committee is necessary to conduct a hearing or any other business to come before the Committee.

3.   In the event any member of the Committee has a personal interest in the case or has any knowledge of the case other than what has been provided to all Committee members, he/she shall withdraw from hearing the case. In the event that the Chair shall withdraw,

the Commission Chair shall appoint another Committee member to act as Chair of the Committee.

Section C: Role and Function

1.   The Ethics Committee is responsible for:

   a.   Educating the certificants as to the Commission's Code of Professional Ethics for Rehabilitation Counselors;

   b.   Periodically reviewing and recommending changes in the Code of Professional Ethics for Rehabilitation Counselors as well as the Guidelines and Procedures for Processing Complaints;

   c.   Receiving and processing complaints of alleged violations of the Code of Professional Ethics for Rehabilitation Counselors; and

   d.   Receiving and processing questions.

2.   The Committee shall meet in person or by telephone conference a minimum of four (4) times per year for processing complaints.

3.   In processing complaints of alleged violations, the Committee will compile an objective, factual account of the dispute in question and make the best possible recommendation for the resolution of the case. The Committee, in taking any action, shall do so only for cause, shall only take the degree of disciplinary action that is reasonable, shall utilize these procedures with objectivity and fairness, and, in general, shall act only to further the interests and objectives of the Commission and its certificants.

4.   If a Committee member excuses himself/herself from a complaint and insufficient members are available to conduct business, the Chair shall appoint a former CRCC Commissioner, who is a CRC, to act as a member of the Committee.

Section D: Responsibilities of the Committee Members

1.   The Committee members have an obligation to act in an unbiased manner, to work expeditiously, to safeguard the confidentiality of the Committee's activities, and to follow procedures established to protect the rights of all individuals involved.

Section E: Responsibilities of the Committee Administering the Complaint

1.   The responsibilities of the Committee will include, but not be limited to, the following:

   a.   Review complaints that have been received;

   b.   Determine whether the alleged behavior, if true, would violate CRCC's Code of Professional Ethics for Rehabilitation Counselors, and whether the Committee should review the complaint under these rules;

c. Notify the complainant that the Committee has determined that no action will be taken; or, if action is to be taken, notifying the complainant and the accused certificant of receipt of the case via certified mail, return receipt requested, and marked "Personal and Confidential";

d. Request additional information from the complainant, accused certificant, or others;

e. Arrange for legal advice with the assistance of the CRCC Chief Executive Officer; and

f. Prepare and send, via certified mail, return receipt requested, and marked "Personal and Confidential," communications to the complainant and accused certificant on the decisions of the Commission.

Section F: Jurisdiction

1. The Committee will consider whether an individual has violated the CRCC Code of Professional Ethics for Rehabilitation Counselors if the individual is a current certificant of the CRCC.

2. Should a respondent attempt to relinquish CRCC certification during the course of any case, CRCC reserves the right to continue the matter for a final and binding resolution according to these rules.

Section G: Eligibility to File Complaints

1. The Committee will accept complaints that a CRCC certificant has violated one or more sections of the CRCC Code of Professional Ethics for Rehabilitation Counselors from the following:

a. Members of the general public who have reason to believe that a CRCC certificant has violated the CRCC Code of Professional Ethics for Rehabilitation Counselors.

b. CRCC certificants or members of other helping professions who have reason to believe that a CRCC certificant has violated the CRCC Code of Professional Ethics for Rehabilitation Counselors.

c. The Chair of the Committee when the Committee has reason to believe through information received through materials in the public domain that a CRCC certificant has violated the CRCC Code of Professional Ethics for Rehabilitation Counselors.

Section H: Time Lines

1. The time lines set forth in these standards are guidelines only and have been established to provide a reasonable framework for processing complaints.

2. Complainants or accused certificants may request extensions of deadlines when appropriate. Extensions of deadlines will be granted by the Committee only when justified by unusual circumstances.

3. CRCs are pledged, in accordance with the CRCC Code of Professional Ethics for Rehabilitation Counselors, to cooperate with proceedings of the CRCC for any alleged violation of the Code of Professional Ethics for Rehabilitation Counselors. If the accused voluntarily relinquishes certification or if the accused or complainant fails to cooperate with an ethical inquiry in any way, the CRCC shall, at its discretion, continue its investigation, noting in its final report the circumstances of the accused's failure to cooperate. The Committee may terminate the complaint of an uncooperative complainant.

Section I: Nature of Communication

1. Only signed, written communications regarding ethical complaints against certificants will be accepted. If telephone inquiries from individuals are received regarding the filing of complaints, responding to complaints, or providing information regarding complaints, the individuals calling will be informed of the signed, written communication requirement and asked to comply.

2. All correspondence related to a complaint must be addressed to the Ethics Committee, CRCC, 1835 Rohlwing Road, Suite E, Rolling Meadows, IL 60008, and must be marked "Confidential." This process is necessary to protect the confidentiality of the complainant and the accused certificant.

Section J: Management of Filed Complaints

1. Upon receipt of complaints, the Committee will communicate in writing with complainants. Receipt of the complaint and confirmation of certification status of the accused certificant will be acknowledged to the complainant.

2. The Committee will determine whether the complaint, if true, would violate one or more sections of the Code of Professional Ethics for Rehabilitation Counselors. If not, the complaint will not be accepted and the complainant so informed.

3. If the Committee determines that there is insufficient information to make a fair determination of whether the behavior alleged in the complaint would be cause for action by the Committee, the Committee may request further information from the complainant or others.

4. When complaints are accepted, the complainant will be so informed.

Section K: Notification of Accused Certificant

1. Once the complaint has been accepted, the accused certificant will be sent a copy of the complaint via certified mail, return receipt requested, and marked "Personal and Confidential."

2. The accused certificant will be asked to respond in writing to the complaint against him/her, addressing each of the following areas:

   a. Acknowledge the section of the CRCC Code of Professional Ethics for Rehabilitation Counselors which he/she has been accused of having violated;

b. Submit all evidence and documents which he/she wishes to be considered by the Committee in reviewing the complaint; and

c. State if he/she requests a hearing before the Committee.

The accused certificant will be informed that if he/she wants to respond, he/she must do so in writing within thirty (30) days from the date of notification. Failure to respond in writing within thirty (30) days could result in revocation of his/her certification.

3. Should the Committee request further information from the accused certificant, the accused certificant shall be given thirty days (30) days from the date of the request to respond.

4. The Committee may, in its discretion, delay or postpone its review of the case.

Section L: Disposition of Complaints

1. After receiving the response of the accused certificant, Committee members will be provided copies of the response and supporting evidence and documents provided by the accused certificant and others.

2. At the next meeting or teleconference of the Committee, the Committee will discuss the complaint, response, and supporting documentation, if any, and determine the outcome of the complaint if no hearing was requested.

3. Based on the information provided, the Committee will determine whether the accused violated any of the provisions of the Code of Professional Ethics for Rehabilitation Counselors.

4. In the event it is determined that any portion of the CRCC Code of Professional Ethics for Rehabilitation Counselors has been violated, the Commission will impose one or a combination of the possible sanctions allowed.

Section M: Withdrawal of Complaints

1. If the complainant and accused certificant agree to discontinue the complaint process, the Committee may, at its discretion, complete the adjudication process if available evidence indicates that this is warranted.

Section N: Possible Sanctions

1. Reprimand. Remedial requirements may be stipulated by the Committee.

2. Probation for a specified period of time subject to Committee review of compliance. Remedial requirements may be imposed to be completed within a specified period of time.

3. Suspension from CRCC certification for a specified period of time subject to Committee review of compliance. Remedial requirements may be imposed to be completed within a specified period of time.

4. Revocation of CRCC certification.

5. The penalty for failing to fulfill, in a satisfactory manner, a remedial requirement imposed by the Commission as a result of a probation sanction will be automatic suspension until the requirement is met, unless the Committee determines that the remedial requirement should be modified based on good cause shown prior to the end of the probationary period.

6. The penalty for failing to fulfill, in a satisfactory manner, a remedial requirement imposed by the Commission as a result of a suspension sanction will be automatic revocation unless the Committee determines that the remedial requirement should be modified based on good cause shown prior to the end of the suspension period.

7. Other corrective action.

Section O: Notification of Results

1. The accused certificant shall be given written notice of Commission decisions regarding complaints against him/her.

2. If a violation has been found and the accused's certification has been suspended or revoked, counselor licensure, certification, or registry boards; other mental health licensure, certification, or registry boards; voluntary national certification boards; and appropriate professional associations will also be notified of the results.

3. If a violation has been found and the accused's certification has been suspended or revoked, a notice of the Commission action that includes the section(s) of the CRCC Code of Professional Ethics for Rehabilitation Counselors that were found to have been violated and the sanctions imposed will be published in the CRCC newsletter.

Section P: Hearings

1. A hearing shall be initiated:

   a. If, within thirty (30) days from the date of the notification of the complaint, the accused certificant requests a hearing;

   b. At any time at the request of the Committee.

2. The Committee Chair shall schedule a hearing on the case at the next scheduled Committee meeting and notify the complainant and the accused certificant of their right to attend the hearing.

3. The hearing will be held before the Committee.

Section Q: Hearing Procedures

1. Purpose:

   a. A hearing will be conducted to determine whether a violation of the Code of

Professional Ethics for Rehabilitation Counselors has occurred and, if so, to determine appropriate disciplinary action.

b. The Committee shall be guided in its deliberations by principles of basic fairness and professionalism, and will keep its deliberations as confidential as possible, except as provided herein.

2. Notice:

a. The accused certificant shall be advised in writing by the Chair administering the complaint of the time and place of the hearing.

b. If the accused certificant fails to appear at the hearing, the Committee shall decide the complaint and determine what testimony it will hear on record. Failure of the accused certificant to appear at the hearing shall not be viewed by the Committee as sufficient grounds alone for taking disciplinary action.

3. Conduct of the Hearing:

a. The location of the hearing shall be determined at the discretion of the Committee. The Committee shall provide a private room to conduct the hearing and no observers or recording devices other than a recording device used by the Committee shall be permitted.

b. The Chair administering the complaint shall preside over the hearing and deliberations of the Committee. At the conclusion of the hearing and deliberations of the Committee, the Chair shall promptly issue written notice to the accused certificant of the Commission's decision.

c. A record of the hearing shall be made and preserved, together with any documents presented in evidence, at CRCC's administrative office. The record shall consist of a summary of testimony received or a verbatim transcript, at the discretion of the Committee.

d. The accused certificant shall be entitled to have legal counsel present to advise and represent him/her throughout the hearing. Legal counsel for CRCC may also be present at the hearing to advise the Committee and shall have the privilege of the floor.

e. Either party shall have the right to call witnesses to substantiate his/her version of the case.

f. The Committee shall have the right to call witnesses it believes may provide further insight into the matter.

g. Witnesses shall not be present during the hearing except when they are called upon to testify and shall be excused upon completion of their testimony and any cross-examination.

h. The Chair administering the complaint shall allow questions to be asked of any witness by the opposition or members of the Committee if such questions and testimony are relevant to the issues in the case.

i. The Chair administering the complaint will determine what questions and testimony are relevant to the case. Should the hearing be subject to irrelevant testimony, the Chair may call a brief recess until order can be restored.

j. Both the complainant and the accused, and any witnesses and legal counsel that they may have must pay their own expenses. CRCC shall pay the expenses of the Committee members. Parties initiating telephone contact will assume the expenses related to the calls.

4. Presentation of Evidence:

   a. The Chair administering the complaint shall be called upon first to present the charge(s) made against the accused certificant and to briefly describe the evidence supporting the charge. The Chair shall also be responsible for examining and cross-examining witnesses on behalf of the complainant and for otherwise presenting the matter during the hearing.

   b. The complainant or a member of the Committee shall then be called upon to present the case against the accused certificant. Witnesses who can substantiate the case may be called upon to testify and answer questions of the accused certificant and the Committee.

   c. If the accused certificant has exercised the right to be present at the hearing, he/she may be called upon to present any evidence which refutes the charges against him/her. This includes witnesses as in Subsection 3 above.

   d. The accused certificant will not be found guilty simply for refusing to testify. Once the accused certificant chooses to testify, however, he/she may be cross-examined by the complainant and members of the Committee, subject to the constitutional rights of the accused certificant

   e. Testimony that is merely cumulative or repetitious may, at the discretion of the Chair administering the complaint, be excluded.

   f. All parties providing testimony will be required to attest to the veracity of their statements.

5. Relevancy of Evidence:

   a. The Committee hearing is not a court of law and is not required to observe formal rules of evidence. Evidence that would be inadmissible in a court of law may be admissible in the hearing before the Committee, if it is relevant to the case. Therefore, if the evidence offered tends to explain, clarify, or refute any of the important facts of the case, it should be considered.

   b. The Committee will not consider evidence or testimony for the purpose of supporting any charge that was not set forth in the notice of the hearing or that is not relevant to the issues of the case.

6. Burden of Proof:

   a. The burden of proving a violation of the Code of Professional Ethics for Rehabilitation Counselors is on the complainant and/or the Committee.

b. Although the charge(s) need not be proved "beyond a reasonable doubt," the Committee will not find the accused certificant guilty in the absence of substantial, objective, and believable evidence to sustain the charge(s).

7. Deliberation of the Committee:

    a. After the hearing is completed, the Committee shall meet in a closed session to review the evidence presented and reach a conclusion. CRCC legal counsel may attend the closed session to advise the Committee if the Committee so desires.

    b. The Committee shall be the sole judge of the facts and shall weigh the evidence presented and assess the credibility of the witnesses. The decision of a majority of the members of the Committee present shall be the decision of the Committee and the Commission. The Chair shall vote only to break a tie or when the Committee consists of three members.

    c. Only members of the Committee who were present throughout the entire hearing shall be eligible to vote.

8. Decision of the Committee:

    a. The Committee will first resolve the issue of the guilt or innocence of the accused certificant on each charge. Applying the burden of proof in Subsection 5 above, the Committee will vote by secret ballot, unless all of the members of the Committee entitled to vote consent to an oral vote.

    b. In the event the Committee does not find the accused certificant guilty, the charges will be dismissed. If the Committee finds the accused certificant has violated the Code of Professional Ethics for Rehabilitation Counselors, it must then determine what sanctions shall be imposed.

Section R: Appeals

1. Decisions of the CRCC Ethics Committee that an accused certificant has violated the CRCC Code of Professional Ethics for Rehabilitation Counselors may be appealed by the accused certificant found to have been in violation based on one or more of the following grounds:

    a. The Committee violated its policies and procedures for processing complaints of ethical violations; and/or

    b. The decision of the Committee was arbitrary and capricious and was not supported by the materials provided by the complainant and the accused certificant.

2. After the accused has received notification that he/she has been found in violation of one or more sections of the CRCC Code of Professional Ethics for Rehabilitation Counselors, he/she will be given thirty (30) days from the date of notification to notify the Committee in writing via certified mail that he/she is appealing the decision.

3. An appeal must be in writing stating one or more of the grounds of appeal listed in Section R.1, Subsection a or b above, and the reasons for the appeal.

4.   The CRCC Chair will appoint a three (3) person appeals panel consisting of at least one (1) former Commission member, who is currently a CRC, with the balance to be certificants, none of whom served on the Committee at the time the original decision was rendered. The CRCC attorney shall serve as legal advisor and have the privilege of the floor.

5.   The three (3) member appeals panel will be given copies of the materials available to the Committee when it made its decision, a copy of the hearing transcript if a hearing was held, and a copy of the letter filed by the appealing certificant.

6.   The decision of a majority of the members of the appeals panel shall be the final decision. The decision shall be rendered within a reasonable period of time.

7.   The decision of the appeals panel may include one of the following:

   a.   The decision of the Commission is upheld.

   b.   The decision of the Commission is reversed and/or remanded with guidance to the Commission for a new hearing. The reason for this action will be given in detail to the Commission in writing.

8.   When a Commission decision is reversed and/or remanded, the complainant and the accused certificant will be informed in writing and additional information may be requested. The Commission will then render another decision after further hearing.

Section S: Substantial New Evidence

1.   In the event substantial new evidence, which was not available to the accused certificant at the time of the hearing , is presented in a case in which an appeal was not filed, or in a case where a final decision has been rendered, the case may be reopened by the Committee.

2.   The Committee will consider substantial new evidence that was unavailable at the time of the hearing and, if it is found to be substantiated and capable of exonerating an accused certificant whose certification was revoked, the Committee will reopen the case and proceed with the entire complaint process again.

Section T: Records

1.   The records of the Committee regarding complaints are confidential except as provided herein.

   a.   All information concerning complaints against accused certificants shall be confidential except that the Committee may disclose such information when compelled by a validly issued subpoena or when otherwise required by law or valid court order. In addition, the Committee may disclose to any appropriate organizations or individuals that an individual is under ethical investigation in cases deemed to be serious threats to the public welfare and only when to do so before final adjudication appears necessary to protect the public.

   b.   Nothing in this Section shall be construed to prevent the Committee from communicating with the complainant, witnesses, potential members of fact-finding committees, or other sources of information necessary to enable the Committee to carry out its investigative function.

2.   Original copies of complaint records will be maintained in locked files at CRCC's administrative office or at an off-site location chosen by CRCC for a specified period of time as listed below:

a.   Confidential Permanent Files. Permanent files of the Committee shall be confidential and shall be available only to those specifically authorized by the Committee and by the Chief Executive Officer of CRCC.

b.   Files for Revocation. Files concerning an accused certificant whose certification has been revoked shall be maintained indefinitely.

c.   Files for Non-Violations. Except for those cases closed for insufficient evidence, personally identifiable information concerning an accused certificant who has been found not to have violated the Code of Professional Ethics for Rehabilitation Counselors shall be destroyed one (1) year after the Committee has closed the case.

d.   Files for Insufficient Information. In cases where the Committee has closed a case due to evidence insufficient to sustain a complaint of ethical violation, records containing personally identifiable information shall be maintained for five (5) years after the Committee has closed the case.

e.   Files of Lesser Sanctions. In cases where the Committee has found an ethical violation but where the sanction is less than revocation, records containing personally identifiable information shall be maintained for five (5) years after the Committee has closed the case.

f.   Files After Death. All records containing personally identifiable information shall be destroyed one (1) year after the Commission is notified of the death of the accused certificant.

g.   Records for Educational Purposes. Nothing in this Section shall preclude the Committee from maintaining records in a form which prevents identification of the accused certificant so that it may be used for archival, educational, or other legitimate purposes.

3.   Members of the Committee will keep copies of complaint records confidential and will destroy copies of records after a case has been closed or when they are no longer members of the Committee.

Section U: Legal Actions Related to Complaints

1.   Accused certificants are required to notify the Committee if they learn of any type of legal action (civil or criminal) being filed in relation to the complaint.

2.   In the event any type of legal action is filed regarding an accepted complaint, all actions related to the complaint may, at the discretion of the Committee, be stayed until the legal action has been concluded.

3.   If actions on a complaint are stayed, the complainant and the accused certificant will be notified.

4.   When actions on a complaint are continued after a legal action is concluded, the complainant and the accused certificant will be notified.

ACKNOWLEDGEMENT

CRCC wishes to thank ACA for granting permission to adopt its Guidelines and Procedures for Ethical Complaints.

Revised June 1995

References

About Deaf World Web. (1995, August1). [Online]. Available: http://www.com-putel.com/~mernix/deafworld/deaf/deaf.html.

Abramms-Mezoff, B., & Johns, D. (1989, February). Managing a culturally diverse workforce. *Supervisory Management,* pp. 34–38.

Ackoff, R. L. (1970). *A concept of corporate planning.* New York: Wiley Interscience.

Acuña, R. (1988). *Occupied America: A histroy of Chicanos* (3rd ed.). New York: Harper & Row.

Agada, J. (1984). Studies of the personality of librarians. *Drexal Library Quarterly, 20* (2), 24–45.

Aiken, W. J., Smits, S. J., & Lollar, D. J. (1972). Leadership behavior and job satisfaction in state rehabilitation agencies. *Personnel Psychology, 25,* 65–73.

Akabas, S. H., Gates, L. B., & Galvin, D. E. (1992). *Disability management: A complete system to reduce costs, increase productivity, meet employer needs, and ensure legal compliance.* New York: AMACOM.

Albrecht, G. L. (1976). Social policy and the management of human resources. In G. L.

Albrecht, G. L. (Ed.), (1976). *The sociology of physical disability and rehabilitation* (pp. 257–279). Pittsburgh: University of Pittsburgh Press.

Alston, R. J., & McCowan, C. J. (1994). Aptitude assessment and African–American clients: The interplay between culture and psychometrics in rehabilitation. *Journal of Rehabilitation, 60,* 41–46.

Altman, D. (1982). *The homosexualization of America, the Americanization of the homosexual.* New York: St. Martin's.

American Association of Spinal Cord Injury Psychologists and Social Workers. (1992). *Standards for Psychologists and social workers in sci rehabilitation.* Jackson Heights, NY: Au. Available: 95–20 Astoria Boulevard, Jackson Heights, New York 11370–1177.

American Educational Research Association, American Psychological Association, & National Council on Measurement in Education. (1985).

Standards for educational and psychological testing. Washington, DC: American Psychological Association.

American Psychological Association. (1994). *Publication manual of the American Psychological Association* (4th ed.). Washington, DC: Author.

Anastasi, A. (1988). *Psychological testing* (6th ed.). New York: Macmillan.

Anastasi, A. (1992, August). *A century of psychological testing: Origins, problems and progress.* Paper presented at the 100th Annual Convention of the American Psychological Association, Washington, DC.

Anderson, N. B. (1989). Racial differences in stress-induced cardiovascular reactivity and hypertension: Current status and substantive issues. *Psychological Bulletin, 105,* 89–105.

Angove, P. (1927). Administration of vocational rehabilitation by a state. *Proceedings of the fourth national conference on vocational rehabilitation of the disabled citizen.* Washington DC: U.S. Government Printing Office.

Arciniega, G. M., & Newlon, B. J. (1995). Counseling and psychotherapy: Multicultural considerations. In D. Capuzzi & D. Gross (Eds.), *Counseling and psychotherapy: Theories and interventions* (pp. 557–588). New Jersey: Merrill.

Arokiasamy, C., & Millington, M. (1994). ADA and the goose that lays golden eggs. *Rehabilitation Education, 8*(1), 93–95.

Arthur, D. (1991). *Recruiting, interviewing, selecting, and orienting new employees* (2nd ed.). New York: AMACOM.

Associated Press, (October 8, 1993). CDC: Number of disabled workers still too high in the United States. *Southern Illinoisan,* p. 5A.

Atkins, B. J., & Wright, G. N. (1980). Vocational rehabilitation of Blacks. *Journal of Rehabilitation, 46*(2), 40, 42–46

Atkinson, D. R., Morten, G., & Sue, D. W. (1983). *Counseling American minorities: A cross cultural perspective* (2nd ed.). Dubuque, IA: William C. Brown.

Axelson, J. A. (1993). *Counseling and development in a multicultural society.* Pacific Grove, CA: Brooks/Cole.

Baker, H. J., & Spier, N. S. (1990). The employment interview: Guaranteed improvement in reliability. *Public Personnel Management, 19,* 85–90.

Balcaza, P., Hopkins, B. L., & Suarez, Y. (1985/86). A critical objective review of performance feedback. *Journal of Organizational Behavior Management, 7*(3/4), 65–89.

Bandura, A. (1982). Self-efficacy mechanism in human agency. *American Psychologist, 37,* 122–147.

Banja, J. D. (1990). Rehabilitation and empowerment. *Archives of Physical Medicine and Rehabilitation, 71,* 614–615.

Barrett, K., Crimando, W., & Riggar, T. F. (1993). Becoming an empowering organization: Strategies for implementation. *Journal of Rehabilitation Administration, 17*(4), 159–167.

Baumann, N. (1986). Keeping business advisory councils active and involved: The aging in America model. *Journal of Job Placement, 2,* 16–17.

Beardsley, M., Riggar, T. F., & Hafer, M. (1984). Rehabilitation supervision: A case for counselor training: *Clinical Supervisor, 2*(3), 55–63.

Beardsley, M. M., Rubin, S. E., & Gamer, W. E. (1987). A systematic model for designing and implementing staff development and training programs for rehabilitation counselors. *Journal of Applied Rehabilitation Counseling, 18*(2), 11–14.

Beauchamp, T. L., & Childress, J. F. (1983). *Principles of biomedical ethics* (2nd ed). Oxford: Oxford University Press.

Beck, R. J. (1994). Encouragement as a vehicle to empowerment in counseling: An existential perspective. *Journal of Rehabilitation, 60*(3), 6–11.

Beer, M., & Spector, B. (1993). Organizational diagnosis: Its role in organizational learning. *Journal of Counseling and Development, 71,* 642–650.

Belgrave, F. E., & Walker, S. (1991). Differences in rehabilitation service utilization patterns of African Americans and white Americans with disabilities. In S. Walker, F. Belgrave, R. W. Nicholls, & K. A. Turner (Eds.), *Future frontiers in the employment of minority persons with disabilities* (pp. 25–29). Washington, DC: Howard University Research and Training Center.

Benshoff, J. J. (1990). The role of rehabilitation and the issues of employment in the 1990s. In L. Perlman & C. Hansen (Eds.), *Employment and disability: Trends and issues for the 1990s* (pp. 50–59). Alexandria, VA: National Rehabilitation Association.

Benshoff, J. J. (1993). Peer self-help groups. In W. Crimando, & T.F. Riggar (Eds.), *Utilizing community resources: An overview of human services* (pp. 57–66). Winter Park, FL: St Lucie Press.

Bergan, J. R. (1977). *Behavioral consultation.* Columbus, OH: Charles E. Merrill.

Berkeley Systems, Inc. (1995, July 2). outSPOKEN. [Computer program]. Available: Berkeley Systems Inc., 2095 Rose St., Berkeley, CA 94709.

Berkowitz, E. D. (1984, November). *The history of rehabilitation.* Presented at NAPAS training sessions for the CAP program, Dallas, TX.

Berkowitz, E. D. (1985). Social influences on rehabilitation: Introductory remarks. In L. Perlman & G. Austin (Eds.), *Social influences in rehabilitation planning: Blueprint for the 21st century* (pp. 11–18). Alexandria, VA: National Rehabilitation Association.

Berkowitz, E. D. (1987). *Disabled policy: American programs for the handicapped.* New York: Cambridge University Press.

Berkowitz, E. D. (1992). Disabled policy: A personal postscript. *Journal of Disability Policy Studies, 3*(1), 1–16.

Berkowitz, E. D., & McQuaid, K. (1980). Bureaucrats as "social engineers": Federal welfare programs in Herbert Hoover's America. *American Journal of Economics and Sociology, 39*(4), 321–334.

Bernard, J., & Goodyear, R. (1992). *Fundamentals of clinical supervision.* Boston: Allyn & Bacon.

Bertsch, E. (1992). A voucher system that enables persons with severe mental illness to purchase community support services. *Hospital and Community Psychiatry, 43,* 1109–1113.

Bérubé, A. (1990). *Coming out under fire: The history of gay men and women in World War II.* New York: Free press.

Berven, N. (1979). The roles and functions of the rehabilitation counselor revisited. *Rehabilitation Counseling Bulletin, 23,* 84–88.

Berven, N. L. (1980). Psychometric assessment in rehabilitation. In B. Bolton & D. W. Cook (Eds.), *Rehabilitation client assessment* (pp. 46–64). Baltimore: University Park Press.

Berven, N. L. (1994, April). *Ten priority research topics to facilitate assessment in rehabilitation settings.* Paper presented at the Forum on Rehabilitation Research and Practice, held at the meeting of the American Counseling Association, Minneapolis, MN.

Berven, N. L., Possi, M. E., Doran, E. A., Ostby, S. S., & Kaplan, S. P. (1982). Training for cooperating agency supervisors in rehabilitation counselor education. *Rehabilitation Counseling Bulletin, 26,* 47–51.

Betz, N. E., & Fitzgerald, L. F. (1995). Career assessment intervention with radical and ethnic minorities. In F. T. L. Leong (Ed.), *Career development and vocational behavior of racial and ethnic minorities* (pp. 263–279). Mahwah, NJ: Lawrence Erlbaum.

Bieschke, K. J., Bishop, R. M., & Herbert, J. T. (1995). Research interest among rehabilitation doctoral students. *Rehabilitation Education, 9*(1), 51–66.

Biggs, H., Flett, R., Voges, K., & Alpass, F. (1995). Job satisfaction and distress in rehabilitation professionals: The role of organizational commitment and conflict. *Journal of Applied Rehabilitation Counseling, 26*(1), 41–46.

Bitter, J. A. (1979). *Introduction to rehabilitation.* St. Louis, MO: C. V. Mosby.

Bloom, J., Gerstein, L., Tarvydas, V., Conaster, J., Davis, E., Kater, D., Sherrard, P., & Esposito, R. (1990). Model legislation for licensed professional counselors. *Journal of Counseling and Development, 68,* 511–523.

Boone, R. S., & Wolfe, P. S. (1995). Emerging roles of the vocational rehabilitation counselor with regard to the ADA. *Journal of Applied Rehabilitation Counseling, 26*(3), 6–12.

Bordieri, J. E., Crimando, W., Riggar, T. F., & Schmidt, M. J. (1992). Performance appraisal: A primer for rehabilitation managers. *Journal of Rehabilitation Administration, 16,* 77–82.

Bordieri, J. E., & Riggar, T. F. (1989). Identifying and enhancing work incentives for rehabilitation facility direct service staff. *Journal of Rehabilitation Administration, 13,* 98–102.

Bordieri, J. E., Riggar, T. F., Crimando, W., & Matkin, R. E. (1988). Education and training needs for rehabilitation administrators. *Rehabilitation Education, 2,* 9–15.

Bordin, E. S. (1994). Theory and research on the therapeutic working alliance: New directions. In A.O. Horvath & L.S. Greensberg (Eds.), *The working alliance: Theory, research, and practices*(pp. 13–37). New York: Wiley.

Boschen, K. A. (1989). Early intervention in vocational rehabilitation. *Rehabilitation Counseling Bulletin, 32,* 254–265.

Bovard, J. (July, 1995). A law that is disabling our courts. *American Spectator,* reprinted in *Reader's Digest,* 47(Oct.), 205–206.

Bowe, F. G. (1993). Statistics, politics, and employment of people with disabilities. *Journal of Disability Policy Studies, 4*(2), 83–91.

Bozarth, J. D., & Emener, W. G. (1981). A person-centered approach to administration and supervision in rehabilitation. *Rehabilitation Counseling Bulletin, 24,* 299–303.

Brabham, R. E., & Emener, W. G. (1988). Human resource development in rehabilitation administration: Futuristic perspectives. *Journal of Rehabilitation Administration, 12,* 124–129.

Brodwin, M., & Brodwin, S. (1993). Rehabilitation: A case study approach. In M. Brodwin, F., Tellez, & S. Brodwin (Eds.), *Medical, psychological and vocational aspects of disability* (pp. 1–19). Athens, GA: Elliot & Fitzpatrick.

Brower, A. M., & Nurius, P. S. (1993). *Social cognition and individual change: Current theory and counseling guidelines.* Newbury Park, CA: Sage.

Brown, C., McDaniel, R., Couch, R., & McClanahan, M. (1994). *Vocational evaluation systems and software: A consumer's guide.* Menomonie: University of Wisconsin-Stout, Stout Vocational Rehabilitation Institute, Materials Development Center.

Brown, D. (1993). Training consultants: A call to action. *Journal of Counseling and Development, 72,* 139–143.

Brown, D., Pryzwansky, W. B., & Schulte, A. C. (1995). *Psychological consultation: Introduction to theory and practice* (3rd ed.). Boston: Allyn & Bacon.

Brown, D., Wyne, M. D., Blackburn, J., & Powell, C. (1979). *Consultation: Strategy for improving education.* Boston: Allyn & Bacon.

Brown, M., Gordon, W. A., & Diller, L. (1983). Functional assessment and outcome measurement: An integrative review. In E. L. Pan, T. E. Backer, & C. L. Vash (Eds.), *Annual review of rehabilitation: Vol. 3* (pp. 93–120). New York: Springer Publishing Co.

Brown University. (1986). *The American university and the pluralistic ideal, A report of the visiting committee on minority life and education at Brown University,* p. ix. Providence, RI: Brown University Press.

Brubaker, D. (1981). Rehabilitation counseling in the 1980's: A discussion with Daniel Sinick. *Journal of Applied Rehabilitation Counseling, 12*(4), 179–185.

Bruhn, J. G., & Fuentes, R. G. (1977). Cultural factors affecting utilization of services by Mexican Americans. *Psychiatric Annals, 7*(12), 608–613.

Bunderson, C. V., Inouye, D. K., & Olsen, J. B. (1989). The four generations of computerized educational measurement. In R. L. Linn (Ed.), *Educational measurement* (3rd ed., pp. 367–407). New York: Macmillan.

Burkhead, E. J., & Sampson, J. P., Jr. (1985). Computer-assisted assessment in support of the rehabilitation process. *Rehabilitation Counseling Bulletin, 28,* 262–274.

Burma, J. H. (1970). *Mexican-Americans in the United States: A reader.* Cambridge, MA: Schenkman Publishing Co., distributed by Canfield Press.

Byrd, E. K., Lesnik, M. J., & Byrd, P. D. (1981). A role play model for teaching supervision in rehabilitation settings. *Journal of Rehabilitation Administration, 5,* 137–141.

California Workers' Compensation Institute (1991). *Vocational rehabilitation: The California Experience 1975–1989.* San Francisco: Author.

Campbell, L. R. (1991). Enhancing diversity: A multicultural employment per-specitve. In S. Walker, F. Belgrave, R. W. Nicholls, & K. A. Turner (Eds.), *Future frontiers in the employment of minority persons with disabilities* (pp. 38–49). Washington, DC: Howard University Research and Training Center.

Caplan, G. (1970). *The theory and practice of mental health consultation.* New York: Basic Books.

Carlsen, M. B. (1988). *Meaning-making: Therapeutic processes in adult development.* New York: Norton.

Case Management Society of America. (1995). Standards of practice for case management. *Journal of Case Management, 1*(3), 7, 9–12, 15–16.

Casper, M. (1995). Book Review(s). *Journal of Disability Policy Issues, 6*(1), 91–95.

Cassell, J. L., Colvin, C. R., & Hannum, M. C. (1991). Microcomputer technology in rehabilitation continuing education. *Rehabilitation Education, 5,* 289–296.

Cassell, J. L., & Mulkey, S. W. (1985). *Rehabilitation caseload management: Concepts and practices.* Austin, TX: PRO-ED.

Cassell, J. L., & Mulkey, S. W. (1992). Caseload management in the rehabilitation curriculum. *Rehabilitation Education, 6,* 151–158.

CCM certification guide. (1995). Commission for Case Management Certification. Rolling Meadows, IL: Author.

Chapa, J., & Valencia, R. R. (1993). Latino population growth, demographic characteristics, and educational stagnation: An examination of recent trends. *Hispanic Journal of Behavioral Sciences, 15,* 165–187.

Christian, W. P. (1981). Programming quality assurance in residential rehabilitation settings: A model for administrative work performance standards. *Journal of Rehabilitation Administration, 5,* 26–33.

Clark, H. B., Wood, R., Kuehnel, T., Flanagan, S., Mosk, M., & Northrup, J. T. (1985). Preliminary validation and training of supervisory interactional skills. *Journal of Organizational Behavior Management, 7*(1/2), 95–133.

Clayton, S., & Bongar, B. (1994). The use of consultation in psychological practice: Ethical, legal, and clinical considerations. *Ethics and Behavior, 4,* 43–57.

Coffey, D. D., & Hansen, G. (1978). Vocational evaluation role clarification. *Vocational Evaluation and Work Adjustments Bulletin, 11*(4), 22–28.

Cohen, E. D. (1990). Confidentiality, counseling, and clients who have AIDS: Ethical foundations of a model rule. *Journal of Counseling and Development, 68,* 282–286.

Collignon, F., Barker, L., & Vencill, M. (1992). The growth and structure of the proprietary rehabilitation sector. *American Rehabilitation, 18,* 7–10, 43.

Commission on Rehabilitation Counselor Certification. (1988). *Code of professional ethics for rehabilitation counselors.* Rolling Meadows, IL: Author.

Commission on Rehabilitation Counselor Certification (CRCC). (1994). *CRCC certification guide.* Rolling Meadows, IL: Author.

Condeluci, A. (1991). *Interdependence.* Winter Park, FL: St. Lucie Press.

Condeluci, A. (1995). *Beyond difference.* Winter Park, FL: St. Lucie Press.

Conger, J. A. (1989). Leadership: The art of empowering others. *The Academy Management Executive, 3,* 17–24.

Conger, J. A., & Kanungo, R. N. (1988). The empowerment process: Integrating theory and practice. *Academy of Management Review, 13,* 471–482.

Conour, T. D. (1982). Comments on the Matkin, Sawyer, Lorenz, Rubin research article. *Journal of Rehabilitation Administration, 6*(4), 183–184.

Cook, A.M., & Hussey, S.M. (1995). *Assistive technologies: Principles and practice.* St. Louis, MO: Mosby.

Cook, D., & Bolton, B. (1992). Rehabilitation counselor education and case performance: An independent replication. *Rehabilitation Counseling Bulletin, 36,* 37–43.

Cook, J. S., & Fritts, G. G. (1994). Planning process determines results. *Health Care Strategic Management, 12*(12), 19–21.

Cooper, S. E., & O'Connor, R. M. (1993). Standards for organizational consultation assessment and evaluation instruments. *Journal of Counseling and Development, 71,* 651–660.

Copp, T. (1937). Federal–state cooperation tested in vocational rehabilitation. *American Labor Legislation Review, 27*(4), 163–166.

Copp, T. (1944). New concepts of disablement and rehabilitation. *Social Service Review, 18*(3), 318–324.

Corey, G. (1991). *Theory and practice of counseling and psychotherapy.* Pacific Grove, CA: Cole.

Corey, G., Corey, M. S., & Callanan, P. (1993). *Issues and ethics in the helping professions.* Pacific Grove, CA: Brooks/Cole.

Cottone, R., & Cottone, L. (1986). A systematic analysis of vocational evaluation in the state–federal rehabilitation system. *Vocational Evaluation and Work Adjustment Bulletin, 19*(2), 47–54.

Cottone, R., & Emener, W. (1990). The psychomedical paradigm of vocational rehabilitation and its alternatives. *Rehabilitation Counseling Bulletin, 34,* 91–102.

Coudroglou, A., & Poole, D. L. (1984). *Disability, work, and social policy,* New York: Springer Publishing Co.

Council on Rehabilitation Education (CORE). (1991a). *Accreditation manual for rehabilitation counselor education programs.* Champaign–Urbana, IL: Author.

Council on Rehabilitation Education (CORE). (1991b). *CORE policy and procedures manual.* Champaign–Urbana, IL: Author.

Council of State Administrators of Vocational Rehabilitation (1993, September). *Recommendations for a model service delivery system for public vocational rehabilitation.* Washington, DC: Author.

Covey, S. R. (1989). *The seven habits of highly effective people: Restoring the character ethic.* New York: Simon & Schuster.

Cox, T. (Ed.). (1993). *Cultural diversity in organizations: Theory, research, & practice.* San Francisco: Berrett-Koehler.

Crewe, N. M., & Dijkers, M. (1995). Functional assessment. In L. A. Cushman & M. J. Scherer (Eds.), *Psychological assessment in medical rehabilitation* (pp. 101–144). Washington, DC: American Psychological Association.

Crimando, W., & Baker, R. (1984). Computer-assisted instruction on rehabilitation counselor education. *Rehabilitation Counseling Bulletin, 28,* 50–54.

Crimando, W., & Bordieri, J. E. (1991). Do computers make it better? Effects of source on students' perceptions of vocational evaluation report quality. *Rehabilitation Counseling Bulletin, 34,* 332–343.

Crimando, W., & Godley, S. H. (1984). Use of computers in expanding the employment opportunities of persons with disabilities. *Rehabilitation Research Review,* Washington, DC: National Rehabilitation Information Center.

Crimando, W., & Godley, S. H. (1985). The computer's potential in enhancing employment opportunities of persons with disabilities. *Rehabilitation Counseling Bulletin, 28,* 275–282.

Crimando, W., Hansen, G., & Riggar, T. F. (1986). Employee turnover: The scope of a state DVR personnel problem. *Journal of Rehabilitation Administration, 10,* 125–128.

Crimando, W., & Riggar, T. F. (Eds.) (1991). *Utilizing community resources: An overview of human services.* Delray Beach, FL: St. Lucie Press.

Crimando, W., Riggar, T. F., & Bordieri, J. (1988). Proactive change management in rehabilitation: An idea whose time has been. *Journal of Rehabilitation Administration, 12*(1), 20–22.

Crimando, W., Riggar, T. F., & Hansen, G. (1986). Personnel turnover: The plague of rehabilitation facilities. *Journal of Applied Rehabilitation Counseling, 17*(2), 17–20.

Crimando, W., & Sawyer, H. (1983a). Microcomputer applications in adjustment service programming. *Vocational Evaluation and Work Adjustment Bulletin, 16,* 7–12, 34.

Crimando, W., & Sawyer, H. (1983b). Microcomputers in private sector rehabilitation. *Rehabilitation Counseling Bulletin, 27,* 26–31.

Critchley, D. L. (1987). Clinical supervision as a learning tool for the therapist in milieu settings. *Journal of Psychosocial Nursing, 25*(8), 18–22.

Cronbach, L. J. (1990). *Essentials of psychological testing* (5th ed.). New York: HarperCollins.

Cummins, J. (1984). *Bilingualism and specail education: Issues in assessment and pedagogy.* London: Multilingual Matters.

Cummins, J. (1986). Empowering minority students: A framework for intervention. *Harvard Educational Review, 56,* 18–36.

Cummins, J., & Swain, M. (1986). *Bilingualism in education: Aspects of theory, research, and practice.* New York: Longman.

Czerlinsky, T., Jensen, R., & Pell, K. L. (1987). Construct validity of the Vocational Decision-Making Interview (VDMI). *Rehabilitation Counseling Bulletin, 31,* 28–33.

Dale, B. E., & McDonald, A. A., Sr. (1982). Toward a comprehensive philosophy of personnel performance appraisal in rehabilitation facilities. *Journal of Rehabilitation Administration, 6,* 80–88.

Danek, M. M., & Lawrence, R. E. (1982). Client–counselor racial similarity and rehabilitation outcomes. *Journal of Rehabilitation, 48*(3), 54–58.

Das, A. K. (1995). Rethinking multicultural counseling: Implications for counselor education. *Journal of Counseling and Development, 74,* 45–52.

Dean, R. J. N. (1972). *New life for millions: Rehabilitation for America's disabled.* New York: Hastings House.

DeJong, G., & Batavia, A. (1990). The Americans with Disabilities Act and the current state of U.S. disability policy. *Journal of Disability Policy Studies, 1*(3), 65–75.

de la Garza, R. D., Dean, F. D., Bonjean, C. M., Romo, R., & Alvarez, R. (Eds.). (1985). *The Mexican American experience: An interdisciplinary anthology.* Austin: University of Texas Press.

Deloach, C., & Greer, B. (1981). *Adjustment to severe disability: A metamorphosis.* New York: McGraw Hill.

D'Emilio, J. (1983). *Sexual politics, sexual communities: The making of a homosexual minority in the United States, 1940–1970.* Chicago: University of Chicago Press.

Dickinson, G. L. (1961). *The Greek view of life.* New York: Collier Books.

DiMichael, S. G. (1967). New directions and expectations in rehabilitation counseling. *Journal of Rehabilitation, 33,* 38–39.

DiMichael, S. G. (1969). The current scene. In D. Malikin & H. Rusalem (Eds.), *Vocational rehabilitation of the disabled: An overview* (pp. 5–27). New York: New York University Press.

Disabilities Mall (1995, August). [On-line]. Available: http//www.disability.com/dismall.html.

Dowd, E. T., & Emener, W. G. (1978). Lifeboat counseling: The issue of survival decisions. *Journal of Rehabilitation, 44*(3), 34–36.

Dziekan, K. I., & Okacha, A. A. G. (1993). Accessibility or rehabilitation services: Comparison by racial–ethnic status. *Rehabilitation Counseling Bulletin, 36,* 183–189.

Ebener, D., Berven, N., & Wright, G. (1993). Self-perceived abilities of rehabilitation educators to teach competencies for rehabilitation practice. *Rehabilitation Counseling Bulletin, 37,* 6–14.

Egan, G. (1994). *The skilled helper* (5th ed.). Pacific Grove, CA: Brooks/Cole.

Eillien, V. J., Menz, F. E., & Coffey, D. D. (1979). Toward professional identity: The adjustment specialist. *Vocational Evaluation and Work Adjustment Bulletin, 12*(3), 16–23.

Eldredge, G. M. (1995). Distance education: A vision for the future. *Journal of Rehabilitaion Administration, 19,* 329–331.

Eldredge, G. M., Gerard, G., & Smart, J. (1994). A distance education model for rehabilitation counseling. *Journal of Rehabilitation Administration, 18,* 75–79.

Elliott, J., & Santner, D. (n.d.). *How to set up a tickler system that works.* Unpublished manuscript.

Elsasser, G. (September 8, 1989). Senate OK's rights bill for disabled. *Chicago Tribune,* p. 1–1.

Embretson, S. E. (1992). Computerized adaptive testing: Its potential substantive contributions to psychological research and assessment. *Current Directions in Psychological Science, 1,* 129–131.

Emener, W. G. (1978). Clinical supervision in rehabilitation settings. *Journal of Rehabilitation Administration, 2,* 44–53.

Emener, W. G. (1978b). Reconciling personal and professional values with agency goals and processes. *Journal of Rehabilitation Administration, 2,* 166–172.

Emener, W. G. (1986a). Future perspecitves on Rehabilitation in America. *Journal of Private Sector Rehabilitation, 1*(2), 59–70.

Emener, W. G. (1986b). *Rehabilitation counselor preparation and development: Selected critical issues.* Springfield, IL: Charles C Thomas.

Emener, W. G. (1991). An empowerment philosophy for rehabilitation in the 20th century. *Journal of Rehabilitation, 57*(4), 7–12.

Emener, W. G., & Cottone, R. (1989). Professionalization, deprofessionalization, and reprofessionalization of rehabilitation counseling according to the criteria of professions. *Journal of Counseling and Development, 67,* 576–581.

Emener, W. G. (1983). Rehabilitation administration and supervision: A critical component of rehabilitation education. National Council on Rehabilitation Education, *NCRE Report, 9*(4), 2, 4.

Emener, W. G., & Ferrandino, J. (1983). A philosophical framework for rehabilitation: Implications for clients, counselors, and agencies. *Journal of Applied Rehabilitation Counseling, 14*(1), 62–68.

Emener, W. G., & Jernigan, J. C. (1985). Creative leadership in rehabilitation administration. *Journal of Rehabilitation Administration, 9,* 81–88.

Emener, W. G., Patrick, A., & Hollingsworth, D. K. (1984). Selected rehabilitation counseling issues: A historical perspective. In W. Emener, A. Patrick, &

D. Hollingsworth (Eds.), *Critical issues in rehabilitation counseling* (pp. 5–41). Springfield, IL: Charles C Thomas.

Emener, W. G., & Placido, D. (1982). Rehabilitation counselor evaluation: An analysis and critique. *Journal of Rehabilitation Administration, 6,* 72–76.

Emener, W. G., & Rubin, S. E. (1980). Rehabilitation counselor roles and functions and sources of role strain. *Journal of Applied Rehabilitation Counseling 11,* 57–69.

Emener, W. G., & Stephens, J. E. (1982). Improving the quality of working life in a changing (rehabilitation) environment. *Journal of Rehabilitation Administration, 6,* 114–124.

English, W. R., Oberle, J. B., & Byrne, A. R. (1979). Rehabilitation counselor supervision: A national perspective [Special Issue]. *Rehabilitation Counseling Bulletin, 22,* 7–123.

Esser, T. J. (1975). *Client rating instruments for use in vocational rehabilitation agencies.* Menomonie, WI: University of Wisconsin-Stout, Vocational Rehabilitation Institute, Materials Development Center.

Esser, T. J. (1980). *Gathering information for evaluation planning.* Menomonie, WI: University of Wisconsin-Stout, Stout Vocational Rehabilitation Institute.

Estes, C. P. (1992). *Women who run with the wolves.* New York: Ballantine Books.

Estrada, A. L., Treviño, F. M., Ray, L. A. (1990). Health care utilization barriers among Mexican Americans: Evidence from HHANES 1982–84. *American Journal of Public Health, 80*(Suppl.), 27–31.

EUREKA: California career information system (Version 3.10) (1996). [Computer software]. Richmond, CA: EUREKA.

Farrant, D. (1989). Supervising your pals. *Supervisory Management, March,* 35–38.

Farruggia, G. (1986). Job satisfaction among private and public sector rehabilitation practitioners. *Journal of Rehabilitation Administration, 10,* 4–9.

Federal occupational career information system (FOCIS) (Version 4.0) (1992). [Computer software]. Springfield, VA: National Technical Information Service.

Feist-Price, S. (1995). African Americans with disabilities and equity in vocational rehabilitation services: One state's review. *Rehabiliation Counseling Bulletin, 39,* 119–129.

Feldman, D. (1981). The multiple socialization of organization members. *Academy of Management Review, 6,* 309–318.

Feroz, R. F., & Katz-Garris, L. (1984). Incorporating theory Z into rehabilitation administration. *Journal of Rehabilitation Administration, 8,* 84–91.

Fidler, H. L. (1924, February). Opening Session at the National Conference on Vocational Rehabilitation of Civilian Disabled. Washington, DC.

Field, T. F., & Sink, J. M. (1981). *The vocational expert.* Athens, GA: VSB, Inc.

Fobbs, J. M. (1994). *Cultural diversity and disability: A workshop manual.* Knoxville, TN: The University of Tennessee.

Francouer, R. T. (1983). Teaching decision making in biomedical ethics for the allied health student. *Journal of Allied Health, 12,* 202–209.

Frankl, V. E. (1985). *Man's search for meaning.* New York: Washington Square Press.

Freeman, J. B. (1979). Rehabilitation counselor and supervisor perceptions of counselor training needs and continuing education. *Journal of Applied Rehabilitation Counseling, 10,* 154–159.

Frum, D., & Brendan, J. (December, 1993). Grumblers, goldbricks and their attorneys. *Reader's Digest,* pp. 29–32.

Fuqua, D. R., & Kurpius, D. J. (1993). Conceptual models in organizational consultation. *Journal of Counseling and Development, 71,* 607–618.

Gaines, T. F. (1979). Caseload management revisited. *Journal of Rehabilitation Administration, 110,* 112–118.

Galassi, J. P., & Perot, A. R. (1992). What you should know about behavioral assessment. *Journal of Counseling and Development, 70,* 624–631.

Gannaway, T. W., & Sink, J. M. (1979). An analysis of competencies or counselors and evaluators. *Vocational Evaluation and Work Adjustment Bulletin, 12*(3), 3–15.

García, A. (1991). The changing demographic face of Hispanics in the United States. In M. Sotomayor (Ed.), *Empowering Hispanic families: A critical issues for the '90s*(pp. 21–38). Milwaukee, WI: Family Service America.

Garrett, J. F. (1969). Historical background. In D. Malikin and H. Rusalem (Eds.), *Vocational rehabilitation of the disabled.* New York: New York University Press.

Garske, G. G. (1995). Self-reported levels of job satisfaction of vocational rehabilitation professionals: A descriptive study. *Journal of Rehabilitation Administration, 19,* 215–224.

Gatens-Robinson, E., & Rubin, S. E. (1995). Societal values and ethical commitments that influence rehabilitation service delivery behavior. In S. E. Rubin & R. T. Roessler (Eds.), *Foundations of the vocational rehabilitation process* (pp. 157–174). Austin, TX: PRO–ED.

General Accounting Office (1993). Report to the Chairman, Subcommittee on Select Education and Civil Rights, Committee on Education and Labor, House of Representatives. *Vocational rehabilitation evidence for federal program's effectiveness is mixed.* United States General Accounting Office: GAO/PEMD Report No. 93–19. Washington, DC: U.S. Government Printing Office.

Gibson, T. F., & Mazur, D. A. (1995). Preparing for the strategic planning process helps ensure implementation success. *Health Care Strategic Management, 13*(1), 14–17.

Gilbride, D. (1993). Rehabilitation education in the private sector. In L. Pearlman

& C. Hansen (Eds.). *Private sector rehabilitation insurance: Trends and issues for the 21st century* (pp. 22–26). Alexandria, VA: National Rehabilitation Association.

Gilbride, D. & Burr, F. (1993). Self-directed labor market survey: An empowering approach. *Journal of Job Placement, 9*(2), 13–17.

Gilbride, D., Connolly, M., & Stensrud, R. (1990). Rehabilitation education for the private-for-profit sector. *Rehabilitation Education, 4,* 155–162.

Gilbride, D., & Stensrud, R. (1992). Demand-side job development: A model for the 1990s. *Journal of Rehabilitation, 51,* 34–39.

Gilbride, D., & Stensrud, R. (1993). Challenges and opportunities for rehabilitation counselors in the Americans with Disabilities Act era. *NARPPS Journal, 8,* 67–74.

Gilbride, D., Stensrud, R., & Johnson, M. (1994). Current models of job placement and employer development: Research, competencies and educational considerations. *Rehabilitation Education, 7,* 215–239.

Glikman, N. (1984). The war of the languages: Comparisons between language wars of Jewish & Deaf communities. *Deaf American, 36*(6), 25–33.

Glosoff, H., Benshoff, J., Hosie, T., & Maki, D. (1995). The 1994 ACA model legislation for licensed professional counselors. *Journal of Counseling and Development, 74*(2), 209–220.

Goffman, E. (1959). *Presentation of self in everyday life.* New York: Anchor Books.

Goffman, E. (1961). *Asylums.* New York: Anchor Books.

Goffman, E. (1963). *Stigma.* Englewood Cliffs, NJ: Prentice Hall.

Goldman, L. (1971). *Using tests in counseling* (2nd ed.). Pacific Palisades, CA: Goodyear.

Gomez, J. S., & Michaelis, R. C. (1995). An assessment of burnout in human service providers. *Journal of Rehabilitation, 61*(1), 23–26.

Gonzalez, G. (1991). Hispanics in the past two decades, Latinos in the next two: Hindsight and foresight. In M. Sotomayor (Ed.), *Empowering Hispanic families: A critical issue for the '90s* (pp. 1–20). Milwaukee, WI: Family Service America.

Goodwin, Jr., L. R. (1992). Rehabilitation counselor specialization: The promise and the challenge. *Journal of Applied Rehabilitation Counseling, 23*(2), 5–11.

Graham, C. S. (1981). The supervisor's role in the performance appraisal process. *Journal of Rehabilitation Administration, 5,* 170–178.

Grantham, C. E., & Nichols, L. D. (1994–1995, Winter). Distributed work: Learning to manage at a distance. *Public Manager,* pp. 31–34.

Graves, W. H., Coffey, D. D., Habeck, R., & Stude, E. W. (1987). NCRE position paper: Definition of the qualified rehabilitation professional. *Rehabilitation Education, 1*(1), 1–7.

Graves, W. H., & Moore, J. E. (1980). Recruitment: The neglected aspect of rehabilitation personnel management. *Journal of Rehabilitation Administration, 4,* 27–31.

Greenwood, R. (1992). Systematic case load management. In R. T. Roessler & S. E. Rubin (Eds.), *Case management and rehabilitation counseling* (2nd ed.), (pp. 143–154). Austin, TX: PRO–ED.

Groce, N. (1992). *The U.S. role in international disability activities: A history and a look towards the future.* A study commissioned by the World Institute on Disability, the World Rehabilitation Fund, and Rehabilitation International.

Growick, B. (1993). Rehabilitation in workers' compensation: A growth potential. In L. G. Pearlman & C. E. Hansen (Eds.), *Private sector rehabilitation: Insurance, trends & issues for the 21st Century: A report on the 17th Mary E. Switzer Seminar* (pp. 68–70). Alexandria, VA: National Rehabilitation Association.

Gutteridge, T., Leibowitz, Z., & Shore, J. (1993). Career development in the United States: Rethinking careers in the flattened organization. In T. Gutteridge, Z. Leibowitz, & J. Shore. (Eds.). *Organizational career development: Benchmarks for building a world-class workforce.* San Francisco: Jossey-Bass.

Habeck, R. V., Kress, M., Scully, S. M., & Kirchner, K. (1994). Determining the significance of the disability management movement for rehabilitation counselor education. *Rehabilitation Education, 8,* 195–240.

Habeck, R. V., & Munrowd, D. C. (1987). Employer-based rehabilitation practice: An educational perspective. *Rehabilitation Education, 1*(2/3), 95–107.

Habeck, R. V., Williams, C. L., Dugan, K. E., & Ewing, M. E. (1989). Balancing human and economic costs in disability management. *Journal of Rehabilitation, 55*(4), 16–19.

Haber, L. (1985). Trends and demographic studies on programs for disabled persons. In L. Perlman & G. Austin (Eds.), *Social influences in rehabilitation planning: Blueprint for the 21st century* (pp. 27–37). Alexandria, VA: National Rehabilitation Association.

Hagan, F. E., Haug, M. R., & Sussman, M. B. (1975). *Comparative profiles of the rehabilitation counseling graduate: 1965 and 1972* (Second Series, Working Paper #5). Case Western Reserve University, Department of Sociology, Institute on the Family and the Bureaucratic Society.

Hahn, H. (1985). Changing perception of disability and the future of rehabilitation. In L. Perlman & G. Austin (Eds.), *Social influences in rehabilitation planning: Blueprint for the 21st century* (pp. 53–64). Alexandria, VA: National Rehabilitation Association.

Hahn, H. (1993). The political implications of disability definitions and data. *Journal of Disability Policy Studies, 4*(1), 41–52.

Hahn, H., & Stout, R. (1994). *The Internet complete reference.* New York: Osborne McGraw-Hill.

Haimann, T., & Hilgert, R. L. (1977). *Supervision: Concepts and practice of management* (2nd ed.). Cincinnati, OH: South-Western Publishing.

Half, R. (1985). *On hiring.* New York: Crown.

Hall, J. H., & Warren, S. L. (Eds.) (1956). *Rehabilitation counselor preparation.* Washington, DC: National Rehabilitation Association and the National Vocational Guidance Association.

Hall, S. (1991). Door into Deaf culture: Folklore in an American Deaf social club. *Sign Language Studies, 73,* 421–429.

Halpern, A. S., & Fuhrer, M. J. (Eds.). (1984). *Functional assessment in rehabilitation.* Baltimore: Paul H. Brookes.

Hanley-Maxwell, C., & Szymanski, E. M. (1992). School-to-work transition and supported employment. In R. M. Parker & E. M. Szymanski (Eds.), *Rehabilitation counseling: Basics and beyond* (2nd ed.), pp. 135–164). Austin, TX: PRO–ED.

Harrison, D. K., Garnett, J. M., & Watson, A. L. (1981). *Client assessment measures in rehabilitation* (Michigan Studies in Rehabilitation. Utilization Series: 5). Ann Arbor: University of Michigan, Rehabilitation Research Institute.

Harrison, D. K., & Lee, C.C. (1979). Rehabilitation counselor competencies. *Journal of Applied Rehabilitation Counseling, 10,* 135–141.

Harvey, R. F., & Jellinek, H. M. (1982). A team approach to comprehensive medical rehabilitation. *Journal of Rehabilitation Administration, 6,* 134–139.

Haveman, R. H., Halberstadt, V., & Burkhauser, R. V. (1984). *Public policy toward disabled workers.* Ithaca, NY: Cornell University Press.

Havranek, J. E., & Brodwin, M. G. (1994). Rehabilitation couselor curricula: Time for a change. *Rehabilitation Education, 8*(4), 369–379.

Henke, R. O., Connolly, S. G., & Cox, J. S. (1975). Caseload management: The key to effectiveness. *Journal of Applied Rehabilitation Counseling, 6*(4), 217–227.

Henry, T. (October 30, 1995). Retarded students still segregated. *USA Today.*

Henry, W. P., & Strupp, H. H. (1994). The therapeutic alliance as interpersonal process. In A. O. Horvath & L. S. Greensberg (Eds.), *The working alliance: Theory, research, and practice* (pp. 51–84). New York: Wiley.

Herbert, J. T. (in press). Clinical supervision. In A. E. Dell Orto & R. P. Marinelli (Eds.), *Encyclopedia of disability and rehabilitation.* New York: Macmillan.

Herbert, J. T., & Chatman, H. E. (1988). Afrocentricity and the Black disability experience: A theoretical orientation for rehabilitation counselors. *Journal of Applied Rehabilitation Counseling, 19*(4), 50–54.

Herbert, J. T., Hemlick, L. M., & Ward, T. J. (1991). Supervisee perception of rehabilitation counseling practica. *Rehabilitation Education, 5,* 121–129.

Herbert, J. T., & Martinez, M. Y. (1992). Client ethnicity and vocational rehabilitation case service outcome. *Journal of Job Placement, 8*(1), 10–16.

Herbert, J. T., & Ward, T. J. (1989). Rehabilitation counselor supervision a national survey of NCRE graduate training practica. *Rehabilitation Education, 3,* 163–175.

Herbert, J. T., & Ward, T. J. (1990). Supervisory styles among rehabilitation counseling practica supervisors. *Rehabilitation Education, 4,* 203–212.

Herbert, J. T., Ward, T. J, & Hemlick, L. M. (1995). Confirmatory factor analysis of the Supervisory Style Inventory and the Revised Supervision Questionnaire. *Rehabilitation Counseling Bulletin, 38,* 334–349.

Herek, G. M. (1990). The context of anti-gay violence: Notes on cultural and psychological heterosexism. *Journal of Interpersonal Violence, 5,* 316–333.

Herek, G. M. (1991). Stigma, prejudice, and violence against lesbians and gay men. In J. C. Gonsiorek & J. D. Weinrich (Eds.), *Homosexuality: Research implications for public policy* (pp. 60–80). Newbury Park: Sage.

Herek, G. M. (1992). The social context of hate crimes: Notes on cultural heterosexism. In G. M. Herek & K. T. Berrill (Eds.), *Hate crimes: Confronting violence against lesbians and gay men.* Newbury Park: Sage.

Herek, G. M., & Berrill, K. T. (Eds.). (1992). *Hate crimes: Confronting violence against lesbians and gay men.* Newbury Park: Sage.

Herrick, W.L. (1983). Letter to the editor. *Journal of Applied Rehabilitation Counseling, 14*(1).

Hershenson, D. (1990). A theoretical model for rehabilitation counseling. *Rehabilitation Counseling Bulletin, 33,* 268–278.

Herzberg, F. (1966). *Work and the nature of man.* New York: World Publishing.

Hillyer, C. (1956, April). Office memorandum to Mary E. Switzer, Department of Health, Education, and Welfare, Office of Vocational Rehabilitation, Washington, DC.

Hillyer, C. (1959, December). Office memorandum to Mary E. Switzer, Department of Health, Education, and Welfare, Office of Vocational Rehabilitation, Washington, DC.

Hillyer, C. (1960, January). Office memorandum to Mary E. Switzer, Department of Health, Education, and Welfare, Office of Vocational Rehabilitation, Washington, DC.

Holland, J. L. (1973). *Making vocational choices: A theory of careers.* Englewood Cliffs, NJ: Prentice-Hall.

Holland, J. L. (1985a). *The self-directed search professional manual.* Odessa, FL: Psychological Assessment Resources.

Holland, J. L. (1985b). *Vocational preference inventory (VPI).* Odessa, FL: Psychological Assessment Resources.

Holmes, G. E. (1993). The historical roots of the empowerment dilemma in vocational rehabilitation. *Journal of Disability Policy Studies, 4,* 1–20.

Holmes, G. E., Hull, L., & Karst, R. H. (1989). Litigation avoidance through conflict resolution: Issues for state rehabilitation agencies. *American Rehabilitation, 15*(3), 12–15.

Holmes, G. E., & Karst, R. H. (1989). Case record management: A professional skill. *Journal of Applied Rehabilitation Counseling, 20*(1), 36–40.

Holmes, S. A. (October 23, 1994). In 4 years, disabilities act hasn't improved jobs rate. *New York Times,* p. 18.

Hong, G. K. (1993). Rehabilitation counseling for Asian Americans: Psychological and social considerations. *Proceedings from the National Association of Multicultural Rehabilitation Concerns.*

Horton, M. (1990). *The long haul.* New York: Doubleday.

Horvath, A. O., & Greenberg, L. S. (1994). Introduction. In A. O. Horvath & L. S. Greenberg (Eds.), *The working alliance: Theory, research, and practice* (pp. 1–9). New York: Wiley.

Hosie, T. W. (1995). Counseling specialties: A case of basic preparation rather than advanced specialization. *Journal of Counseling & Development, 74,* 177–180.

House, R. B. (1995). Comments on McLaren. *Journal of Rehabilitation Administration, 19*(4), 269–270.

House of Representatives Report 101–544. (1990). Report to Accompany HR 1013, the Individuals with Disabilities Education Act Amendments of 1990.

House of Representatives Report 101–787. (1990). Conference report to Accompany S. 1824, the Individuals with Disabilities Education Act Amendments of 1990.

Hutchinson, J. D., Luck, R. S., & Hardy, R. E. (1978). Training needs of a group of vocational rehabilitation agency administrators. *Journal of Rehabilitation Administration, 2,* 156–159, 178.

Irons, T. R. (1989). Professional fragmentation in rehabilitation counseling. *Journal of Rehabilitation, 55,* 41–45.

Jacobs, K. (1995). Marketing ergonomic consultation. In K. Jacobs & E. M. Bettencoun (Eds.), *Ergonomics for therapists* (pp. 205–216). Newton, MA: Butterworth-Heinemann.

Jaques, M. E. (1959). *Critical counseling behavior in rehabilitation settings.* Iowa City, IA: State University of Iowa, College of Education.

Jaques, M. E. (1970). *Rehabilitation counseling: Scope and services.* Boston: Houghton Mifflin.

Jaques, M. E., & Kauppi, D. R. (1983). Vocational rehabilitation and its relationship to vocational psychology. In W. B. Walsh & S. H. Osipow (Eds.), *Handbook of vocational psychology* (pp. 207–256). Hillsdale, NJ: Lawrence Erlbaum.

Jenkins, W., Patterson, J. B., & Szymanski, E. M. (1992). Philosophical, historical, and legislative aspects of the rehabilitation counseling profession. In R. M. Parker & E. M. Szymanski (Eds.), *Rehabilitation counseling: Basics and beyond* (2nd ed., pp. 1–40). Austin, TX: PRO–ED.

JobHunt. (1995, July 12). [Online]. Available: http://rescomp.stanford.edu/jobs.html.

Johnson, S. (1976). *The history of Rasselas, Prince* of Abyssinia. In Stevenson, B. (Ed.) (1967). *The home book of quotations,* Chapter 4. NY: Dood, Mean & Co.

Kanner, L. (1964). *A history of the care and study of the mentally retarded.* Springfield, IL: Charles C Thomas.

Kaplan, I., & Hammond, N. (1982). Projects with industry: The concept and the realization. *American Rehabilitation, 8,* 3–7.

Kaplan, R. M., & Saccuzzo, D. P. (1993). *Psychological testing: Principles, applications, and issues.* Pacific Grove, CA: Brooks/Cole.

Karp, H. B. (1989, June). Supervising the plateaued worker. *Supervisory Management,* pp. 35–40.

Katsinas, R. P., Phillips, J. S., & Sawyer, H. W. (1987). Decision-making strategies within groups. *Journal of Rehabilitation Administration, 11,* 133–137.

Keefe, S. E., & Padilla, A. M. (1987). *Chicano ethnicity.* Albuquerque: University of New Mexico Press.

Keith-Spiegel, P., & Koocher, G. P. (1985). *Ethics in psychology.* New York: Random House.

Kelley, S. D. M., & Satcher, J. (1992). An organizational support model for rehabilitation agencies. *Journal of Rehabilitation Administration, 16,* 117–121.

Kessler, H. H. (1947). *Rehabilitation of the physically handicapped.* New York: Columbia University Press.

Kiernan, W., Sanchez, R., & Schalock, R. (1989). Economics, industry, and disability in the future. In W. Kiernan & R. Schalock (Eds.), *Economics, industry, and disability* (pp. 365–374). Baltimore: Paul H. Brookes.

Kilborn, P. (November 26, 1994). EEOC choking on bureaucracy, mounting backlog of cases. *State Journal-Register* (IL).

Kilbury, R. F., Benshoff, J. J., & Riggar, T. F. (1990). The expansion of private sector rehabilitation: Will rehabilitation education respond? *Rehabilitation Education, 4,* 163–170.

Kirk, F., & La Forge, J. (1995). The National Rehabilitation Counseling Association: Where we've been, where we're going. *Journal of Rehabilitation, 61*(3), 47–50.

Kitchener, K. S. (1984). Intuition, critical evaluation and ethical principles: The foundation for ethical decisions in counseling psychology. *Counseling Psychologist, 12*(3), 43–55.

Kitzinger, C. (1991). Lesbians and gay men in the workplace: Psychosocial issues. In M. J. Davidson & J. Earnshaw (Eds.), *Vulnerable workers: Psychosocial and legal issues* (pp. 223–240). New York: Wiley.

Knippen, J. T., & Green, T. B. (1989). Directing employee efforts through goal setting. *Supervisory Management, April,* 32–36.

Kosciulek, J. (1993). Advances in trait-and-factor theory: A person x environment fit approach to rehabilitation counseling. *Journal of Applied Rehabilitation Counseling, 24*(2), 11–14.

Kramer, J. J., & Conoley, J. C. (Eds.). (1992). *The eleventh mental measurements yearbook.* Lincoln, NE: Buros Institute of Mental Measurements, University of Nebraska–Lincoln.

Kramer, J. J., & Conoley, J. C. (Eds.). (1993). *The eleventh mental measurements yearbood on CD–ROM and master index to test information* [CD–ROM]. Lincoln, NE: Buros Institute of Mental Measurements, University of Nebraska–Lincoln.

Kuehn, M. D. (1991). An agenda for professional practice in the 1990s. *Journal of Applied Rehabilitation Counseling, 22*(3), 6–15.

Kuehn, M. D., Crystal, R. M., & Ursprung, A. (1988). Challenges for rehabilitation counselor education. In S. Rubin & N. Rubin (Eds.), *Contemporary challenges to the rehabilitation counseling profession* (pp. 273–302). Baltimore, MD: Paul H. Brookes.

Kunce, J. T., & Cope, C. S. (1987). Personal styles analysis. In N.C. Gysbers & E. J. Moore, *Career counseling: Skills and techniques for practitioners,* (pp. 100–130). Englewood Cliffs, NJ: Prentice-Hall.

Kundu, M. M. (1987). Marketing and placing graduates in the private sector. *Rehabilitation Education, 1,* 191–196.

Kurpius, D. J., & Fuqua, D. R. (1993). Fundamental issues in defining consultation. *Journal of Counseling and Development, 71,* 598–600.

Kurpius, D. J., Fuqua, D. R., & Rozecki, T. (1993). The consulting process: A multidimensional approach. *Journal of Counseling and Development, 71,* 601–606.

Kurtz, T. (1989, March). Performance plateauing. *Supervisory Management, March,* 19–22.

LaBuda, J. (Fall, 1995). Counselors counsel; clients sue. *CRC: The Counselor,* pp. 6–7.

LaFramboise, T. D. (1988). American Indian mental health policy. *American Psychologist, 43,* 388–397.

Lakein, A. (1973). *How to get control of your time and your life.* New York: Signet.

Lansing, R. L. (1989, January). Training new employees. *Supervisory Management,* pp. 16–20.

Latta, J. (1981). Toward a more effective management philosophy. *Journal of Rehabilitation Administration, 5,* 51–57.

Lawrie, J. (1989, May). Steps toward an objective appraisal. *Supervisory Management,* pp. 17–24.

Leahy, M. M. (1994). *Validation of essential knowledge dimensions in case management.* The Foundation for Rehabilitation Certification, Education and Research, Rolling Meadows, IL.

Leahy, M. J. (1994). *Validation of essential knowledge dimensions in case management.* Rolling Meadows, IL: Foundation for Rehabilitation Certification, Education and Research,

Leahy, M. J., & Holt, E. (1993). Certification in rehabilitation counseling: History and process. *Rehabilitation Counseling Bulletin, 37,* 71–80.

Leahy, M. J., Shapson, P. R., & Wright, G. N. (1987). Rehabilitation practitioners competencies by role and setting. *Rehabilitation Counseling Bulletin, 31,* 119–131.

Leahy, M. J., & Szymanski, E. M. (1995). Rehabilitation counseling: Evolution and current status. *Journal of Counseling and Development, 74,* 163–166.

Leahy, M. J., Szymanski, E. M., & Linkowski, D. C. (1993). Knowledge importance in rehabilitation counseling. *Rehabilitation Counseling Bulletin, 37,* 130–145.

Leal-Idrogo, A. (1995). Further thoughts on "The use of interpreters and translators in delivery of rehabilitation services". *Journal of Rehabilitation, 61*(2), 21–23.

Leibowitz, H. H., Johnson, W. O, & Pilsk, A. (1973, March). *Proceedings at the State of the Art Editorial Seminar* (Monograph 3), Youth Projects, Inc. and Department of Health, Education, and Welfare, Social and Rehabilitation Service. Washington, DC: U.S. Government Printing Office.

Leong, F. T. L. (Ed.). (1995). *Career development and vocational behavior of racial and ethnic minorities.* Mahwah, NJ: Lawrence Erlbaum.

Leung, P. (1993). A changing demography and its challenge. *Journal of Vocational Rehabilitation, 3*(1), 3–11.

Levers, L. L., & Maki, D. R. (1995). African indigenous healing and cosmology: Toward a philosophy of ethnorehabilitation. *Rehabilitation Education, 9,* 127–145.

Lewis, J. W. (1970, September/October). Excerpt of correspondence to Robert M. Long, Administrator of Georgia Rehabilitation Center in Warm Springs, GA. *Rehabilitation Record, 9.*

Linkowski, D. L., & Szymanski, E. M. (1993). Accreditation in rehabilitation counseling: Historical and current content and process. *Rehabilitation Counseling Bulletin, 37,* 81–91.

Linkowski, D. C., Thoreson, R. W., Diamond, E. E., Leahy, M. J., Szymanski, E. M., & Witty, T. (1993). Instrument to validate rehabilitation counseling accreditation and certification knowledge areas. *Rehabilitation Counseling Bulletin, 37*(2), 123–129.

Lippitt, G., & Lippitt, R. (1986). *The consulting process in action* (2nd ed.). San Diego, CA: University Associates.

Lofquist, L. H., & Dawis, R. V. (1969). *Adjustment to work: A psychological view of man's problems in a work-oriented society.* New York: Appleton-Century-Crofts.

Lorenz, J. R. (1979). Setting performance objectives and evaluating individual performance in rehabilitation settings. *Journal of Rehabilitation Administration, 3,* 5–12.

Lorenz, J. R., Larsen, L., & Schumacher, B. (1981). Prologue to the future. In W. G. Emener, R. S. Luck, & S. J. Smits (Eds.) *Rehabilitation administration and supervision* (pp. 355–370). Baltimore: University Park Press.

Lorenz, J. R., Nelipovich, M., & Wainwright, C. O. (1984). NRAA membership profile & attitudes toward certification of administrators and supervisors in rehabilitation. *Journal of Rehabilitation Administration, 8,* 13–20.

Lowrey, L. (1983). Cultural diversity in management. *Journal of Rehabilitation Administration, 7,* 45–51.

Lubove, R. (1965). *The professional altruist.* Cambridge, MA: Harvard University Press.

Luck, R. S. (1978) Rehabilitation supervisor: Technical expert and trainer. *Journal of Rehabilitation Administration, 2,* 66–72.

Lui, J. (1993). Trends and innovation in private sector rehabilitation for the 21st Century. In L. Pearlman & C. Hansen (Eds.). *Private sector rehabilitation insurance: Trends and issues for the 21st century* (pp. 47–50). Alexandria, VA: National Rehabilitation Association.

Luther, D. B. (1995). Put strategic planning to work. *Association Management, 47*(1), 73–76.

Lynch, R. K. (1983). The vocational expert. *Rehabilitation Counseling Bulletin, 27,* 18–25.

Lynch, R. K., Lynch, R. T., & Beck, R. (1992). Rehabilitation counseling in the private sector. In R. Parker and E. Szymanski (Eds.) *Basics and beyond* (2nd ed.) (pp. 73–101). Austin, TX: PRO–ED.

Lynch, R., & Martin, T. (1982). Rehabilitation counseling: A training needs survey. *Journal of Rehabilitation, 48,* 51–52, 73.

Mabe, A. R., & Rollin, S. A. (1986). The role of a code of ethical standards in counseling. *Journal of Counseling and Development, 64,* 294–297.

Macan, T. H., & Dipboye, R. L. (1990). The relationship of interviewers' preinterview impressions to selection and recruitment outcomes. *Personnel Psychology, 43,* 745–768.

MacDonald, M. E. (1949, December). Review of the annual report of the Federal Security Agency: Office of Vocational Rehabilitation. *Social Service Review,* pp. 541–542.

MacDonald, M. E. (1948, March). Review of the book *Rehabilitation of the physically handicapped. Social Service Review,* pp. 105–106.

Maki, D. (1986). Foundations of applied rehabilitation counseling. In T.F. Riggar, D. Maki, & A. Wolf (Eds.) *Applied rehabilitation counseling.* (pp. 3–11). New York: Springer Publishing Co.

Maki, D., & Delworth, U. (1995). Clinical supervision: A definition and model for the rehabilitation counseling profession. *Rehabilitation Counseling Bulletin, 38*(4), 282–293.

Maki, D., McCracken, N., Pape, D., & Scofield, M. (1978). The theoretical model of vocational rehabilitation. *Journal of Rehabilitation, 44,* 26–28.

Maki, D. R., McCracken, N., Pape, D. A., & Scofield, M. E. (1979). A systems approach to vocational assessment. *Journal of Rehabilitation, 45*(1), 48–51.

Maki, D., & Murray, G. (1995). Philosophy of rehabilitation. In A. Dell Orto, & R. Marenelli (Eds.), *Encyclopedia of disability and rehabilitation.* New York: Macmillan.

Manning, A. (1994, July 21). Disabled say legislation only a start to better life. *USA Today,* p. 5D.

Margolin, R. J. (1964). How an employer can aid mental patients. *Rehabilitation Record, 5*(3), 33–36.

Mariani, M. (1995). Beyond psychobabble: Careers in psychotherapy. *Occupational Outlook Quarterly, 39*(1), 13–25.

Marrin, A. (1958). Office memorandum to Mary E. Switzer, Director, Office of Vocational Rehabilitation, Washington, DC.

Marshall, C. A., Martin, W. E., Thompson, T. S., Jr., & Johnson, M. J. (1991). Multiculturalism and rehabilitation counselor training: Recommendations for providing culturally appropriate counseling services to American Indians. *Journal of Counseling and Development, 70,* 225–234.

Marshall, K. T., & Oliver, R. M. (1995). *Decision making and forecasting.* New York: McGraw-Hill.

Matarazzo, J. D. (1987). There is only one psychology, no specialties, but many applications. *American Psychologist, 42,* 893–903.

Matkin, R. E. (1980). Supervisory responsibilities relating to legal and ethical issues in rehabilitation settings. *Journal of Rehabilitation Administration, 4,* 133–143.

Matkin, R. E. (1982). Preparing rehabilitation counselors to perform supervisory and administrative responsibilities. *Journal of Applied Rehabilitation Counseling, 13*(3), 21–24.

Matkin, R. E. (1983a). Credentialing and the rehabilitation profession. *Journal of Rehabilitation, 49,* 25–28, 67.

Matkin, R. (1983b). The roles and functions of rehabilitation specialists in the private sector. *Journal of Applied Rehabilitation Counseling, 14,* 14–27.

Matkin, R. E. (1985). *Insurance rehabilitation: Service applications in disability compensation systems.* Austin, TX: PRO–ED.

Matkin, R. (1987). Content areas and recommended training sites of insurance rehabilitation specialists. *Rehabilitation Education, 1,* 233–246.

Matkin, R. E. (1995). Private sector rehabilitation. In S. E. Rubin & R. T. Roessler (Eds.), *Foundations of the vocational rehabilitation process* (4th ed., pp. 375–398). Austin, TX: PRO–ED.

Matkin, R. E., & Bauer, L. L. (1993). Assessing predeterminants of job satisfaction among certified rehabilitation counselors in various work settings. *Journal of Applied Rehabilitation Counseling, 24*(1), 26–33.

Matkin, R. E., Bauer, L. L., & Nickles, L. E. (1993). Personality characteristics of certified rehabilitation counselors in various work settings. *Journal of Applied Rehabilitation Counseling, 24*(3), 42–53.

Matkin, R. E., & Riggar, T. F. (1986). The rise of private sector rehabilitation and its effects on training programs. *Journal of Rehabilitation, 52*(2), 50–58.

Matkin, R. E., & Riggar, T. F. (1991). *Persist and publish: Hints for academic writing and publishing.* Niwot, CO: University Press of Colorado.

Matkin, R. E., Sawyer, H. W., Lorenz, J. R., & Rubin, S. E. (1982). Rehabilitation administrators and supervisors: Their work assignments, training needs, and suggestions for preparation. *Journal of Rehabilitation Administration, 6,* 170–183.

May, R. (1973). *Man's search for himself.* New York: Delta.

May, R. (1989). *The art of counseling.* Lake Worth, FL: Gardner Press.

May, R. (1991). *The cry for myth.* New York: Delta.

McArthur, C. (1954). Analyzing the clinical process. *Journal of Counseling Psychology, 1,* 203–208.

McCarthy, P., DeBell, C., Kanuha, V., & McLeod, J. (1988). Myths of supervision: Identifying the gaps between theory and practice. *Counselor Education and Supervision, 28,* 22–28.

McDonald, A., & Lorenz, J. (1977). Graudate curriculum and training delivery preference of practicing rehabilitation facility administrators. *Journal of Rehabilitation Administration, 1,* 12–22.

McFarlane, F. R., & Turner, T. (1995). A glimpse into the future for technology and distance education. *Journal of Rehabilitation Administration, 19*(4), 327–328.

McGinn, F., Flowers, C. R., & Rubin, S. E. (1994). In quest of an explicit multicultural emphasis in ethical standards for rehabilitation counselors. *Rehabilitation Education, 7,* 261–268.

McKee, B. G., & Chiavaroli, K. S. (1984). Computer-assisted career guidance with hearing-impaired college students. *Journal of Counseling and Development, 63,* 162–167.

McLaren, M. B. (1995). Distance learning: Expanding educational opportunities. *Journal of Rehabilitation Administration, 19*(4), 261–268.

McMahan, R. S. (1979). An economist looks at the business of rehabilitation. *Journal of Rehabilitation Administration, 3,* 161–167.

McMahon, B. T., Shaw, L. R., & Mahaffey, D. P. (1988). Preservice graduate education for private sector rehabilitation counselors. *Rehabilitation Counseling Bulletin, 27*(1), 54–60.

McNutt, P. (1942). Office memorandum to Franklin D. Roosevelt, Washington, DC.

Meili, P. (April/May, 1993). The rehabilitation market. *Rehabilitation Management,* pp. 96–102.

Meier, S. T., & Davis, S. R. (1993). *The elements of counseling* (2nd ed.). Pacific Grove, CA: Brooks/Cole.

Menz, F. E., & Bordieri, J. E. (1986). Rehabilitation facility administrator training needs: Priorities and patterns for the 1980's. *Journal of Rehabilitation Administration, 10,* 89–98.

Menz, F. E., & Bordieri, J. E. (1987). Training experiences and perceptions of rehabilitation facility administrators. *Journal of Rehabilitation Administration, 11,* 60–67.

Meyer, J., & Donaho, M. (1979). *Get the right person for the job.* Englewood Cliffs, NJ: Prentice-Hall.

Millington, M. J., Asner, K., Linkowski, D. L. & Der-Stepian, J., (1996). Employers and job development: The business perspective. In E. M. Szymanski, & R. M. Parker (Eds.), *Work and disability: Issues and strategies in career development and job placement.* pp. 277–308. Austin, TX: PRO–ED.

Millington, M., Szymanski, E., & Johnston-Rodriguez, S. (1995). A context–stage model of employment selection. *Journal of Job Placement, 11*(1), 31–36.

Mitchell, K. (1995, June). *The politics of incapacity: Working with the employer organization as the client.* Paper presented at the Michigan State University Disability Managers' Training Conference, East Lansing, MI.

Mittra, S. S. (1986). *Decision support system.* New York: Wiley.

Morales, R., & Bonilla, F. (Eds.). (1993). Latinos in a changing U. S. economy: Comparative perspectives on growing inequality. Newbury Park: Sage.

Morelock, K., Roessler, R., & Bolton, B. (1987). The employability maturity interview: Reliability and construct validity. *Vocational Evaluation and Work Adjustment Bulletin, 20,* 3–59.

Moriarty, J. (1987). Rearranging chairs on the Titanic: Decline and fall of vocational rehabilitation 1973–1995. *Fourteenth Institute on Rehabilitation Issues,* 1–18.

Moriarty, J. B., Walls, R. T., & McLaughlin, D. E. (1987). The preliminary diagnostic questionnaire (PDQ): Functional assessment of employability. *Rehabilitation Psychology, 32,* 5–15.

Morrill, W. H., Oefting, E. R., & Hurst, J. C. (1974). Dimensions of counselor functioning. *Personnel and Guidance Journal, 52,* 354–359.

Morris, K. (1973). Welfare reform 1973: The social services dimension. *Science, 181,* 515–522.

Morrissey, P. A. (1995). Consumerism and choice: Basic standards for judging efforts and expectations in the vocational rehabilitation process [Monograph 18]. In L. G. Perlman & C. E. Hansen (Eds.), *Vocational rehabilitation: Preparing for the 21st century* (pp. 16–21). Alexandria, VA: National Rehabilitation Association.

Morrow, K. A., & Deidan, C. T. (1992). Bias in the counseling process: How to recognize and avoid it. *Journal of Counseling and Development, 70,* 571–577.

Mount, B. (1988). *What we are learning about circles of support.* New Haven, CT: Graphic Futures.

Mullahy, C. M. (1995). *The case manager's handbook.* Gaithersburg, MD: Aspen.

Murphy. L. L., Conoley, J. C., & Impara, J. C. (Eds.). (1994). *Tests in print IV.* Lincoln, NE: Buros Institute of Mental Measurements, University of Nebraska–Lincoln.

Murray, R. (1992). Enhancing interdependent relationships between counselors and consumers: A conceptual model. *Journal of Vocational Rehabilitation, 2*(3), 39–45.

Murray, S. O. (1979). The institutional elaboration of a quasi-ethnic community. *International Review of Modern Sociology, 9,* 165–177.

Muthard, J. E., & Salamone, P. (1969). The roles and functions of the rehabilitation counselor. *Rehabilitation Counseling Bulletin, 13,* 81–168.

Nagler, M., & Wilson, W. (1995). Disability. In A. Dell Orto, & R. Marenelli (Eds.), *Encyclopedia of disability and rehabilitation* (pp.257–260). New York: Macmillan.

NAMI. (1995, July 14). [On-line]. Available: http://www-leland.stanford.edu/~llurch/nami.html.

Nathanson, R. (1979) Counseling persons with disabilities: Are the feelings, thoughts, and behaviors of helping professionals helpful? *Personnel and Guidance Journal, 58,* 233–237.

National Center for Medical Rehabilitation Research. (1993). *National Center for Medical Rehabilitation Research Plan.* Washington, DC: National Institutes of Health.

National Council on the Handicapped (1986). *Toward independence: An assessment of federal laws and programs affecting persons with disabilities—with legislative recommendations.* Washington, DC: Author.

National Council on Rehabilitation Education (1995–1996). *Membership directory.* Logan, UT: Author.

National Hispanic Reporter (1992, August). The state of Hispanic health 1992. *National Hispanic Reporter: An Independent Monthly Newspaper Addressing National Hispanic Issues III*(8), 12.

National Rehabilitation Association. (1950). *Proceedings from the NRA conference.* New York: Author.

Neely, C. (1974). Rehabilitation counselor attitudes: A study to compare the attitudes of general and special counselors. *Journal of Applied Rehabilitation Counseling, 5,* 153–158.

Nester, M. A. (1993). Psychometric testing and reasonable accommodation for persons with disabilities. *Rehabilitation Psychology, 38,* 75–83.

Newman, I., & Benz, C. R. (In press). *Qualitative-quantitative research methodology exploring the interactive continuum.* Carbondale, IL: Southern Illinois University Press.

Nezu, A. M., & Nezu, C. M. (1993). Identifying and selecting target problems for clinical interventions: A problem-solving model. *Psychological Assessment, 5,* 254–263.

Nichtern, S. (1974). *Helping the retarded child.* New York: Grossett and Dunlap.

Noble, B. P. (November 6, 1994). Still in the dark on diversity. *New York Times,* p. 27.

Noble, J. H. (1985). Employment in the context of disability policy. In R. Habeck, W. Frey, D. Galvin, L. Chadderdon, & D. Tate (Eds.), *Economics and equity in employment of people with disabilities* (pp. 95–105). East Lansing, MI: Michigan State University Center for International Rehabilitation.

Nosek, M. A. (1992). Independent living. In R. M. Parker & E. M. Szymanski (Eds.), *Rehabilitation counseling: Basics and beyond* (2nd ed., pp. 103–133). Austin, TX: PRO–ED.

Nwachuku, U. T., & Ivey, A. E. (1991). Culture specific counseling: An alternative training model. *Journal of Counseling and Development, 70,* 106–111.

Obermann, C. E. (1965). *A history of vocational rehabilitation in America.* Minneapolis, MN: T. S. Denison & Co.

Occupational Access System (OASYS)-Job Match (Version 1.61–2) (1996). [Computer software]. Bellevue, WA: VERTEK.

Office of Vocational Rehabilitation. (1959, February). *A broadening concept of the role of the rehabilitation counselor in the total community rehabilitation effort: OVR and the rehabilitation counseling training programs panel discussion.* Third Rehabilitation Counselor Training Workshop. New York: Department of Health, Education, and Welfare.

Olney, M. F., & Salomone, P. R. (1992). Empowerment and choice in supported employment: Helping people to help themselves. *Journal of Applied Rehabilitation Counseling, 23*(3), 41–44.

Olshansky, S. (1971, November/December). Breaking workshop exit barriers. *Rehabilitation Record,* pp. 27–30.

Olshesky, J. A. (1993). Comments on Buys. *Journal of Rehabilitation Administration, 17,* 14.

Oncken, W., Jr., & Wass, D. L. (1974). Management time: Who's got the monkey? *Harvard Business Review, 52*(6), 75–80.

Ong, M. A. (1993). Asian American cultural dimensions in rehabilitation counseling. [Monograph]. In *Rehabilitation cultural diversity initiative.* San Diego: San Diego State University.

Padden, C. (1980). The Deaf community and the culture of deaf people. In S. Baker & M. Battison (Eds.), *Sign language & the deaf community.* Silver Spring, MD: National Association of the Deaf.

Padden, C. (1988). *Deaf in America: Voices from a culture.* Cambridge, MA: Harvard University Press.

Page, J. M. (1993). Ethnic identity in deaf Hispanics of New Mexico. *Sign Language Studies, 72,* 185–221.

Page, R. C., & Bailey, J. B. (1995). Addictions counseling certification: An emerging counseling specialty. *Journal of Counseling & Development, 74,* 167–171.

Parker, R., & Szymanski, E. (1992). *Rehabilitation counseling: Basics and beyond* (2nd ed.). Austin, TX: PRO–ED.

Parsons, T. (1951). *Social systems.* Glencoe, IL: Free Press.

Patrick, D. C., & Riggar, T. F. (1985). Organizational behavior management:

Applications for program evaluation. *Journal of Rehabilitation Administration, 9,* 100–105.

Patterson, C. H. (1957). Counselor or coordinator? *Journal of Rehabilitation, 23*(3), 13–15.

Patterson, C. H. (1966). The rehabilitation counselor: A projection. *Journal of Rehabilitation, 32,* 31, 49.

Patterson, C. H. (1967). Specialization in rehabilitation counseling. *Rehabilitation Counseling Bulletin, 10,* 147–154.

Patterson, J. B. (1989). Ethics and rehabilitation supervision. *Journal of Rehabilitation, 55,* 44–49.

Patterson, J. B. (1992). Ethics and ethical decision making in rehabilitation counseling. In R. M. Parker & E. M. Szymanski (Eds.), *Rehabilitation counseling: Basics and beyond* (2nd ed., pp. 165–193). Austin, TX: PRO-ED.

Patterson, J. B., & Fabian, E. (1992). Mentoring and other career enhancement relationships for women in rehabilitation. *Journal of Rehabilitation Administration, 16,* 131–135.

Patterson, J. B., & Pankowski, J. (1988). Preparing the consumer of rehabilitation administration, management, and supervision: Preservice, inservice, and continuing education issues. *Journal of Rehabilitation Administration, 12,* 117–121,

Patterson, L. E., & Welfel, E. R. (1994). *The counseling process* (4th ed.). Pacific Grove, CA: Brooks/Cole.

Pedersen, P. (1982). The intercultural context of counseling and therapy. In A. Marsella & G. White (Eds.), *Cultural conceptions of mental health and therapy,* (pp. 333–358). Dordrecht, Holland: D. Reidel.

Pedersen, P. (1985). *Handbook of cross-cultural counseling and therapy.* Westport, CT: Greenwood Press.

Pedersen, P. (Ed.). (1991). Multiculturalism as a fourth force in counseling [special issue]. *Journal of Counseling and Development, 70.*

Pedersen, P. (1994). *A handbook for developing multicultural awareness* (2nd ed.). Alexandria, VA: American Counseling Association.

Pedersen, P., & Ivey, A. (1993). *Culture-centered counseling and interviewing skills.* Westport, CN: Praeger.

Pedersen, P. B. (1991). Introduction to the special issue on multiculturalism as a fourth force in counseling. *Journal of Counseling & Development, 70,* 4.

Pepinsky, H. B., & Pepinsky, N. (1954). *Counseling theory and practice.* New York: Ronald Press.

Percy, S. L. (1989). *Disability, civil rights, and public policy: The politics of implementation.* Tuscaloosa, AL: University of Alabama Press.

Perez, S. M., & Salazar, D. De La R. (1993). Economic, labor force, and social implications of Latino educational and population trends. *Hispanic Journal of Behavioral Sciences, 15,* 188–229.

Phillips, J. S., Bordieri, J. E., Buys, N. J., & Sabin, M. C. (1987). A national survey of performance appraisal systems. *Journal of Rehabilitation Administration, 11,* 80–86.

Phillips, J. S., Puckett, F. D., Smith, S. L, & Tenney, F. E. (1985). Performance appraisal: Legal concerns, interpersonal factors, and a proposed format. *Journal of Rehabilitation Administration,9,* 18–25.

Phillips, J. S., & Wainwright, C. O. (1986). The National Rehabilitation Administration Association. *Journal of Rehabilitation, 52,* 47–50.

Polanyi, M. (1962). *Personal knowledge.* Chicago: The University of Chicago Press.

Pope, A., & Tarlov, A. (1991). *Disability in America: Toward a national agenda for prevention.* Washington, DC: Institute of Medicine, National Academy Press.

Porter, T. L., & Jenkins, W. (1979). Reflections by three significant contributors: Interviews with James Garrett, Craig Mills, and E. B. Whitten. *Journal of Rehabilitation, 45*(4), 28–33.

Powell, S. K., & Wekell, P. M. (1996). *Nursing case management.* Philadelphia: Lippincott.

Power, P. W. (1991). *A guide to vocational assessment* (2nd Ed.). Austin, TX: PRO–ED.

Puckett, F. D. (1996). Rehabilitation engineering/technology services. In W. Crimando, & T. F. Riggar (Eds.), *Utilizing community resources: An overview of human resources* (pp. 167–176). Delray Beach, FL: St. Lucie Press.

Rasch, J. D. (1979). The case for an independent association of rehabilitation counselors. *Journal of Applied Rehabilitation Counseling, 10,* 171–176.

Reagles, K. W. (1981). Perspectives on the proposed merger of rehabilitation organizations. *Journal of Applied Rehabilitation Counseling, 12,* 75–79.

Redfield, R., Linton, R., & Herskovits, J. (1936). Memorandum for the study of acculturation. *American Anthropologist, 38,* 149–152.

Reeves, T. (1994). *Managing effectively: Developing yourself through experience.* Oxford, England: The Institute of Management, Butterworth Heinemann.

Rehabilitation Engineering. (1995, July 2). [Online] Available: http://fourier. bme.med.ualberta.ca/ BJA-work.html.

Rehabilitation Services Administration. (1993). A synopsis of the Rehabilitation Act Amendments of 1992. Washington, DC: United States Department of Education.

Rest, J. R. (1984). Research on moral development: Implications for training psychologists. *Counseling Psychologist, 12*(3), 19–29.

Rice, J. M. (1981). Behavioral applications to rehabilitation administration: An examination of four relevant concepts. *Journal of Rehabilitation Administration, 5,* 5–10.

Riggar, T. F. (1985). *Stress burnout: An annotated bibliography.* Carbondale, IL: Southern Illinois University Press.

Riggar, T. F, Crimando, W., & Bordieri, J. E. (1991). Human resource needs: The staffing function in rehabilitation—Part II. *Journal of Rehabilitation Administration, 15,* 135–140.

Riggar, T. F., Crimando, W., Bordieri, J., & Phillips, J. S. (1988). Rehabilitation administration preservice education: Preparing the professional rehabilitation administrator, manager and supervisor. *Journal of Rehabilitation Administration, 12*(4), 93–102.

Riggar, T. F., Crimando, W., Bordieri, J. E., & Phillips, J. S. (1990). Matrix management: Increasing applicability for rehabilitation administration. *Journal of Rehabilitation Administration, 14,* 113–118.

Riggar, T. F., Eckert, J. M., & Crimando, W. (1993). Cultural diversity in rehabilitation: Management strategies for implementing organizational pluralism. *Journal of Rehabilitation Administration, 17,* 53–61.

Riggar, T. F., Garner, W. E., & Hafer, M. (1984). Rehabilitation personnel burnout: Organizational cures. *Journal of Rehabilitation Administration, 8,* 94–104.

Riggar, T. F., Godley, S. H., & Hafer, M. (1984). Burnout and job satisfaction in rehabilitation administrators and direct service providers. *Rehabilitation Counseling Bulletin , 27,* 151–160.

Riggar, T. F., & Hansen, G. (1986). Problem solving, performance based continuing education: A new RCEP paradigm. *Journal of Applied Rehabilitation Counseling, 17*(2), 47–50.

Riggar, T. F., Hansen, G., & Crimando, W. (1987). Rehabilitation employee organizational withdrawal behavior. *Rehabilitation Psychology, 32,* 121–124.

Riggar, T. F., & Lorenz, J. (Eds.). (1986). *Reading in rehabilitation administration.* Albany: State University of New York Press.

Riggar, T. F., Maki, D., & Flowers, C. (1991). Civil Rights Act of 1991. *Journal of Applied Rehabilitation Counseling, 22*(4), 36–43.

Riggar, T. F., & Matkin, R. E. (1984). Rehabilitation counselors working as administrators: A pilot investigation. *Journal of Applied Rehabilitation Counseling, 15*(1), 9–13.

Riggar, T. F., & Patrick, D. (1984). Case management and administration. *Journal of Applied Rehabilitation Counseling, 15*(3), 29–33.

Rinas, J., & Clyne-Jackson, S. (1988). *Professional conduct and legal concerns in mental health practice.* Norwalk, CT: Appleton & Lange.

Rittenhouse, R. K., Johnson, C., Overton, B., Freeman, S., & Jaussi, K. (1991). The black and deaf movements in America since 1960: Parallelism an agenda for the future. *American Annals of the Deaf, 136,* 392–400.

Rockwood, G. F., (1993). Edgar Schein's process versus content consultation models. *Journal of Counseling and Development, 71,* 636–638.

Roessler, R. (1990). A quality of life perspective on rehabilitation counseling. *Rehabilitation Counseling Bulletin, 34*(2), 82–90.

Roessler, R. T., & Rubin, S. E. (Eds.). (1992). *Case management and rehabilitation counseling* (2nd ed.). Austin, TX: PRO–ED.

Roessler, R. T., & Schriner, K. F. (1991). The implications of selected employment concerns for disability policy and rehabilitation practice. *Rehabilitation Counseling Bulletin, 35*(1), 52–67.

Ross, C. K. (1979). Supervision theory: A prescription for practice. *Journal of Rehabilitation Administration, 3,* 14–19.

Roth, W. (1985). The politics of disability: Future trends as shaped by current realities. In L. Perlman & G. Austin (Eds.), *Social influences in rehabilitation planning: Blueprint for the 21st century* (pp. 41–48). Alexandria, VA: National Rehabilitation Association.

Rothman, R. A. (1987). *Working: Sociological perspectives.* Englewood Cliffs, NJ: Prentice Hall.

Rothstein, M. A. (1991). The law–medicine interface in assessing vocational capacity. In S. J. Scheer (Ed.), *Medical perspectives in vocational assessment of impaired workers* (pp. 407–422). Gaithersburg, MD: Aspen.

Rotter, J. B. (1966). Generalized expectancies for internal versus external control of reinforcement. *Psychological Monographs, 80*(1), 1–28.

Rotter, J. B. (1975). Some problems and misconceptions related to the construct of internal versus external control of reinforcement. *Journal of Consulting and Clinical Psychology, 43,* 56–57.

Rubin, S. E., Matkin, R. E., Ashley, J., Beardsley, M. M., May, V. R., Onstott, K., & Puckett, F. D. (1984). Roles and functions of certified rehabilitation counselors. *Rehabilitation Counseling Bulletin, 27,* 199–224, 238–245.

Rubin, S. E., & Millard, R. P. (1991). Ethical principles and American public policy on disability. *Journal of Rehabilitation, 57*(1), 13–16.

Rubin, S. E., & Roessler, R. T. (1978). *Foundations of the vocational rehabilitation process.* Baltimore: University Park Press.

Rubin, S. E., & Roessler R. T. (1995). *Foundations of the vocational rehabilitation process* (4th ed.). Austin, TX: PRO–ED.

Rubin, S. E., Wilson, C. A., Fischer, J., & Vaughn, B. (1991). *Ethical practices in rehabiliation: A series of instructional modules for rehabilitation education programs.* Carbondale, IL: Southern Illinois University–Carbondale, Rehabilitation Institute.

Rusalem, H., & Malikin, D. (1976). *Contemporary vocational rehabilitation.* New York: New York University.

Sample, J. A. (1984). A model for the collaborative development and use of BARS in appraising the performance of rehabilitation supervisors and counselors. *Journal of Rehabilitation Administration, 8,* 105–110.

Santiago, A. M. (1988). Provision of vocational rehabilitation services to blind and visually impaired Hispanics: The case of New Jersey. *Journal of Applied Rehabilitation Counseling, 19*(4), 11–15.

Sartain, A., & Baker, A. (1978). *The supervisor and the job* (3rd ed.). New York.

Sawyer, H., & Schumacher, B. (1980). Stress and the rehabilitation administrator. *Journal of Rehabilitation Administration, 4,* 49–55.

Scalia V. A., & Wolfe, R. R. (1984). Rehabilitation counselor education. *Journal of Applied Rehabilitation Counseling, 15*(3), 34–38.

Scheck, A. (1990). Rehab engineers vote for two certification levels. *Team Rehab, 1*(2), 30–31.

Schein, E. H. (1969). *Process consultation: Its role in organization development.* Reading, PA: Addison-Wesley.

Schein, E. H. (1986). A critical look at current career development theory and research. In D. T. Hall & Associates, *Career development in organizations* (pp. 310–331). San Francisco: Jossey-Bass.

Schein, E. H. (1991). Process consultation. *Consulting Psychology Bulletin, 43*, 16–18.

Schein, J., & Delk, M. (1974). *The deaf population in the United States.* Silver Spring, MD: National Association of the Deaf.

Schoemaker, P. J. H. (1995). Scenario planning: A tool for strategic thinking. *Sloan Management Review, 36*(2), 25–40.

Schriner, K. F. (1990). Why study disability policy? *Journal of Disability Policy Studies, 1*(1), 1–7.

Scofield, M., Berven, N., & Harrison, R. (1981). Competence, credentialing, and the future of rehabilitation. *Journal of Rehabilitation, 47*, 31–35.

Scofield, M., Pape, D., McCracken, N., & Maki, D. (1980). An ecological model for promoting acceptance of disability. *Journal of Applied Rehabilitation Counseling, 11*(4), 183–187.

Scotch, R. K. (1984). *From good will to civil rights: Transforming federal disability policy.* Philadelphia: Temple University Press.

Scotch, R. K., & Berkowitz, E. D. (1990). One comprehensive system? A historical perspective on federal disability policy. *Journal of Disability Policy Studies, 1*(3), 1–19.

Segall, M. H. (1984). More than we need to know about culture, but are afraid not to ask. *Journal of Cross-Cultural Psychology, 15*,111–138.

Seitel, F. (1984). *The practice of public relations.* Columbus, Ohio: Charles E. Merrill.

Shapiro, J. (1993). *No pity.* New York: Times Books.

Shapson, P. R., Wright, G. N., & Leahy, M. J. (1987). Education and the attainment of rehabilitation competencies. *Rehabilitation Counseling Bulletin, 31*, 131–145.

Shaw, L. R., MacGillis, P. W., & Dvorchik, K. M. (1994). Alcoholism and the Americans With Disabilities Act: Obligations and accommodations. *Rehabilitation Counseling Bulletin, 38*(2), 108–123.

Shepherd, C. (1989). *Does it make a difference?: Multi-cultural counseling issues.* Paper presented at the Michigan Rehabilitation Association Annual Conference. Grand Rapids, MI.

Sheppard, C., Bunton, J., Menifee, S., Rocha, G. (1995). Rehabilitation service providers: A minority perspective. *Journal of Applied Rehabilitation Counseling, 26*(2), 36–40.

Sherman, S., & Robinson, N. (Eds.). (1982). *Ability testing of handicapped people: Dilemma for government, science, and the public.* Washington, DC: National Academy Press.

Silva, F. (1993). *Psychometric foundations and behavioral assessment.* Newbury Park, CA: Sage.

Simon, S. E. (1982). Productivity measurement and evaluation in rehabilitation and social service agencies. *Journal of Rehabilitation Administration, 6,* 161–166.

Simon, S. E. (1987). Productivity, efficiency and effectiveness: Simple indicators of agency performance. *Journal of Rehabilitation Administration, 11,* 4–10.

Sink, J., & Porter, T. (1978). Convergence and divergence in rehabilitation counseling and vocational evaluation. *Rehabilitation Counseling Bulletin, 2,* 5–20.

Smart, J. F., & Smart, D. W. (1995). The use of translators/interpreters in rehabilitation. *Journal of Rehabilitation, 61*(2), 14–20.

Smith, C. A., & Bordieri, J. E. (1988). The provision of training and perceived training needs of rehabilitation facility production staff. *Journal of Rehabilitation Administration, 12,* 67–71.

Smith, E., & Vasquez, M. (1985). Cross cultural counseling: An introduction. *Counseling Psychologist, 13*(4), 531–536.

Smith, E. J. (1973). *Counseling the culturally different black youth.* Columbus, OH: Charles E. Merrill.

Smits, S. J. (1972). Counselor job satisfaction and employment turnover in state rehabilitation agencies: A follow-up study. *Journal of Counseling Psychology, 19,* 512–517.

Smits, S. J. (1978). The two faces of rehabilitation supervision [Editorial]. *Journal of Rehabilitation Administration, 2,* 40–42.

Smits, S. J., Rossini, F. A., & Davis, L. M. (1987). Managing the present from the future: The challenge of preparing for technology in rehabilitation. *Journal of Rehabilitation Administration, 11,* 120–130.

Snipp, C. M. (1989). *American Indians: The first of this land.* New York: Russell Sage Foundation.

Snipp, C. M., & Summers, G. F. (1992). American Indians and economic poverty. In C. M. Dunkin (Ed.), *Rural poverty in America* (pp. 155–176). New York: Auburn House.

Spaniol, L. (1977). A program evaluation model for rehabilitation agencies and facilities. *Journal of Rehabilitation Administration, 1,* 4–13.

Spanos, W. J. (Ed.) (1966). *A casebook on existentialism.* New York: Thomas Y. Crowell Company.

Standards of practice for case managers. (1995). Case Management Society of America, Little Rock, AR.

Starr, P. (1982). *The social transformation of American medicine.* New York: Vintage.

Steenbarger, B. N. (1992). Toward science-practice integration in brief counseling and therapy. *Counseling Psychologist, 20,* 403–450.

Stensrud, R., & Gilbride, D. (1994). Revitalizing employer development: Placement in the ADA era. *Journal of Job Placement, 9,* 12–15.

Stephens, J. E., & Emener, W. G. (1988). Preparing the professional rehabilitation administrator, manager and supervisor: In-service and continuing education issues and approaches. *Journal of Rehabilitation Administration, 12,* 106–114.

Stephens, J. E., & Kneipp, S. (1981). Managing human resource development in rehabilitation. In W. G. Emener, R. S. Luck, & S. J. Smits (Eds.), *Rehabilitation Administration & Supervision* (pp. 87–103). Baltimore: University Park Press.

Stoltenberg, C., & Delworth, U. (1987). *Supervising counselors and therapists.* San Fransico, CA: Jossey-Bass.

Strohmer, D. C., Pellerin, M. F., & Davidson, K. J. (1995). Rehabilitation counselor hypothesis testing: The role of negative information, client disability, and counselor experience. *Rehabilitation Counseling Bulletin, 39*(2), 82–93.

Strohmer, D. C., Shivy, V. A., & Chiodo, A. L. (1990). Information processing strategies in counselor hypothesis testing: The role of selective memory and expectancy. *Journal of Counseling Psychology, 37,* 465–472.

Stubbins, J. (1982). *The clinical attitude in rehabilitation: A cross cultural view.* (Rehabilitation Monograph No. 6). New York: World Rehabilitation Fund.

Sue, D. W., & Sue, D. (1990). *Counseling the culturally different* (2nd ed.). New York: Wiley.

Sundberg, N. D. (1977). *Assessment of persons.* Englewood Cliffs, NJ: Prentice-Hall.

Sundberg, N. D., & Tyler, L. E. (1962). *Clinical psychology.* New York: Appleton-Century-Crofts.

Swan, W. (1989). *Swan's how to pick the right people program.* New York: Wiley.

Switzer, M. E. (1956, June). Correspondence with Mr. Sokolik, Director, Department of Social Rehabilitation, Jerusalem, Israel.

Switzer, M. E. (1959, February). Presentation at the Second Session of the Third Rehabilitation Counselor Training Workshop, New York: Department of Health, Education, and Welfare, Office of Vocational Rehabilitation.

Switzer, M. E. (1965). New novel, Monday Voices, gives drama of rehabilitation. *Rehabilitation Record, 6*(6), 18–19.

Switzer, M. E. (1965, September). *The comfort of the shared burden.* 1965 Donald Dabelstein Memorial Lecture presented at the annual conference of the National Rehabilitation Association.

Switzer, M. E. (1966, August). *Rehabilitation: Hope for recovery.* Presentation at the 52nd Annual National Hadassah Convention, Boston, MA.

Switzer, M. E. (1967, May). *The impact of Rehabilitation Amendments Act of*

1965 on psychiatric rehabilitation. Presentation at the 123rd Annual Meeting of the American Psychiatric Association, Detroit, MI.

Switzer, M. E. (1968, March/April). Rehabilitation: An act of faith. *Rehabilitation Record,* 1–4.

Switzer, M. E. (1969, April). *Changing missions of the helping professions.* First Distinguished Lecture, State University of New York at Buffalo, School of Health Related Professions, Buffalo, NY.

Switzer, M. E. (1970, May/June). Some of the great ones. *Rehabilitation Record,* 1–6.

Szufnarowski, J. (1972). Case development: An organized system of steps and functions for the rehabilitation counselor. In T. J. Ruscio & J. P. Atsaides (Eds.), *Case development in rehabilitation—what, why, how?* (pp. 19–27). Springfield, MA: Rehabilitation Services Department of Springfield College.

Szymanski, E. M. (1985). Rehabilitation counseling: A profession with a vision, an identity, and a future. (Presidential address). *Rehabilitation Counseling Bulletin, 29*(1), 2–5.

Szymanski, E. M. (1988). Comments on Stephens and Emener. *Journal of Rehabilitation Administration, 12,* 116.

Szymanski, E. M. (1991). The relationship of the level of rehabilitation counselor education to rehabilitation client outcome in the Wisconsin Division of Vocational Rehabilitation. *Rehabilitation Counseling Bulletin, 35,* 23–37.

Szymanski, E. M., & Danek, M. M. (1992). The relationship of rehabilitation counselor education to rehabilitation client outcome: A replication and extension. *Journal of Rehabilitation, 58,* 49–56.

Szymanski, E. M., Herbert, J., Parker, R. M., & Danek, M. M. (1992). State vocational rehabilitation agency counselor education and performance in Pennsylvania, Maryland, and Wisconsin. *Journal of Rehabilitation Administration, 16,* 109–113.

Szymanski, E. M., & King, J. (1989). Rehabilitation counseling in transition planning and preparation. *Career Development for Exceptional Individuals, 12,* 3–10.

Szymanski, E. M., Leahy, M. J., & Linkowski, D. C. (1993). Reported preparedness of certified counselors in rehabilitation counseling knowledge areas. *Rehabilitation Counseling Bulletin, 37,* 146–162.

Szymanski, E. M., Linkowski, D. C., Leahy, M. J., Diamond, E. E., & Thoreson, R. W. (1993). Validation of rehabilitation counseling accreditation and certification knowledge areas: Methodology and initial results. *Rehabilitation Counseling Bulletin, 37,* 109–122.

Szymanski, E. M., & Parker, R. M. (1989). Relationship of rehabilitation client outcome to level of rehabilitation counselor education. *Journal of Rehabilitation, 55,* 32–36.

Takaki, R. T. (1989). *Strangers from a different shore: A history of Asian Americans.* New York: Penguin Books.

Tarvydas, V. M. (1987). Decision-making models in ethics: Models for increased clarity and wisdon. *Journal of Applied Rehabilitation Counseling, 18*(4), 50–52.

Tarvydas, V. M., & Cottone, R. R. (1991). Ethical responses to legislative, organizational and economic dynamics: A four level model of ethical practice. *Journal of Applied Rehabilitation Counseling, 22*(4), 11–18.

Tarvydas, V., & Leahy, M. J. (1993). Licensure in rehabilitation counseling: A critical incident in professionalization. *Rehabilitation Counseling Bulletin, 37,* 92–108.

Tarvydas, V. M., & Pape, D. A. (1988). A unified code of ethics for rehabilitation counselors. *Rehabilitation Counseling Bulletin, 32,* 322–326.

Taylor, S., Lehman, C. M., & Forde, C. M. (1989, August). How employee self-appraisals can help. *Supervisory Management,* pp. 32–41.

Tenth Institute of Rehabilitation Issues. (1983). *Functional assessment.* Dunbar: West Virginia Research and Training Center, West Virginia University.

Terborg, J. R. (1977). Women in management: A research review. *Journal of Applied Psychology, 62,* 647–664.

The 'far out' success of teleworking. (1995). *Supervisory Management, January,* 1, 6.

Thomas, K. R. (1987). Warning!: Certification and accreditation may be hazardous to rehabilitation counseling's health. *Journal of Rehabilitation, 53,* 19–22.

Thomas, K. R. (1991a). The future of rehabilitation counseling. In K.R. Thomas and Associates, *Rehabilitation counseling: A profession in transition* (pp. 170–194). Athens, GA: Elliot & Fitzpatrick.

Thomas, K. R. (1991b). *Rehabilitation counseling: A profession in transition.* Athens, GA: Elliot & Fitzpatrick.

Thomas, K. R. (1993). Professional credentialing: A doomsday machine without a failsafe. *Journal of Applied Rehabilitation Counseling, 24*(4), 74–76.

Thomas, K., Butler, A., & Parker, R. (1987). Psychosocial counseling. In R. M. Parker (Ed.), *Rehabilitation counseling: Basics and beyond* (pp. 65–95). Austin, TX: PRO–ED.

Thomas, K. R., & Parker, R. M. (1984). Counseling interventions. *Journal of Applied Rehabilitation Counseling, 15*(3), 15–19.

Thomas, P. L., & Thomas, J. G. (1989). Retaining your good employees. *Supervisory Management, 34,* 9–11.

Thompson, A. (1990). *Guide to ethical practice in psychotherapy.* New York: Wiley.

Thornhill, H. L., Weiss, L., & Anderson, A. D. (1970, September/October). Rehabilitation in a black ghetto hospital. *Rehabilitation Record,* pp. 5–9.

Tombazian, C. M. (1994). Looking to your future: Managing change through strategic planning. *Managers Magazine, 69*(9), 16–21.

Tooman, M. (1986). The job placement division. *Journal of Rehabilitation, 52,* 35–38.

Triandis, H., Lambert, W., Berry, J., Lonner, W., Heron, A., Brislin, R., & Draguns, J. (Eds.). (1980). *Handbook of cross-cultural psychology: Vols. 1–6.* Boston: Allyn & Bacon.

Trueba, H. T. (1993). Castification in multicultural America. In H. T. Trueba, C. Rodriguez, Y. Zou, & J. Cintron (Eds.), *Healing multicultural America: Mexican immigrants rise to power in rural California* (pp. 29–51). Philadelphia: Falmer.

Trueba, H. T., Rodriguez, C., Zou, Y., & Cintron, J. (Eds.). (1993). *Healing multicultural America: Mexican immigrants rise to power in rural California.* Philadelphia: Falmer.

Tucker, C. M., McNeil, P., Abrams, J. M., & Brown, J. G. (1988). Characteristics important to an effective supervisor: Perceptions of vocational rehabilitation staff. *Journal of Rehabilitation Administration, 12,* 40–43.

Tucker, C. M., Parham, G. D., McNeill, P., & Knopf, L. G. (1988). Characteristics important for effective vocational rehabilitation administration: Views of supervisors and administrators in a state VR agency. *Journal of Rehabilitation Administration, 12,* 61–64.

Turk, D. C., & Salovey, P. (1985). Cognitive structures, cognitive processes, and cognitive-behavior modification: II. Judgements and inferences of the clinician. *Cognitive Therapy and Research, 9,* 19–33.

Tversky, A., & Kahneman, D. (1974). Judgement under incertainty: Heuristics and biases. *Science, 185,* 1124–1131.

U.S. Bureau of the Census. (1986, November). Projections of Hispanic population, 1983–2080. *Current population reports.* Washington, DC: U.S. Government Printing Office.

U.S. Bureau of the Census. (1990). *Current population reports.* Washington, DC: U.S. Government Printing Office.

U.S. Bureau of the Census. (1991, March). *Current population reports.* Washington, DC: U.S. Government Printing Office.

U.S. Bureau of the Census. (1993, November). We the American . . . Hispanics. *Current population reports.* Washington, DC: U.S. Government Printing Office.

U.S. Bureau of the Census. (1993, December). Americans with disabilities: 1991–92. *Current population reports.* Washington, DC: U.S. Government Printing Office.

U. S. Department of Commerce, Bureau of the Census. (1992). *Statistical abstract of the United States.* Washington, DC: U.S. Government Printing Office.

U.S. Department of Labor, Employment and Training Administration. (1991). *Dictionary of occupational titles* (4th ed., rev., vols. 1–2). Washington, DC: Author.

U.S. Office of Personnel Management. (1990). *Qualification standards for positions under the general schedule* (Handbook X–118). Washington, DC: U.S. Government Printing Office.

Vandergoot, D. (1987). Review of placement research literature: Implications for research and practice. *Rehabilitation Counseling Bulletin, 21,* 243–272.

Vandergoot, D. (1992). The marketing responsibilities of placement professionals. *Journal of Job Placement, 8,* 6–9.

Vandergoot, D. (1993). Reactions to "Current models of job placement and employer development: Research, competencies, and educational considerations". *Rehabilitation Education, 7*(4), 269–271.

Van Hoose, W. H., & Kottler, J. A. (1985). *Ethical and legal issues in counseling and psychotherapy.* San Francisco: Jossey-Bass.

Viranyi S., Crimando, W., Riggar, T. F., & Schmidt, M. J. (1992). Promoting mentoring relationships in rehabilitation. *Journal of Rehabilitation Administration, 16,* 56–61.

Vocational Evaluation and Work Adjustment Association. (1975). Vocational evaluation project final report. *Vocational Evaluation and Work Adjustment Bulletin, 8* (Special Issue).

Vocational Rehabilitation Administration. (1965). *Excerpts from recommendations of rehabilitation counseling advisory panel regarding educational preparation of personnel for vocational rehabilitation counseling, Division of Training.* Washington, DC: U.S. Government Printing Office.

Vontress, C. E. (1988). An existential approach to cross-cultural counseling. *Journal of Mulitcultural Counseling and Development, 16,* 78–83.

Wainwright, C. O., Newman, J. P., & Phillips, J. S. (1995). The National Rehabilitation Association. *Journal of Rehabilitation, 61,* 43–46.

Wainwright, C. O., & Sanders, R. W. (1988). Human resource development in rehabilitation administration: Historical and current perspectives. *Journal of Rehabilitation Administration, 12,* 87–90.

Walker, M. (1995). Rehabilitation counseling. In A. Dell Orto & R. Marenelli (Eds.), *Encyclopedia of disability and rehabilitation* (pp. 618–623). New York: Macmillan.

Walker, M. L. (1985). *Beyond bureaucracy: Mary Elizabeth Switzer and rehabilitation.* Lanham, MD: University Press of America.

Walker, R. A. (1968, May/June). The disadvantaged enter rehabilitation: Are both ready? *Rehabilitation Record,* pp. 1–4.

Walker, S., Turner, K. A., Haile-Michael, M., Vincent, A., & Miles, M. D. (Eds.). (1995). *Disability and diversity: New leadership for a new era.* Washington, DC: President's Committee on Employment of People with Disabilities.

Washburn, W. (1992). *Worker compensation disability and rehabilitation: An alert to claimants.* Arlington, VA: CEDI.

Weaver, C. L. (1994). Privatizing vocational rehabilitation. *Journal of Disability Policy Studies, 5*(1), 53–74.

Webb, N. B. (1983). Developing competent clinical practitioners: A model with guidelines for supervisors. *Clinical Supervisor, 1,* 41–51.

Webber, R. A. (1975). *Management: Basic elements of managing organizations.* Homewood, IL: Richard D. Irwin.

Weinburger, T. J. (1977). The design and implementation of a uniform staff performance evaluation instrument. *Journal of Rehabiltation Administration,1,* 26–30.

Weiss, D. J. (1985). Adaptive testing by computer. *Journal of Consulting and Clinical Psychology, 53,* 774–789.

Weiss, D. J., & Vale, C. D. (1987). Adaptive testing. *Applied Psychology: An International Review, 36,* 249–262.

Welcome to online AA resources. (1995, July 14). [Online]. Available: http:// www. casti.com/aa/.

Welcome to the ARC's World Wide Web site. (1995, July 8). [Online]. Available: http://www.metronet.com/~thearc/welcome.html.

Wells, G. K. (1978). The identity conflict of the first-line supervisor. *Journal of Rehabilitation Administration, 2,* 160–164.

Wendover, R. (1989). *Smart hiring.* Englewood Cliffs, NJ: Prentice-Hall.

West, J. F., & Idol, L. (1993). The counselor as consultant in the collaborative school. *Journal of Counseling and Development, 71,* 678–683.

Wheaton, J. E. (1995). Vocational rehabilitation acceptance rates for European Americans and African Americans: Another look. *Rehabilitation Counseling Bulletin, 38,* 224–231.

Whitehead, C. (1989). Influencing employment through federal and state policy. In W. Kiernan & R. Schalock (Eds.), *Economics, industry, and disability* (pp. 27–36). Baltimore: Paul H. Brookes.

Whiteside, K. A. (1995). *Computer use for cognitive rehabilitation of head injured patients.* [Unpublished master's paper]. Carbondale, IL: Southern Illinois University.

Whitfield, D. (1994). Toward an integrated approach to improving multicultural counselor education. *Journal of Multicultural Counseling and Development,* 22(4), 239–252.

Whitten, E. B. (1974). Rehabilitation in review: E. B. Whitten interviews Corbett Reedy. *Journal of Rehabilitation,* 34–38.

Whitten, E. B. (1980). *A poor man's lobby: History of the National Rehabilitation Association.* Unpublished manuscript.

Willey, D. A. (1978). Caseload management for the vocational rehabilitation counselor in a state agency. *Journal of Applied Rehabilitation Counseling,* 9(4), 156–158.

Will, M. (1984). *OSERS programming for the transition of youth with severe disabilities: Bridges from school to working life.* Washington, DC: Office of Special Education and Rehabilitative Services, U.S. Department of Education.

Willingham, W. W., Ragosta, M., Bennett, R. E., Braun, H., Rock, D. A., & Powers, D. E. (1988). *Testing handicapped people.* Boston: Allyn & Bacon.

Winn, R. (Ed.) (1960). *Dictionary on existentialism.* New York: Philosophical Library.

Wolfensberger, W. (1972). *Normalization.* Toronto: National Institute of Mental Retardation.

Wolfensberger, W. (1983). *Passing.* Toronto: National Institute of Mental Retardation.

Woodruff, D. M. (1989). Seven steps to better employee relations. *Supervisory Management, January,* 35–38.

Wright, B. A. (1983). *Physical disability—A psychosocial approach* (2nd ed.). New York: Harper & Row.

Wright, B. A. (1986). *Physical disability: A psychological approach.* New York: Harper & Row.

Wright, G. N. (1980). *Total rehabilitation.* Boston: Little Brown.

Wright, G. N. (1982). Contemporary rehabilitation counselor education. *Rehabilitation Counselor Bulletin, 2–5,* 254–256.

Wright, G. N., & Fraser, R. T. (1975). *Task analysis for the evaluation, preparation, classification and utilization of rehabilitation counselor track personnel.* [Monograph] *Wisconsin Studies in Vocational Rehabilitation, 22,*(3).

Wright, G. N., Leahy, M., & Sharpson, P. (1987). Rehabilitation skills inventory: Importance of counselor competencies. *Rehabilitation Counseling Bulletin, 31,* 107–118.

Wright, G. N., Reagles, K. W., & Butler, A. J. (1970). An expanded program of vocational rehabilitation: Methodology and description of client population [Monograph]. *Wisconsin Studies in Vocational Rehabilitation, 11*(2).

Wright, T. J. (1988). Enhancing the professional preparation of rehabilitation counselors for improved services to ethnic minorities with disabilities. *Journal of Applied Rehabilitation Counseling, 19*(4), 4–10.

Wright, T. J. (1993). African Americans and the public vocational rehabilitation system. *Journal of Vocational Rehabilitation, 3*(1), 20–26.

WVRRTC's Project Enable and Dial-JAN. [Online]. Available: http://www.icdi. wvu.edu/Enable.htm.

Yate, M. (1987). *Hiring the best.* Boston: Bob Adams.

Zadney, I., & James, L. (1977). Time spent on placement. *Rehabilitation Counseling Bulletin, 21,* 31–38.

Zola, I. K. (1989). Aging and disability: Toward a unified agenda. *Journal of Rehabilitation, 55*(4), 6–8.

Zolla, I. (1986). The medicalization of aging and disability. In C. Mahoney, C. Estes, & J. Heumann (Eds.), *Toward a unified agenda.* Berkeley, CA: World Institute on Disability.

Zuckerman, M. (1990). Some dubious premises in research and theory on racial differences: Scientific, social, and ethical issues. *American Psychologist, 45,* 1297–1303.

Index